T0264164

Treatment of Fingertip Injuries and Nail Deformities

Editor

AVIRAM M. GILADI

HAND CLINICS

www.hand.theclinics.com

Consulting Editor
KEVIN C. CHUNG

February 2021 • Volume 37 • Number 1

ELSEVIER

1600 John F. Kennedy Boulevard • Suite 1800 • Philadelphia, Pennsylvania, 19103-2899

http://www.theclinics.com

HAND CLINICS Volume 37, Number 1
February 2021 ISSN 0749-0712, ISBN-13: 978-0-323-79098-7

Editor: Lauren Boyle
Developmental Editor: Kristen Helm

© **2021 Elsevier Inc. All rights reserved.**

This periodical and the individual contributions contained in it are protected under copyright by Elsevier, and the following terms and conditions apply to their use:

Photocopying

Single photocopies of single articles may be made for personal use as allowed by national copyright laws. Permission of the Publisher and payment of a fee is required for all other photocopying, including multiple or systematic copying, copying for advertising or promotional purposes, resale, and all forms of document delivery. Special rates are available for educational institutions that wish to make photocopies for non-profit educational classroom use. For information on how to seek permission visit www.elsevier.com/permissions or call: (+44) 1865 843830 (UK)/(+1) 215 239 3804 (USA).

Derivative Works

Subscribers may reproduce tables of contents or prepare lists of articles including abstracts for internal circulation within their institutions. Permission of the Publisher is required for resale or distribution outside the institution. Permission of the Publisher is required for all other derivative works, including compilations and translations (please consult www.elsevier.com/permissions).

Electronic Storage or Usage

Permission of the Publisher is required to store or use electronically any material contained in this periodical, including any article or part of an article (please consult www.elsevier.com/permissions). Except as outlined above, no part of this publication may be reproduced, stored in a retrieval system or transmitted in any form or by any means, electronic, mechanical, photocopying, recording or otherwise, without prior written permission of the Publisher.

Notice

No responsibility is assumed by the Publisher for any injury and/or damage to persons or property as a matter of products liability, negligence or otherwise, or from any use or operation of any methods, products, instructions or ideas contained in the material herein. Because of rapid advances in the medical sciences, in particular, independent verification of diagnoses and drug dosages should be made.

Although all advertising material is expected to conform to ethical (medical) standards, inclusion in this publication does not constitute a guarantee or endorsement of the quality or value of such product or of the claims made of it by its manufacturer.

Hand Clinics (ISSN 0749-0712) is published quarterly by Elsevier Inc., 360 Park Avenue South, New York, NY 10010-1710. Months of publication are February, May, August, and November. Business and Editorial Offices: 1600 John F. Kennedy Blvd., Ste. 1800, Philadelphia, PA 19103-2899. Customer Service Office: 3251 Riverport Lane, Maryland Heights, MO 63043. Periodicals postage paid at New York, NY and at additional mailing offices. Subscription price is $439.00 per year (domestic individuals), $1039.00 per year (domestic institutions), $100.00 per year (domestic students/residents), $501.00 per year (Canadian individuals), $1086.00 per year (Canadian institutions), $562.00 per year (international individuals), $1086.00 per year (international institutions), $256.00 (international students/residents), and $100.00 (Canadian students/residents). Foreign air speed delivery is included in all *Clinics* subscription prices. All prices are subject to change without notice. **POSTMASTER:** Send address changes to *Hand Clinics*, Elsevier Health Sciences Division, Subscription Customer Service, 3251 Riverport Lane, Maryland Heights, MO 63043. Customer Service (orders, claims, online, change of address): Elsevier Health Sciences Division, Subscription **Customer Service, 3251 Riverport Lane, Maryland Heights, MO 63043. Tel: 1-800-654-2452 (U.S. and Canada); 314-447-8871 (outside U.S. and Canada). Fax: 314-447-8029. E-mail: journalscustomerservice-usa@elsevier.com (for print support); journalsonlinesupport-usa@elsevier.com (for online support).**

Reprints. For copies of 100 or more of articles in this publication, please contact the Commercial Reprints Department, Elsevier Inc., 360 Park Avenue South, New York, New York 10010-1710. Tel.: 212-633-3874; Fax: 212-633-3820; E-mail: reprints@elsevier.com.

Hand Clinics is covered in *MEDLINE/PubMed (Index Medicus)*, *Current Contents/Clinical Medicine*, *EMBASE/Excerpta Medica*, and *ISI/BIOMED*.

Contributors

CONSULTING EDITOR

KEVIN C. CHUNG, MD, MS
Charles B. G. de Nancrede Professor of
Surgery, Professor of Plastic Surgery and
Orthopaedic Surgery, Chief of Hand Surgery,
Michigan Medicine, Assistant Dean for Faculty
Affairs, Associate Director of Global REACH,
University of Michigan Medical School, Ann
Arbor, Michigan, USA

EDITOR

AVIRAM M. GILADI, MD, MS
Hand Surgery and Plastic Surgery, Research
Director, The Curtis National Hand Center,
MedStar Union Memorial Hospital, Baltimore,
Maryland, USA

AUTHORS

JOSHUA M. ADKINSON, MD
Assistant Professor of Surgery, Adjunct
Assistant Professor of Orthopaedic Surgery,
Chief of Hand Surgery, Division of Plastic
Surgery, Chief of Plastic Surgery, Sidney and
Lois S. Eskenazi Hospital, Indiana University
School of Medicine, Indianapolis, Indiana,
USA

ERIC ASTACIO, MD
Hand Fellow, UPMC Hamot, Erie,
Pennsylvania, USA; Hospital Metropolitano,
San Juan, Puerto Rico

DIANE J. ATKINS, OTR
Department of Physical Medicine and
Rehabilitation, Baylor College of Medicine,
Houston, Texas, USA

ABDO BACHOURA, MD
Hand Surgeon, University of Central Florida/
HCA Healthcare, Ocala, Florida, USA

**CHRISTOPHER M. BASCHUK, MPO, CPO,
FAAOP(D)**
Handspring Clinical Services, Salt Lake City,
Utah, USA

BRYAN BOURLAND, DO
Hand Fellow, UPMC Hamot, Erie,
Pennsylvania, USA; Texas Tech University
Health Sciences Center, Lubbock, Texas, USA

BRIAN L. CHANG, MD
The Curtis National Hand Center, MedStar
Union Memorial Hospital, Baltimore, Maryland,
USA; Department of Plastic Surgery, MedStar
Georgetown University Hospital, Washington,
DC, USA

KEVIN C. CHUNG, MD, MS
Charles B. G. de Nancrede Professor of
Surgery, Professor of Plastic Surgery and
Orthopaedic Surgery, Chief of Hand Surgery,
Michigan Medicine, Assistant Dean for Faculty

Affairs, Associate Director of Global REACH, University of Michigan Medical School, Ann Arbor, Michigan, USA

SOUMEN DAS DE, MBBS, FRCS, MPH
Consultant, Department of Hand and Reconstructive Microsurgery, National University Hospital, Singapore

CHRISTOPHER C. DUNCAN, MD
Department of Physical Medicine and Rehabilitation, University of Utah School of Medicine, Craig H. Neilsen Rehabilitation Hospital, Salt Lake City, Utah, USA

MAJ JOHN C. DUNN, MD
Department of Orthopaedic Surgery, William Beaumont Army Medical Center, El Paso, Texas, USA; Uniformed Services University of the Health Sciences, Bethesda, Maryland, USA

KATE ELZINGA, MD
Clinical Lecturer, Section of Plastic Surgery, University of Calgary, Calgary, Alberta, Canada

AVIRAM M. GILADI, MD, MS
Hand Surgery and Plastic Surgery, Research Director, The Curtis National Hand Center, MedStar Union Memorial Hospital, Baltimore, Maryland, USA

EMILY M. GRAHAM, BSN
Division of Plastic Surgery, Department of Surgery, University of Utah School of Medicine, Salt Lake City, Utah, USA

JESSICA B. HAWKEN, MD
Resident, Orthopaedic Surgery, Medstar Orthopaedic Institute at Union Memorial Hospital, Baltimore, Maryland, USA

RUSSELL HENDRYCKS, BS
Division of Plastic Surgery, Department of Surgery, University of Utah School of Medicine, Salt Lake City, Utah, USA

MIN KI HONG, MD
Department of Plastic and Reconstructive Surgery, Gwangmyeong Sungae General Hospital, Gwangmyeong, Korea

RYAN D. KATZ, MD
The Curtis National Hand Center, MedStar Union Memorial Hospital, Baltimore, Maryland, USA

LANA KEIZER, OTR, CHT
Department of Occupational Hand Therapy, University of Utah, Salt Lake City, Utah, USA

JIN SOO KIM, MD, PhD
Department of Plastic and Reconstructive Surgery, Gwangmyeong Sungae General Hospital, Gwangmyeong, Korea

MAJ NICHOLAS A. KUSNEZOV, MD
Department of Orthopaedic Surgery, Blanchfield Army Community Hospital, Fort Campbell, Kentucky, USA

SUNG HOON KOH, MD, PhD
Department of Plastic and Reconstructive Surgery, Gwangmyeong Sungae General Hospital, Gwangmyeong, Korea

DONG CHUL LEE, MD
Department of Plastic and Reconstructive Surgery, Gwangmyeong Sungae General Hospital, Gwangmyeong, Korea

KYUNG JIN LEE, MD
Department of Plastic and Reconstructive Surgery, Gwangmyeong Sungae General Hospital, Gwangmyeong, Korea

NIKOLA LEKIC, MD
Hand Surgery Fellow, Department of Orthopaedics, Baylor College of Medicine, Houston, Texas, USA

JANICE C.Y. LIAO, MBBS, MRCS, FAMS
Associate Consultant, Department of Orthopaedic Surgery, Ng Teng Fong General Hospital, Department of Hand and Reconstructive Microsurgery, National University Hospital, Singapore

SCOTT N. LOEWENSTEIN, MD
Chief Resident, Division of Plastic Surgery, Integrated Plastic Surgery Residency Program, Indiana University School of Medicine, Indianapolis, Indiana, USA

JOHN D. LUBAHN, MD
Program Director for Hand Fellowship, UPMC Hamot, Erie, Pennsylvania, USA

KENNETH R. MEANS Jr, MD
The Curtis National Hand Center, MedStar Union Memorial Hospital, Baltimore, Maryland, USA

SHAUN D. MENDENHALL, MD
Division of Plastic Surgery, Department of
Surgery, University of Utah School of Medicine,
Salt Lake City, Utah, USA

LTC LEON J. NESTI, MD
Department of Orthopaedic Surgery,
Walter Reed National Military Medical
Center, Uniformed Services University of
the Health Sciences, Bethesda, Maryland,
USA

DAVID NETSCHER, MD
Clinical Professor of Plastic Surgery and
Orthopedic Surgery, Program Director Hand
Fellowship, Baylor College of Medicine,
Adjunct Professor of Clinical Surgery, Weill
Cornell Medical College, New York, New York,
USA

**MICHAEL W. NEUMEISTER, MD, FRCSC,
FACS**
Chair and Professor, Department of Surgery,
Institute for Plastic Surgery, Southern Illinois
University School of Medicine, Springfield,
Illinois, USA

JIN HA PARK, MD
Department of Plastic and Reconstructive
Surgery, Gwangmyeong Sungae General
Hospital, Gwangmyeong, Korea

MITCHELL A. PET, MD
Division of Plastic and Reconstructive Surgery,
Washington University in St. Louis, St Louis,
Missouri, USA

SI YOUNG ROH, MD, PhD
Department of Plastic and Reconstructive
Surgery, Gwangmyeong Sungae General
Hospital, Gwangmyeong, Korea

REBECCA J. SAUNDERS, PT, CHT
The Curtis National Hand Center, MedStar
Union Memorial Hospital, Baltimore, Maryland,
USA

CPT JOHN P. SCANALIATO, MD
Department of Orthopaedic Surgery, William
Beaumont Army Medical Center, Texas Tech
University Health Sciences Center, El Paso,
Texas, USA

LUIS SCHEKER, MD
Kleinert Institute for Hand and Microsurgery,
Associate Professor of Hand Surgery,
Department of Plastic Surgery, University of
Louisville, Louisville, Kentucky, USA

AMELIA C. VAN HANDEL, MD
Division of Plastic and Reconstructive Surgery,
Washington University in St. Louis, St Louis,
Missouri, USA

CPT MATTHEW E. WELLS, DO
Department of Orthopaedic Surgery, William
Beaumont Army Medical Center, Department
of Orthopaedic Surgery, Texas Tech University
Health Sciences Center, El Paso, Texas, USA

JAMES N. WINTERS, MD
Resident Physician, Institute for Plastic
Surgery, Southern Illinois University School of
Medicine, Springfield, Illinois, USA

Contents

Appropriate management of the acute fingertip and nail bed injury is critical for optimizing patient outcomes. Mismanaged injuries can lead to chronic pain and deformity. Subungual hematomas may be treated with simple trephination for pain relief. Nail bed lacerations may be repaired using dissolvable suture or octyl-2-cyanoacrylate, and in most cases with no need to replace the nail plate or stent the fold. Amputations, partial or complete, can be treated with a wide variety of techniques, but many distal injuries can be left to heal by secondary intention with excellent results.

The volar fingertip is a unique anatomic structure, delicate yet durable, that allows us to navigate the world, acquire information from our surroundings, and express ourselves. Injuries to the volar finger can cause permanent dysfunction and should be taken seriously. In treating injuries of the volar fingertip, the surgeon has an opportunity to choose from a host of reconstructive options and provide the patient with an outcome suitable to their needs. In doing so, the hand surgeon is well-positioned to aim for the reconstructive ideal of restoring both structure and function.

Acute tendon and bony injuries of the distal phalanx are challenging injuries because they may result in chronic pain, hypersensitivity, stiffness, and deformity if they are not adequately treated. Flexor tendon avulsions require early surgical repair. Conversely, most extensor tendon injuries and fractures heal well with nonoperative treatment. However, surgery is indicated in selected patients, and meticulous technique is required to achieve good postoperative outcomes. In this article, we outline the pertinent clinical anatomy of the distal phalanx, review the current literature regarding treatment options, and highlight key management points to ensure good clinical outcomes while minimizing complications.

Following a fingertip amputation, if vessels are present and of adequate condition, microsurgical replantation is the preferred technique for management. Composite grafting has a limited role in the management of fingertip amputations due to its unreliable nature but can be an option when an amputated fingertip is not replantable and the patient desires restoration of fingertip length and aesthetics. When composite grafting is selected as the treatment of choice for a particular patient, there are methods of optimizing the chances of graft revascularization and survival, including early grafting, graft cooling, and a moist wound healing environment.

Amelia C. Van Handel and Mitchell A. Pet

Fingertip replantation is technically challenging, but in a motivated patient excellent aesthetic and functional outcomes can be achieved. Fingertip microanatomy by zone is described to facilitate the classification and treatment of these injuries. In this article, we outline our preferred techniques for fingertip replantation and review the current body of evidence surrounding indications, techniques, and outcomes while highlighting opportunities for future study.

Michael W. Neumeister and James N. Winters

This article reviews the nomenclature, anatomic components, and physiologic growth involving the perionychium. Fingertip and nailbed injuries are commonly encountered problems in hand surgery. This article focuses primarily on dealing with chronic nailbed deformities following traumatic injury such as nonadherence, split nails, avulsion loss, and hook nails. Nail deformities secondary to pincer nail, mass effect, and pigmented lesions are reviewed as well. The underlying pathology and treatment options are examined for each deformity. The senior author highlights technical pearls and surgical planning for his preferred methods of reconstruction.

Nikola Lekic, Luis Scheker, and David Netscher

Delayed finger and thumb tip reconstruction should try to optimally reconstruct perioncyhial aesthetic and functional units by replacing tissue as closely resembling the original loss as possible. Avoid thinking in terms of a "reconstructive ladder" but rather going directly to the reconstructive choice that seems most suited to the task. Some reconstructive choices may seem more attractive because of their simplicity, but may not necessarily give the best functional and aesthetic result. Free flaps and the newer advancements with vascular island flaps give many more and versatile reconstructive options.

Min Ki Hong, Jin Ha Park, Sung Hoon Koh, Dong Chul Lee, Si Young Roh, Kyung Jin Lee, and Jin Soo Kim

Fingertip injuries occur commonly owing to trauma in everyday life. Performing amputation or stump revision for a fingertip injury can make it possible to quickly return to daily life, but causes functional and cosmetic problems. We believe that free flaps are the ideal way to minimize donor site morbidity and provide satisfactory reconstruction. Fingertips have different anatomic characteristics on the dorsum, volar aspect, and pulp, so it is necessary to select the appropriate free flap. Sometimes for larger defects, composite tissue transfer can be considered for reconstruction. This article discusses various free flap options for different fingertip defects.

Pediatric Fingertip Injuries

Scott N. Loewenstein and Joshua M. Adkinson

Pediatric fingertip injuries are common and peak at 2 years of age. These injuries most frequently result from a crush mechanism and half sustain an associated fracture. The presence of a physis results in unique injury patterns and management considerations in the growing child. Due to a substantial healing potential in children, an initial conservative approach to management for many soft tissue and nail bed injuries is recommended. This article reviews the evidence and approach for treating pediatric fingertip injuries and amputations.

Fingertip Injuries in Athletes, Musicians, and Other Special Cases

Bryan Bourland, Eric Astacio, Abdo Bachoura, and John D. Lubahn

Management of fingertip injuries in athletes is optimized by consideration of the sport, the playing position, the timing within the season, the level of competition, and the patient's goals. Mallet and jersey fingers are common injuries in athletes and may be treated in several different ways, based on the nature of the injury and the timing of presentation, as well as the athlete's demands. Management of fingertip injuries in musicians is optimized by consideration of how the musician handles his or her instrument and the specific requirements of the injured digit in the context of musical performance.

Understanding and Measuring Long-Term Outcomes of Fingertip and Nail Bed Injuries and Treatments

Kenneth R. Means Jr. and Rebecca J. Saunders

There are many outcome measures to choose from when caring for or studying fingertip and nail bed trauma and treatments. This article outlines general outcome measures principles as well as guidelines on choosing, implementing, and interpreting specific tools for these injuries. It also presents recent results from the literature for many of these measures, which can help learners, educators, and researchers by providing a clinical knowledge base and aiding study design.

The Burden of Fingertip Trauma on the US Military

Matthew E. Wells, John P. Scanaliato, Nicholas A. Kusnezov, Leon J. Nesti, and John C. Dunn

Fingertip injuries in the military are common and often hinder the fighting force and support personnel. Injuries range from small subungual hematomas to proximal finger amputations. Treatment modalities are dictated by injury patterns, anatomic considerations, and the need to return to duty. Nail bed injuries should be repaired when possible and exposed bone or tendon is treated with appropriate soft tissue coverage. If soft tissue coverage is unobtainable, revision amputation should be performed with attention given to maintaining as much finger length as possible. Antibiotics may not be required, however they are often utilized in the deployed setting.

Emily M. Graham, Russell Hendrycks, Christopher M. Baschuk, Diane J. Atkins, Lana Keizer, Christopher C. Duncan, and Shaun D. Mendenhall

Partial hand amputations are the most common upper extremity amputations and affect individuals across a spectrum of socioeconomic and geographic backgrounds. Prosthetic devices can provide straightforward solutions to the devastating aesthetic, functional, psychological, and social deficits caused by these injuries. However, because of the recent development of multiple partial hand prosthetic devices, many hand providers remain unaware of their applicability in practice. This article highlights the various classes of partial hand prostheses currently available, including passive functional, body-powered, and externally powered options. Familiarity with these partial hand prostheses will better enable providers to care for partial hand amputees.

HAND CLINICS

SERIES OF RELATED INTEREST:

Clinics in Plastic Surgery
https://www.plasticsurgery.theclinics.com/

Orthopedic Clinics of North America
https://www.orthopedic.theclinics.com/

Physical Medicine and Rehabilitation Clinics of North America
https://www.pmr.theclinics.com/

THE CLINICS ARE AVAILABLE ONLINE!
Access your subscription at:
www.theclinics.com

Preface

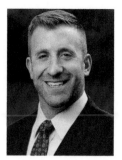

Aviram M. Giladi, MD, MS
Editor

Although perhaps not as controversial or exciting as many of the other frequently reviewed topics in hand surgery, managing fingertip injuries and nail deformities is an integral part of all hand surgery practice. Anyone who has sustained a minor crush or small laceration to their fingertip is aware of the incredible discomfort and functional limitation that can come from a seemingly unimpressive insult. Yet, for such a commonly injured and relatively impactful part of the body, academic pursuits around fingertip care, from the simplest problems to the most complex injuries and treatment options, remain sparse. Treatment decisions are often guided by anecdotal teaching, and recent innovation has overall been limited. However, there are many incredibly talented and thoughtful surgeons working on the problems of fingertip injuries and nail deformities, and in this issue of *Hand Clinics*, we have an opportunity to learn from many of them.

Appropriate management of acute injuries as well as the long-term sequelae is critical to reducing patient and health system burden. Through this issue, we look at all aspects of treating fingertip and nail trauma. We review management of the acute injury, including emergency room procedures, bone and tendon repairs and reconstruction, grafting, and flap reconstruction options. We also approach the complexities of distal replantation, with a synthesis of the incredible work presented in case series and cohort studies to give a comprehensive roadmap to these daunting procedures. We focus on the challenging issues around nail and nailbed injuries, including acute management as well as secondary reconstruction for deformities. Knowing that measuring outcomes after these injuries is critical in understanding what treatments and approaches are most successful, we include a thorough review of how to best obtain and interpret proper outcomes measures for fingertip injuries. We then review treatment approaches for special populations, including children, musicians, athletes, and the military. And we finish with a look at current prosthetic approaches, and the growing list of options for novel distal finger prostheses.

It has been an honor to work with and learn from the incredible authors in this issue of *Hand Clinics*. My deepest thanks to all the contributors and to the dedicated *Hand Clinics* staff who supported this entire process with skill, kindness, and flexibility, especially as the manuscript deadlines and initial edits occurred during the peak of the COVID-19 pandemic. And thank you to my mentor, Dr Kevin Chung, for his guidance, teachings, and endless support, and for privileging me with the opportunity to curate this issue. We hope that these articles are a valuable educational and clinical resource for all providers tasked with treating fingertip and nailbed trauma.

Aviram M. Giladi, MD, MS
Hand Surgery and Plastic Surgery
3333 N. Calvert Street
JPB 2nd floor
Baltimore, MD 21218, USA

E-mail address:
giladi@curtishand.com

Hand Clin 37 (2021) xiii
https://doi.org/10.1016/j.hcl.2020.09.014
0749-0712/21/© 2020 Published by Elsevier Inc.

Primary Management of Nail Bed and Fingertip Injuries in the Emergency Department

Jessica B. Hawken, MD[a], Aviram M. Giladi, MD, MS[b,*]

KEYWORDS

- Nail bed injury • Nail bed laceration • Fingertip injury • Subungual hematoma
- Fingertip amputations

KEY POINTS

- Systematically evaluate each injury in the same manner every time.
- Consider trephination with a heated blunt instrument to drain any subungual hematoma that covers more than 50% of the nail, or even smaller if notably painful.
- When visualization or access are limited but nail bed laceration repair is required, gently remove the nail plate to fully expose the injury and facilitate well-approximated repair with fine absorbable suture or adhesives.
- Although commonly described and reported in the literature, nail fold stenting after nail plate removal may not be needed or indicated for most injuries.
- Distal fingertip avulsions and amputations can be successfully managed conservatively using dressings alone with good restoration of aesthetics, function, and sensation.

INTRODUCTION

Hands are our way of communicating, feeling, and navigating the world. The fingertip and nail play a critical role in sensation, durability, and cosmetic appearance of the hand, and contribute to strength and function. Recreational and work-related activities place the fingertips at risk daily because they are often the first part of the hand exposed to various obstacles and machines, including doors, saws, lawnmowers, and many others. Fingertip injuries are a frequent cause for emergency department visits. When someone's hand is injured, there is a risk for substantial time away from work and recreational activities, ranging from 1 week to several months.[1,2] There is also risk of chronic deformity and disability if the injury is managed inappropriately.

Although fingertip injuries are common, providers with experience in managing them are not always available. Mismanagement and inadequate repair can lead to chronic deformity, and treatment of these deformities often requires a more difficult secondary reconstructive procedure with less reliable outcomes than a well-managed initial repair. Anyone providing care for these injuries in the emergency room or urgent care setting must understand and have experience with various management approaches and techniques, and know when to refer a patient with a complex injury to a more experienced provider. This article reviews the emergency medicine and hand surgery

[a] Orthopaedic Surgery, Medstar Orthopaedic Institute at Union Memorial Hospital, Baltimore, MD, USA;
[b] Hand Surgery and Plastic Surgery, The Curtis National Hand Center, MedStar Union Memorial Hospital, 3333 N. Calvert Street, JPB 2nd floor, Baltimore, MD 21218, USA
* Corresponding author.
E-mail address: giladi@curtishand.com

Hand Clin 37 (2021) 1–10
https://doi.org/10.1016/j.hcl.2020.09.001

0749-0712/21/© 2020 Elsevier Inc. All rights reserved.

literature and details the current recommendations for acute nonsurgical (aside from suture closure) emergency department management of fingertip injuries ranging from subungual hematomas to amputations.

ANATOMY

The fingertip is composed of numerous structures, all of which play a role in function and aesthetics (**Fig. 1**). Identifying the various anatomic components after injury is a difficult but critical step in assessing the traumatized nail and fingertip.[3]

The distal phalanx lies in the dorsal one-half of the fingertip and is the underlying bony foundation of the nail. The periosteum is connected to the skin by fibrous septae, which anchor the skin to the bone. The pulp of the fingertip also has septae that divide the fibroadipose tissue and tether the glabrous skin to assist with traction during grip.

The perionychium consists of the paronychium and the nail bed; and includes the nail plate, nail bed, and the hyponychium. The paronychium are the ulnar and radial walls of the nail. The eponychium is the proximal fold, which is a continuation of the dorsal skin of the hand.

The nail bed itself consists of the germinal matrix and sterile matrix. The lunula is the white crescent visible under the nail plate, just distal to the eponychial fold. The extensor tendon insertion is approximately 5 mm proximal to the lunula.[4] The germinal matrix extends from its origin 1.2 to 1.4 mm distal to the extensor tendon insertion, under the dorsal skin/eponychium, and out to its most distal margin that forms the lunula, with approximately 1 mm showing in the most proximal aspect of the nail plate. The germinal matrix is a critical structure, responsible for 90% of the nail growth by secreting the keratinous material from which the nail plate is made. The sterile matrix begins at the lunula and extends out to the hyponychium. The sterile matrix is responsible for adhering the nail plate to the nail bed.

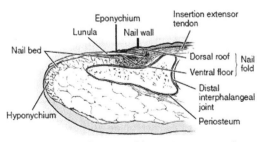

Fig. 1. Anatomic drawing of fingertip anatomy. (*From* Peterson SL, Peterson EL, Wheatley MJ. Management of fingertip amputations. *J Hand Surg Am.* 2014 Oct;39(10):2093-101, with permission.)

The hyponychium is the junction of the sterile matrix and the fingertip skin. The nail plate is nonadherent at this point. Fortunately, the hyponychium has a rich supply of white blood cells; it is the first barrier to external infectious organisms, such as bacteria and fungi.

The nail plate is quite adherent to the nail bed and removing an intact nail plate from the nail bed can be difficult. During procedures, care must be taken when removing the adherent nail plate to avoid iatrogenic injury to the bed. And if an injury results in disruption of the nail plate, this should raise suspicion that more extensive nail bed trauma has occurred.

NATURE OF THE PROBLEM

Hand and fingertip injuries account for 4.8 million emergency room visits annually.[5] For many fingertip injuries, the emergency room is the location of definitive management. This includes treatment of subungual hematomas, simple or stellate lacerations, avulsions, open fractures, and amputations. Whether management is performed by the emergency department provider or a specialist is based on practitioner comfort level and services readily available via consultation.

EVALUATION

Evaluating each fingertip injury should be done systematically. Radiographs should be taken of the injured digit to assess for fracture or dislocation. Remove any dressings that are on the patient when they arrive. Arterial bleeding may be controlled with direct pressure, or if visualization is difficult, pressure can be applied proximal to the injury to slow or stop bleeding. A tourniquet may also be used if needed for examination visualization, as a last option. The level of injury is then noted. Vascularity should be determined first by checking capillary refill and confirmed with use of a doppler on the pulp or remnant digit distal to the injury. The digit should be evaluated for sensation, for both fine touch sensation and 2-point discrimination, radially and ulnarly, proximal and distal to the injury. Two-point discrimination can be assessed by using various objects regularly available in most emergency departments, including the 2 ends of a bent paperclip or two 25-gauge needles.

Once sensation and vascularity have been determined, a digital block may be performed. There are numerous techniques, but the authors' preferred technique is tumescence of the dorsal metacarpophalangeal region first, followed by infiltration of each webspace from a dorsal approach with a total of 5 to 10 mL of lidocaine. Some authors advocate use of lidocaine with epinephrine to provide appropriate hemostasis with no increased risk to the finger.[6] This option may be appropriate for some patients, especially if a tourniquet is not available, as long as the finger does not have notable vascular compromise owing to injury, and the patient has no specific medical reasons that epinephrine should be avoided. Any gross contamination should then be removed with irrigation and the digit should be cleansed. This technique can simply be performed by gently submerging the digit in a mixture of water and betadine or water and peroxide and allowing the digit to soak as preparations are made for a procedure. Before the procedure, we copiously irrigate once more and then use a final betadine swab. If necessary for the procedure, a digital tourniquet may be applied; a bloodless field facilitates an excellent repair. For a tourniquet, we often use available materials such as a Penrose drain or a glove. Always tag the tourniquet as a reminder to remove it when the procedure is done. Once appropriate analgesia has been achieved, the injury may be addressed by whatever technique is deemed appropriate.

SUBUNGUAL HEMATOMAS

Subungual hematomas are an accumulation of blood under the nail plate. This accumulation is usually the result of direct crushing trauma to the fingertip, which injures the nail bed, although the nail plate remains intact. The collection of blood under the nail is painful owing to pressure in a confined space. This injury often requires decompression by making a hole in the nail plate ("trephinate").[7] The amount of the nail that is involved with the hematoma has traditionally dictated whether to intervene or monitor. Typically, if 50% or more of the nail is involved, or if there is a very painful hematoma, trephination is indicated.[8]

There are numerous methods described to trephinate the nail. These include using a punch biopsy, electrocautery, or a presterilized needle to bore a hole in the nail plate. One electrocautery tool available in many emergency departments is a single-use, battery powered, handheld device with a blunt tip that decreases the risk of incidental injury to the nail bed that could more easily occur with a sharp tip. The device tip heats to approximately 1200°F in less than 1 second and glows red when heated. This instrument can then be used to carefully cauterize through the nail plate only and express the hematoma. The critical part of the procedure, whichever device is used, is avoiding injuring the nail bed underneath the plate

by remaining superficial.[9,10] We prefer using blunt heated instruments whenever possible because even a slight overshot with a sharp tip can cause substantial nail bed trauma.

Complete nail plate removal can also be used, although this carries increased risk of iatrogenic nail bed injury that can be avoided if treated with trephination alone. Nail plate removal was advocated after Garcia-Rodriguez[11] performed a study of 47 patients with subungual hematomas involving more than 25% of the nail plate. When the nail was removed for exploration of the wound, Garcia-Rodriguez[11] found a 60% incidence of 3 mm or greater fissures in the nail bed as a result of the initial injury. The incidence increased to 95% when there was an associated distal phalanx fracture. It was therefore recommended to remove the plate and fix these injuries.

However, more recent evidence indicates that removal of the nail, although facilitating exposure of an injured nail bed, can result in more scarring and risks iatrogenic damage to the nail bed. Trephination alone decreases these risks as well as the cost, without notable increased risk of worse outcomes. Meek and White[12] looked at 94 subungual hematomas treated with trephination alone and found 85% excellent and very good results using Zook's criteria (excellent = normal; very good = minor deformity). Seaberg and colleagues[13] looked at 45 children with fingertip injuries with more than one-half having subungual hematomas in more than 50% of the nail bed surface area. All were treated with trephination alone and at 10 months revealed no complications. Gellman[14] compared 53 patients with subungual hematomas, one-third of which had greater than 75% of the nail involved. Twenty-six consecutive patients received formal nail plate removal and nail bed repair and 27 underwent trephination or no treatment. There was no difference in outcomes at the 2-year follow-up other than cost of treatment, which was substantially higher for the repair group. Therefore, to prevent unnecessary iatrogenic injury, trephination alone is recommended when there is not an obvious or extensive disruption in the nail bed.

When a subungual hematoma is associated with a fracture, it is typically a crush injury resulting in a fracture of the distal phalanx (**Figs. 2** and **3**). These fractures reliably heal without intervention unless there is substantial comminution, displacement, instability, or intra-articular extension. If not amenable to nonoperative treatment, then a Kirschner wire or a screw may be needed to stabilize the bone for optimal nail regrowth.[15] In a prospective study by Da Cruz and associates,16 crush injuries associated with a fracture had worse

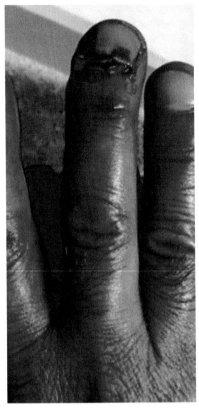

Fig. 2. Clinical photograph of a subungual hematoma with associated eponychial fold injury.

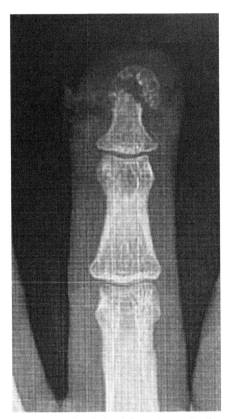

Fig. 3. Radiograph of the injury demonstrating displaced tuft fracture.

outcomes, including persistent pain, nail bed deformity, and stiffness. Only 17% of the patients in their study had fully recovered at 6 months when there was a tuft fracture.[16] Patients with these more severe injuries should be counseled as to their expected recovery.

NAIL BED LACERATIONS

Nail bed lacerations with associated fracture and splitting of the nail plate are commonly the result of sharp or crush injuries to the fingertip. Nail bed lacerations are classified by their shape, namely, simple, complex, and stellate.[7] Management of the laceration begins with proper analgesia, cleaning the wound with an antimicrobial solution such as betadine, and establishing a bloodless field, often by using a tourniquet or lidocaine with epinephrine as mentioned elsewhere in this article.

The damaged nail is removed to expose the underlying bed laceration(s), typically with the aid of a flat elevator such as a freer. If a sharp-edged instrument is used, the sharp side should be used to push up on the plate rather than down on the bed to prevent further injury to the nail bed.

Additionally, the plate is often adherent to the underside of the eponychial fold, which also requires gentle removal. Once the plate is off the nail bed is then approached. The segments of the nail bed are reapproximated, typically using fine absorbable sutures, such as 5-0, 6-0, or 7-0 chromic gut. Minimal debridement should be performed so as not to place the repair under additional tension. If the nail bed segments seem to be robust, for example, with a linear laceration and minimal surrounding trauma and edema, they can be gently elevated to allow for mobilization and reapproximation. Repair of injured segments with restoration of the nail bed architecture, whether the laceration is simple or complex, facilitates the best results. Zook and colleagues[17] reported 90% good-to-excellent results in 300 nail bed injuries treated with nail plate removal and nail bed repair with 7-0 chromic gut suture. When indicated, they also performed reduction and pinning of unstable distal phalanx fractures. Of note, worse outcomes were associated with crush and avulsion-type injuries and infection, indicating it is perhaps not the repair, but rather the injury itself that is the most impactful factor in determining the outcome. **Figs. 4** and **5** demonstrate a nail bed laceration before and after repair.

The use of alternative methods of repair has also been investigated. Topical glue has recently been considered as an acceptable alternative to suture repair of the nail bed.[18] It is reportedly simpler, quicker, and, according to some authors, allows for a more standardized approach to nail issues by eliminating variability in repair technique.[19] Strauss and colleagues[20,21] evaluated 40 adult patients with nail bed lacerations in a prospective, randomized study reporting no significant differences in patient satisfaction, physician assessment of nail appearance, or functional outcome between patients who had nail bed repair with octyl-2-cyanoacrylate (Dermabond, Ethicon, Inc., Somerville, NJ) compared with patients who had repair with 6-0 absorbable sutures.

Stenting the fold after nail bed repair has traditionally been done under the belief that it will prevent scarring between the bed and the underside of the fold, maintaining appropriate nail plate growth and progression. However, replacement of the nail or other material as a stent for the eponychial fold is controversial. This is especially true when the injury does not involve the eponychium. The replacement of the nail plate itself was first recommended by Schiller in 1957. This recommendation has transitioned in many institutions to splinting the nail fold with foil from the suture packaging and, more recently, transitioning to using something softer like xeroform. O'Shaughnessy and colleagues[22] compared 10 patients where the nail was replaced as a stent after nail bed repair with 54 patients where no stent was used. There was no significant difference in the appearance of the nail or the rate of regrowth, but crush injuries were worse in both groups. This finding again indicates that injury mechanism plays a substantial role in determining the outcome. Zook and colleagues[17] also found there was no difference in outcomes after nail plate replacement as a fold stent compared with no replacement.

Our recommendation and practice regarding nail plate replacement or other stent after nail bed repair is that it is generally unnecessary if there is no injury to the nail fold. Injuries that also involve the nail fold have not been adequately studied. If the fold itself is injured, it is possible

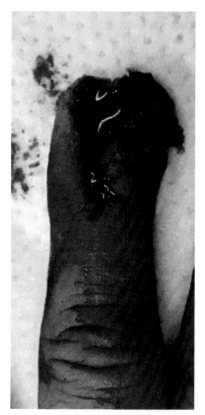

Fig. 4. Injury photograph of a complex nail bed laceration.

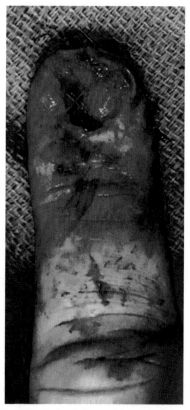

Fig. 5. Repair of the injury without replacement of nail or stent.

that the risk of scarring and synechiae compromising subsequent nail growth is higher; however, there are no robust data to support or refute this idea. As a result, many providers still advocate use of a nail fold stent, either hard (plate or foil) or soft (xeroform or other petroleum gauze) for these injuries. Although not yet rigorously studied, we recommend a soft stent when possible to avoid unnecessary trauma to the perionychium with sharp or hard stents.

Replantation and Amputations

When the distal digit sustains an amputation injury, there are various treatment algorithms that can help to guide management. Many classifications exist for distal fingertip amputations. The most commonly used is the Tamai classification, which divides fingertip injuries into 2 zones (**Fig. 6**).[23] Zone I is from the distal fingertip to the lunula, and zone II extends from the lunula to the distal interphalangeal joint. If the injury is a relatively clean laceration and meets indications, the distal part can be considered for replantation. This procedure is highly technically demanding and requires the availability of microsurgical instruments and presence and size of adequate arteries (and perhaps veins) in the distal amputation segment. These techniques and details are

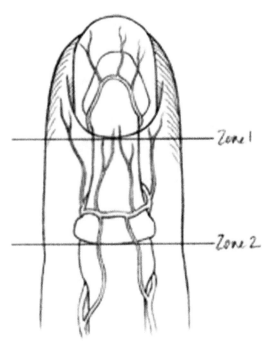

Fig. 6. Tamai classification of fingertip amputations. (*From* Peterson SL, Peterson EL, Wheatley MJ. Management of Fingertip Amputations. J Hand Surg Am. 2014 Oct;39(10):2093-101. With permission.)

not discussed in this article. If replantation is not possible, grafting is a consideration. The dorsal side of the hand has thinner, more mobile skin that is, therefore, more amenable to skin grafting. Volar pulp sensation is of such high value that skin grafting the volar fingertip is avoided if possible. Additionally, there are surgical procedures for volar defect closure, especially of volar oblique injuries with extensive soft tissue loss, including V–Y advancement flaps, cross-finger flaps, thenar flaps, and heterodigital or homodigital island flaps among others. These techniques are also not discussed in this article, because we are focusing on nonsurgical management in the emergency department.

In the emergency department evaluation, there is a treatment decision to make for distal tip amputation (or partial amputation/avulsion) injuries. The options are usually between closure of the wound, often with minimal shortening of the tip/bone to get closure, versus allowing for healing by secondary intention. For some authors, fingertip injuries with small pulp defects (<1 cm^2) and/or simple skin lacerations are ideal for debridement and repair.[24] An important variable in this decision-making step is presence of remnant nail tissue. With remnant germinal matrix but loss of sterile matrix and bone and volar tissue, there is risk of a nonadherent nail deformity because the germinal matrix will produce nail, but the bed will be injured or even absent. With remnant germinal and sterile matrix with associated bone loss, there is risk of a hook nail deformity because the nail continues to grow but the distal and volar support is gone and the sterile matrix often scars over the injured tip, carrying the nail plate with it as the plate grows. Both of these nail deformities are associated with pain and diminished function of the finger, with a high likelihood of needing associated secondary procedures to address the deformity. Nail ablation should be considered in these scenarios.[25]

Another variable is the amount of remnant tissue. When closure is too tight over prominent distal bone, the site can become thinned and painful. When bone removal is required to obtain appropriate closure, this results in loss of length, which has associated cosmetic and sometimes functional challenges for patients.[7,26]

Taking these variables into consideration when assessing the injury is critical in achieving optimal outcomes. When amenable, the skin should be loosely approximated after performing a thorough irrigation and debridement with removal of any contamination. Loose closure allows for drainage of any remaining contaminants during the healing process. This strategy can allow for the quickest recovery with minimal downtime.[24]

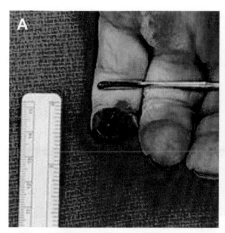 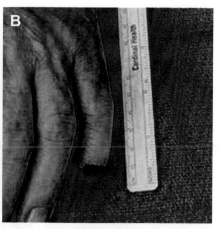

Fig. 7. (A) Volar and (B) dorsal injury photographs taken of an adult with a distal tip amputation of the small finger.

If the patient is amenable or the wound is too complex to close, allowing it to heal by secondary intention is an excellent option rather than pursuing one of the more complex options listed. Recently, owing to various reassuring case series publications, the indications for this conservative treatment approach have expanded, including complete tip amputations, avulsion injuries, and even amputations that result in small amounts of distal phalanx exposure. When there is exposed bone or tendon, an additional procedure to facilitate closure has traditionally been recommended. However, the need for covering or cutting back

exposed bone may not be absolute, as shown by Hoigne and colleagues,[27] who treated a series of 19 fingertip amputations distal to the distal interphalangeal joint with semiocclusive dressing alone and observed regeneration of soft tissue thickness to nearly 90% of the baseline.

Conservative treatment is initiated by thoroughly cleansing the wound and removing any debris. A moist occlusive dressing is then applied. Options for lubrication and prevention of the dressing sticking to the wound include petroleum jelly (Vaseline), silver sulfadiazine (Silvadene), or xeroform. Patients are then instructed to elevate their affected

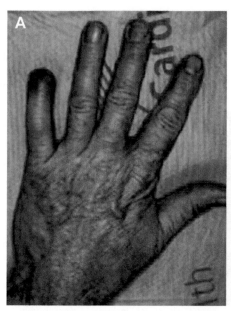 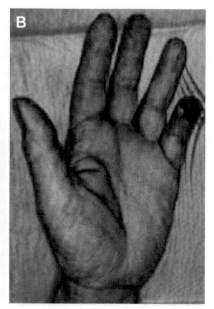

Fig. 8. (A) Dorsal and (B) volar 2-week visit photographs taken of the same injury, managed with dressing changes and local wound care.

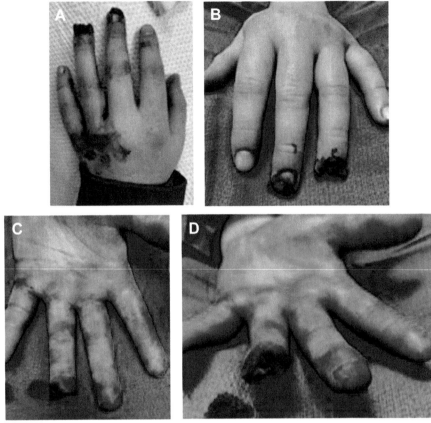

Fig. 9. Clinical photographs of a pediatric fingertip avulsion injury of the middle and ring finger at time of presentation, and after the wounds were irrigated and minimally debrided. (*A*) Dorsal, arrival of patient in the emergency department (*B*). Dorsal, after irrigation and gentle debridement. (*C*) Volar, after irrigation and debridement. (*D*) Distal axial image of the injury.

extremity. Timing of the initial dressing change varies from 2 to 5 days later. A tip protector can help the patient return to work more rapidly than if they had no protection on the end of the sensitive digit.[2,28] The outcomes of nonprocedural wound care treatment of these injuries have been reported to be overall very good to excellent, with appropriate functional and cosmetic restoration for many injury types and patterns.

Additionally, healing by secondary intention allows for overall better recovery of sensation as compared with surgical interventions.[29,30]

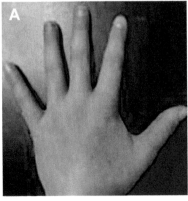
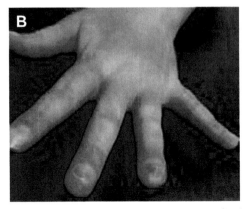

Fig. 10. (*A*) Dorsal (*B*) volar final visit photographs taken 16 weeks after injury with treatment of only dressings and local wound care.

Although Weichman and colleagues[31] found a small number of a cohort of nonsurgically treated fingers to have decreased 2-point discrimination, other studies have found 2-point discrimination comparable with the uninjured hand in most patients.[7] Secondary intention healing also has the benefit of facilitating motion shortly after injury, which may prevent the postoperative stiffness that can occur after surgical interventions.[26] Lee and colleagues[1] treated 156 consecutive patients with a fingertip cap alone and had satisfactory outcomes in all patients, with the majority reporting a near normal fingertip.

Figs. 7–10 demonstrate 2 fingertip avulsion injuries that were treated conservatively. **Figs. 7** and **8** show appearance at 1 week and 3 weeks after injury in a 46-year-old male smoker, illustrating the progress of recovery in the early weeks. **Figs. 8–10** show the injury and 16-week follow up in a 10-year-old boy, demonstrating the excellent cosmetic outcome of this treatment method.

A drawback to secondary intention healing is the length of time it takes for the patient to recover. Healing using conservative measures alone can routinely take more than 4 weeks, but smaller wounds with no bony involvement are often healed down to small residual scabs within 2 weeks. Complete resolution of all healing and sensitivity can take longer. Ma and colleagues[30] compared secondary intention healing against various flaps and had excellent results of conservative management with an average time to heal of 28 days and return to work at 41 days. Another drawback to this treatment is scar tenderness and hook nail deformity. Scar tenderness resolves typically around 3 months.[32] Loss of bone results in inadequate support for the nail, which can then become further distorted by wound contracture, and can result in a hook nail deformity. To prevent this complication when using secondary intention healing to treat an injury resulting in some distal phalanx loss, it is suggested that the nail bed be excised to a level 2 mm proximal to the shortened bone.[25]

SUMMARY

Management of fingertip injuries is as variable as the injuries themselves. Subungual hematomas can be trephinated if the patient is uncomfortable or the injury involves a substantial amount of the nail plate (traditionally >50%). Nail bed lacerations with obvious disruption of the nail plate should have the nail removed and the laceration repaired as anatomically as possible with either Dermabond or chromic suture, with a nail fold stent only if the eponychium is injured. Although distal tip amputations can undergo replantation, flap coverage, or primary closure, the indications for allowing these injuries to heal by secondary intention are expanding with overall excellent outcomes reported.

CLINICS CARE POINTS

- Trephination can easily be achieved with an electrocautery pen.
- Simple nailbed lacerations can be repaired with dermabond.
- Nail plate stenting is not always necessary.
- Conservative management of distal amputations can lead to excellent results in appropriate patients.

DISCLOSURE

The authors have nothing to disclose.

REFERENCES

1. Lee LP, Lau PY, Chan CW. A simple and efficient treatment for fingertip injuries. J Hand Surg Br 1995;20B:63–71.
2. Muhldorfer-Fodor M, Hohendorff AS, Vorderwindkler K-P, et al. Treatment of fingertip defect injuries with a semi-occlusive dressing according to Mennen and Wiese (German). Oper Orthop Traumatol 2013;25:104–14.
3. Zook EG. The perionychium: anatomy, physiology, and care of injuries. Clin Plast Surg 1981;8:21–31.
4. Shum C, Bruno RJ, Ristic S, et al. Examination of the anatomic relationship of the proximal germinal nail matrix to the extensor tendon insertion. J Hand Surg Am 2000;25(6):1114–7.
5. Sindhu K, DeFroda SF, Harris AP, et al. Management of partial fingertip amputation in adults: operative and non operative treatment. Injury 2017;48(12):2643–9.
6. Chowdry S, Seidenstricker L, Cooney D, et al. Do not use epinephrine in digital blocks: myth or truth? Part II. A retrospective review of 1111 cases. Plast Reconstr Surg 2010;126(6):2031–4.
7. Lee DH, Mignemi ME, Crosby SN. Fingertip injuries: an update on management. J Am Acad Orthop Surg 2013;21(12):756–66.
8. Roser SE, Gellman H. Comparison of nail bed repair versus nail trephination for subungual hematomas in children. J Hand Surg Am 1999;24(6):1166–70.
9. Salter SA1, Ciocon DH, Gowrishankar TR, et al. Controlled nail trephination for subungual hematoma. Am J Emerg Med 2006;24(7):875–7.
10. Simon RR, Wolgin M. Subungual hematoma: association with occult laceration requiring repair. Am J Emerg Med 1987;5(4):302–4.

11. Garcia-Rodriguez JA. Draining a subungual hematoma: procedures and assessments video series. Can Fam Physician 2013;59(8):853.

12. Meek S, White M. Subungual hematomas: is simple trephining enough? J Accid Emerg Med 1998;15(4):269–71.

13. Seaberg DC, Angelos WJ, Paris PM. Treatment of subungual hematomas with nail trephination: a prospective study. Am J Emerg Med 1991;9(3):209–10.

14. Gellman H. Fingertip-nail bed injuries in children: current concepts and controversies of treatment. J Craniofac Surg 2009;20(4):1033–5.

15. Gaston RG, Chadderdon C. Phalangeal fractures: displaced/nondisplaced. Hand Clin 2012;28(3):395–401, x.

16. Da Cruz DJ, Slade RJ, Malone W. Fractures of the distal phalanges. J Hand Surg Br 1988;13:350–2.

17. Zook EG, Guy RJ, Russell RC. A study of nail bed injuries: causes, treatment, and prognosis. J Hand Surg Am 1984;9(2):247–52.

18. Hallock GG, Lutz DA. Octyl-2-cyanoacrylate adhesive for rapid nail plate restoration. J Hand Surg Am 2000;25:979–81.

19. Yam A, Tan SH, Tan AB. A novel method of rapid nail bed repair using 2-octyl cyanoacrylate (Dermabond). Plast Reconstr Surg 2008;121:148e–9e.

20. Strauss EJ, Weil WM, Jordan C, et al. A prospective, randomized, controlled trial of 2-octylcyanoacrylate versus suture repair for nail bed injuries. J Hand Surg Am 2008;33(2):250–3.

21. Fehrenbacher V, Blackburn E. Nail bed injury. J Hand Surg Am 2015;40(3):581–2.

22. O'Shaughnessy M, McCann J, O'Connor TP. Nail regrowth in fingertip injuries. Ir Med J 1990;83(4):136–7.

23. Tamai S. Twenty years' experience of limb replantation: review of 293 upper extremity replants. J Hand Surg Am 1982;7(6):549–56.

24. Alwis W. Fingertip injuries. Emerg Med Australas 2006;18(3):229–37.

25. Pandya AN. Prevention of parrot beak deformity in fingertip injuries. Hand Surg 2001;6(2):163–6.

26. Allen MJ. Conservative management of finger tip injuries in adults. Hand 1980;12:257–65.

27. Hoigne D, Hug U, Schurch M, et al. Semi-occlusive dressing for the treatment of fingertip amputations with exposed bone: quantity and quality of soft-tissue regeneration. J Hand Surg Eur Vol 2014;39(5):505–9.

28. Farrell RG, Disher WA, Nesland RS, et al. Conservative management of fingertip amputations. JACEP 1977;6(6):243–6.

29. Hattori Y, Doi K, Ikeda K, et al. A retrospective study of functional outcomes after successful replantation versus amputation closure for single fingertip amputations. J Hand Surg Am 2006;31A:811–8.

30. Ma GFY, Cheng LCY, Chan KT, et al. Finger tip injuries—a prospective study on seven methods of treatment on 200 cases. Ann Acad Med Singap 1982;11:207–13.

31. Weichman KE, Wilson SC, Samra F, et al. Treatment and outcomes of fingertip injuries at a large metropolitan public hospital. Plast Reconstr Surg 2013;131:107–12.

32. Krauss EM, Lalonde DH. Secondary healing of fingertips: a review. Hand (N Y) 2014;9(3):282–8.

Locoregional Options for Acute Volar Pulp Fingertip Defects

Brian L. Chang, MD[a,b], Ryan D. Katz, MD[a,*]

KEYWORDS

- Volar fingertip injuries • Fingertip reconstruction • Distal finger amputation • Distal finger resurfacing

KEY POINTS

- It is important to treat each patient and his or her injury on an individualized basis; there is no one best procedure for all distal finger or thumb wounds.
- Fingertip reconstruction is challenging and must consider—and deliver—an appropriate aesthetic contour and, ideally, functional sensation.
- As with most defects elsewhere in the body, treating volar fingertip defects is best accomplished by replacing like with like.

INTRODUCTION

Richly innervated and mobile, the fingertip is a durable yet delicate instrument through which we navigate our environment and acquire information. Even in the absence of sight, data from the external world can be collected in minute detail with the tip of the finger. This article discusses how to approach volar fingertip defects and technical considerations when choosing a reconstructive option.

SURGICAL ANATOMY

"The fingertip" is the portion of the finger distal to the distal interphalangeal joint flexion crease. This aspect of the finger is composed of the distal phalanx, profundus tendon insertion, terminal extensor tendon insertion, volar pulp, nail bed, and nail plate.[1,2]

The volar aspect of the fingertip is covered by glabrous skin characterized by thick epidermis with deep papillary ridges. Meissner corpuscles, the rapid-adapting primary sensory end-organ for moving 2-point discrimination (2PD), reside at the apices of these dermal ridges.[3] The underlying pulp has well-vascularized fibrofatty tissue that is, stabilized by fibrous septa connecting the dermis to periosteum. This pulp structure aids in proper grip, proprioception, and sensation.

The volar fingertip benefits from a rich vascular supply. The proper digital arteries travel with their corresponding digital nerve longitudinally along the radial and ulnar sides of the digit. The ulnar and radial digital arteries communicate via 3 transverse arches: proximal arch at level of C1 pulley, middle at level of C3 pulley, and distal at the distal end of the FDP insertion. These arches supply the flexor tendons via vincula. The proper digital arteries have multiple small branches that supply the phalanges, condyles, and soft tissues.[4] The thumb, compared with the other digits, has a redundant dorsal blood supply. This affords a margin of safety for volar-based reconstructive methods such as the Moberg flap (described elsewhere in this article).

In the finger, the proper digital nerves travel alongside and volar to their corresponding digital arteries. Sensation to the volar pulp is derived from the proper digital nerves. The sensation to the dorsal fingertip is primarily derived from dorsal branches of the same proper digital nerves.[4]

[a] The Curtis National Hand Center, MedStar Union Memorial Hospital, Baltimore, 3333 North Calvert Street, 2nd Floor, Baltimore, MD 21218, USA; [b] MedStar Georgetown University Hospital, Department of Plastic Surgery, 3800 Reservoir Road, Washington, DC 20007, USA
* Corresponding author.
E-mail address: ryankatz1@gmail.com

Hand Clin 37 (2021) 11–26
https://doi.org/10.1016/j.hcl.2020.09.004
0749-0712/21/© 2020 Elsevier Inc. All rights reserved.

In young adults, the average static 2PD is 2.0 to 2.5 mm. This number increases to 3 to 5 mm in elderly patients.[5] Generally, a static 2PD 6 mm or less at the volar fingertip is considered useful.

EVALUATION

The hand injury should not distract from potential life-threatening injuries.

The hand examination should include an assessment of handedness, occupation, and medical comorbidities. Particular attention is paid to a history of smoking, peripheral vascular disease, autoimmune conditions known to affect small to medium blood vessels (Buerger's disease, lupus, CREST syndrome [calcinosis, Raynaud's phenomenon, esophageal dysmotility, sclerodactyly, and telangiectasia], etc), diabetes, or prior injuries to the hand because these risk factors are known for poor healing, infection, suboptimal surgical outcomes, and postsurgical complications.[6–8]

Wound characteristics that should be documented include:

- Presence of contamination
- Location of the soft tissue defect
- Size of the soft tissue defect
- Bone exposure
- Bone loss or fracture
- Nail bed injury or loss
- Tendon exposure

Although fingertip injury classification systems have been proposed and can help guide the surgeon in selecting a method of reconstruction, they are rarely used .[9,10] This article focuses exclusively on volar fingertip injuries.

GOALS OF RECONSTRUCTION

Fingertip reconstruction should be based on the premise of optimizing digital motion, sensation, and aesthetics. This goal can be accomplished by preserving digital length and, whenever possible, selecting a reconstruction that restores sensation to the pulp. The restored volar skin must be durable and should provide volar pulp volume, texture, and aesthetic contour similar to the premorbid digit. Preserving nail elements and minimizing nail deformity will aid in fingertip function (fine manipulation and pulp-to-pulp pinch) and appearance. The risk of developing a hook nail deformity can be minimized by preserving the distal phalanx length and supporting distal nail growth with a sterile matrix.[11] Thus, injuries to the nail matrix should be repaired at the time of injury or, in the setting of nail bed avulsion

injuries, grafted. Nail bed graft can be harvested from the underside of the nail plate (where it is often adherent), from the same or other injured digits, or from a toe.[12,13]

THERAPEUTIC OPTIONS
Secondary Intention

Because this topic is covered in other articles, it is not covered in detail here. Allowing a fingertip wound to heal secondarily is perhaps the simplest and most cost-effective option available.[14–16] Excellent results, including near-normal sensation and cosmesis, can be achieved with this treatment method in healthy patients[15] (**Fig. 1**).

Composite Grafting

A composite graft contains multiple tissues. In the setting of a distal fingertip amputation, the amputated part may be composed of multiple tissues, and may include portions (or all of) the nail bed. Given the low metabolic demands of skin, fat, bone, and nail bed and the relatively rapid rate of neovascularization of the fingertip, composite grafting is a reasonable treatment option for very distal finger wounds or amputations, especially for young patients. Composite grafting to the fingertip carries with it a very favorable risk-to-benefit ratio and carries no donor site morbidity. To improve chances at graft "take," a limited defatting is recommended to further diminish the metabolic demands of the composite graft and to increase the surface area of potential skin contact to the underlying wound bed. The chances of graft survival are higher in younger patients. Although various adjunctive procedures have been tried to increase the chances of graft take, none of these strategies has been proven to deliver a predictable outcome superior to grafting alone.[17,18] Because the success of this technique is not guaranteed, its use is often limited to young, healthy patients.[17,18]

Hypothenar composite grafting has been proposed as an alternative to skin grafting alone, with the advantage of providing more soft tissue padding. Hong and colleagues[19] reported their success with a composite graft of glabrous skin and subcutaneous fat from the hypothenar eminence.

Revision Amputation

Because this topic is covered in other articles, it is not covered in detail here. Revision amputation is an excellent option for patients with fingertip injuries proximal to the lunula who desire no reconstruction or a quick return to work. Although cold

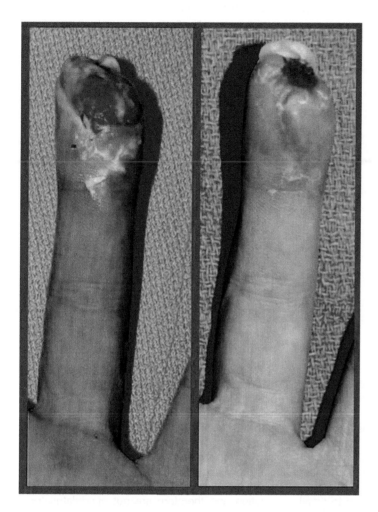

Fig. 1. An example of a large volar finger defect in the process of healing by secondary intention. (*Left*) An extensive wound of the distal phalanx. (*Right*) The appearance of the wound after several weeks of healing by secondary intention.

intolerance and stump hypersensitivity can persist for several years, these symptoms are not expected to last indefinitely[20] (**Fig. 2**).

Skin Grafting

Covering a fingertip wound with a skin graft is a quick and easy way to reconstruct large soft-tissue defects not amenable to healing by secondary intention. Full-thickness skin grafts (FTSG) are preferred to minimize dermal scar burden and secondary contracture. A healthy, well-vascularized wound bed free of devitalized or contaminated tissue is a prerequisite to skin grafting. Typical graft harvest sites include the thenar or hypothenar eminence (glabrous skin), medial brachium, groin, or lateral thigh (supple, nonglabrous skin). Although a contour deformity may be appreciated early in the healing process, the grafted skin tends to remodel once taken on the fingertip and exposed to everyday forces. This technique should provide durable soft tissue coverage with

a pleasing aesthetic contour over time. The drawbacks of skin grafting a fingertip are that it does not provide immediate sensate coverage and is subject to issues such as cold intolerance and fingertip hypersensitivity (**Fig. 3**).

Local Flaps

Multiple local advancement flaps have been described in managing fingertip wounds. The most widely used include the following:

- Atasoy volar V-Y advancement (**Fig. 4**)
- Kutler double opposing V-Y advancements from the radial and ulnar aspect of the finger (**Fig. 5**A and **B**)
- Moberg bipedicled neurovascular island flap for the thumb (**Fig. 6**)

These flaps are single-stage procedures that replace lost tissue with comparable "like" tissue, which, under most circumstances, is immediately sensate. With the exception of the Moberg flap,

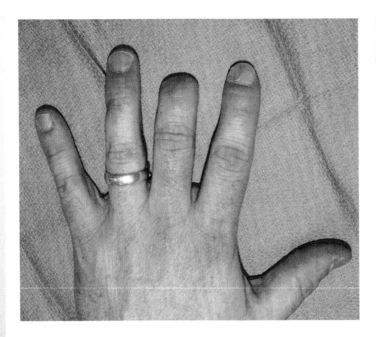

Fig. 2. An example of a finger after a revision amputation. The distal finger is covered with robust and healthy soft tissue.

which sometimes requires a skin graft at the proximal site of advancement, there is no donor defect requiring management. These flaps can often be performed with local anesthesia alone.

The major drawback to these flaps is the limited degree of advancement achievable. Though the Moberg flap can be used to cover a 2-cm defect of the volar distal thumb, the Atasoy and Kutler flaps enjoy less potential distal advancement. Therefore, their use is usually restricted to small distal transverse wounds of the fingertip (≤1 cm).

The Moberg flap is often the treatment of choice for distal thumb defects up to 2 cm. This bipedicled neurovascular island flap is immediately sensate and can provide well-vascularized glabrous tissue for reconstruction of missing thumb pulp. The unique dorsal vascular supply to the thumb allows this flap to be raised without compromising the blood supply to the digit. The nonthumb digits do not have as robust a dorsal circulation and therefore are not candidates for a similar volar bipedicled advancement flap.

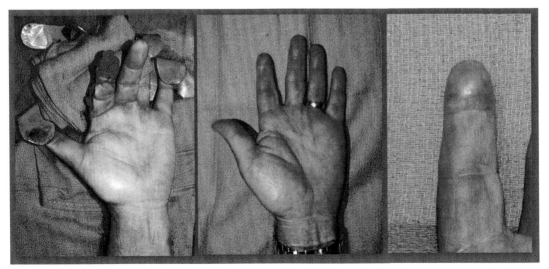

Fig. 3. An example of a volar finger pulp wound treated with a FTSG from the hypothenar eminence. (*Left*) Intraoperative appearance of volar pulp defect. (*Middle*) Suitable soft tissue pulp reconstruction after skin graft incorporation. (*Right*) A close up view demonstrating an excellent color and tissue quality match.

A

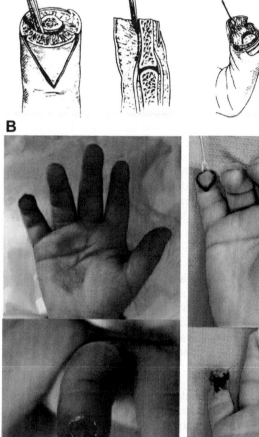

B

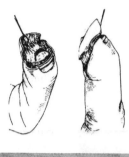

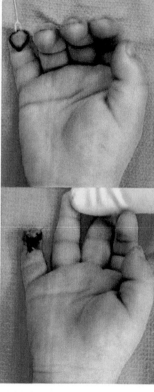

Fig. 4. (A) A drawing depicting the technical aspects of the Atasoy V-Y advancement flap. (*Left*) Palmar and lateral views of the Atasoy flap being raised. (*Right*) A drawing demonstrating the flap being advanced to cover the distal finger. (B) A clinical case showing the usefulness of the Atasoy V-Y advancement flap for distal injuries of the finger. (*Top left*) A photograph demonstrating the distal nature of the injury. (*Bottom left*) A close up view suggests exposed distal phalanx tuft. (*Top right*) The design of the Atasoy V-Y advancement flap is marked on the finger in purple ink. (*Bottom right*) The flap has been advanced and inset allowing for coverage of the distal phalanx. ([A] *From* Atasoy E., Ioakimidis, E., Kasdan, M. L., et al. Reconstruction of the Amputated Finger Tip with a Triangular Volar Flap: A new surgical procedure, *Journal of Bone and Joint Surgery.* 1970;52(5): 921-926; with permission; and [B] *From* Atasoy E., Ioakimidis, E., Kasdan, M. L., et al. Reconstruction of the Amputated Finger Tip with a Triangular Volar Flap: A new surgical procedure, *Journal of Bone and Joint Surgery* 1970;52(5): 921-926; with permission from Wolters Kluwer Health, Inc.; and *Clinical photos provided by Dr. Kevin Chung.*)

Other local flaps have been described.[21–23] All of these flaps share in common the drawbacks of limited size and advancement.

Heterodigital Flaps: Cross-Finger Flap

The cross-finger flap is a powerful reconstructive option that provides durable and supple nonglabrous soft tissue coverage of the fingertip. This 2-stage flap is used to resurface medium-to-large volar soft tissue defects of the distal digit. Because this flap carries its own blood supply in the first stage, it does not require intact paratenon or periosteum at the recipient site to succeed. Thus, the flap works well in the setting of sizable volar finger wounds with exposed tendon or bone. An innervated modification using a branch

of the dorsal digital nerve has been reported[24] (**Fig. 7**).

Drawbacks

- The donor skin is harvested from an adjacent, often uninjured, digit.
- The recipient digit needs to flex at the proximal interphalangeal joint (PIPJ) for flap inset and is thus at risk for stiffness.
- The donor site requires a skin graft. A full-thickness skin graft (FTSG) is recommended.
- The procedure requires 2 stages: flap elevation and initial inset, then flap division and final inset.
- The resultant skin coverage is nonglabrous and initially insensate.

A

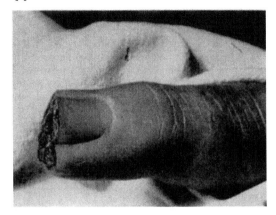

B

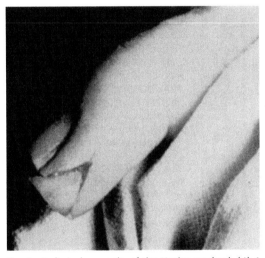

Fig. 5. A clinical example of the Kutler method. (*A*) A photo demonstrating a very distal fingertip wound. (*B*) A lateral view showing 1 of the 2 Kutler V-Y flaps having been raised. Because 2 flaps are used, neither flap requires extensive mobilization. (*From* Fisher, R.H.,The Kutler method of repair of finger-tip amputations. *Journal of Bone & Joint Surgery* 1967;49(2):317-321; with permission.)

- High risk of cold intolerance at the recipient and donor sites.[25,26]

Pearls

1. The transverse markings of the flap can be placed obliquely to allow for a more distal advancement of the flap if needed.
2. The flap is elevated full thickness, taking care to leave the paratenon on the extensor tendon undisturbed. This optimizes skin graft take when FTSG is used to resurface the donor defect.
3. The flap should be inset without tension. This process can be facilitated by gently flexing the injured digit's PIPJ.

4. The donor site FTSG should be protected for at least 1 week with splinting and/or a bolster.
5. The flap is usually divided at postoperative week 3.

Thenar Flap

The thenar flap is a treatment option for large distal volar wounds of the index or middle finger. Similar to the cross-finger flap, this is a 2-stage pedicled flap that can be used in the setting of exposed bone and/or tendon (**Fig. 8**). Because the flap is elevated from the thenar eminence and requires flexing the injured digit at the PIPJ to bring the defect toward the flap, there is a risk of PIPJ contracture. Using this technique to treat injuries to the ring or small finger is not advised.

Drawbacks

- The recipient digit needs to flex at the PIPJ for flap inset and is at risk for stiffness.
- The donor site may require a skin graft, although a modification has been described that allows primary closure.[27]
- The procedure requires 2 stages.
- The resultant skin coverage, although glabrous, is initially insensate, with a final average static 2PD of 7 mm.[28,29]
- The resultant thenar scar is often hypertrophic.

Pearls

1. Design the flap near volar and radial surface of thumb metacarpophalangeal joint to position scar away from main contact surface of the palm.
2. To compensate for primary contraction, the flap is often designed slightly larger than the defect.
3. The flap should be elevated in a full thickness fashion and include a thin layer of fat.
4. The inset should be protected by placing the patient in a dorsal blocking splint until flap division.
5. The flap should be divided at postoperative week 3.

Pedicled (Island) Homodigital and Heterodigital Flaps

Although heterodigital neurovascular island flaps have fallen out of favor, perhaps owing to donor site morbidity and/or the rise of microsurgical reconstructive options, they can be useful when the zone of injury to the injured digit precludes homodigital island flaps and if microvascular

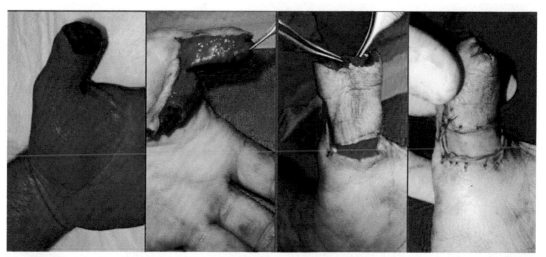

Fig. 6. A case example of a Moberg bipedicle advancement flap demonstrating the advancement gained with a transverse back-cut at the MP flexion crease. (*Far left*) A photo of a sizable distal thumb defect. (*Second from left*) An intraoperative photo showing elevation of the Moberg flap off of the underlying fibroosseous sheath. (*Third from left*) A back cut has been made at the MP flexion crease allowing for greater flap advancement. (*Far right*) The flap has been mobilized to allow complete coverage of the defect. The donor defect from the back cut has been managed with a skin graft. (*Clinical photos courtesy of Dr. Jonas Matzon.*)

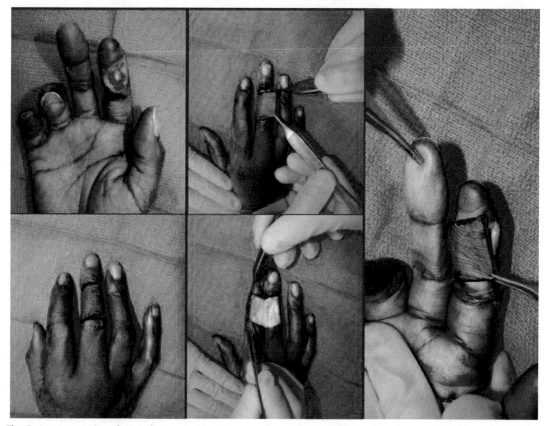

Fig. 7. Intraoperative photos demonstrating the cross-finger flap markings, elevation, and inset for a volar index finger wound. Note the preservation of the paratenon during elevation so as to provide a bed for donor site skin grafting. (*Top left*) A full-thickness wound with exposed tendon exists over the volar middle phalanx of the index finger. (*Bottom left*) The cross-finger flap has been designed over the middle phalanx of the middle finger. (*Top middle*) The cross-finger flap has been elevated off the dorsal aspect of the middle finger. (*Bottom middle*) The mobility of the cross-finger flap is demonstrated. The flap has been left pedicled to the radial aspect of the digit. (*Far right*) The proposed flap inset is demonstrated.

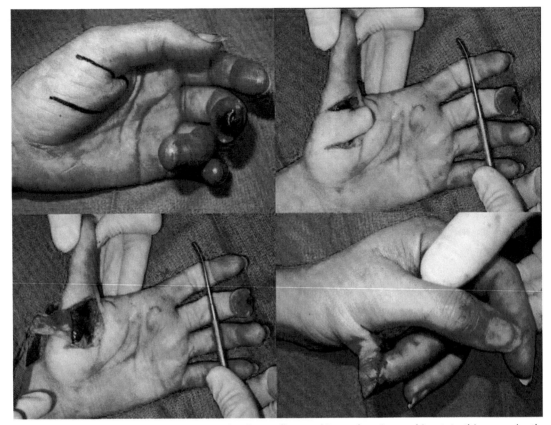

Fig. 8. Intraoperative photos demonstrating the thenar flap markings, elevation and inset. In this example, the flap was used to resurface a distal volar defect of the middle finger. (*Top left*) The middle finger defect and proposed flap design are visible. (*Bottom left*) The thenar flap has been elevated and reflected upon itself. (*Top right*) The thenar flap has been mobilized and the finger wound has been prepared for inset. (*Bottom right*) A clinical photo demonstrating the final inset of the thenar flap.

reconstructive resources are limited or unavailable.

Neurovascular island flaps derive arterial inflow from a proper digital artery. The venous outflow of these flaps has not been well-studied or described but is probably from the perivascular and fibrofatty leash accompanying the pedicle. In the absence of vascular disease or vasospastic syndromes, these flaps are quite reliable and can bring immediately sensate full-thickness glabrous skin to challenging fingertip wounds including those with exposed bone, fractures, hardware, and/or tendon. Because these flaps are dependent on the integrity of a digital artery, a finger Doppler Allen test can be performed to ensure proper digital artery patency before flap elevation. An absent signal in the pulp with the proposed flap pedicle open while the nonpedicle vessel is compressed is a contraindication to proceeding.

Antegrade Homodigital Island Flap

The antegrade homodigital island flap reliably reaches the distal finger and can be used for volar resurfacing in the setting of partial or total pulp loss or for distal finger resurfacing to avoid having to shorten bone.[30] Reported outcomes are excellent. In otherwise healthy patients, the risk of flap loss is low. The static 2PD, in some studies ranging between 3 to 5 mm, approaches near normal (especially with smaller flaps).[31–34] As most patients can return to their premorbid occupation and hobbies, there is high patient satisfaction[31–34] (**Fig. 9**).

Drawbacks

- Because distal flap mobilization is facilitated by flexing the digit, there is potential for PIPJ contracture.
- Isolating the pedicle means taking down dorsal and volar nerve branches. This could lead to periscar dysesthesia, numbness, or hypersensitivity.
- The donor site often has to be skin grafted, although V-Y modifications have been described that can eliminate this need.[35]

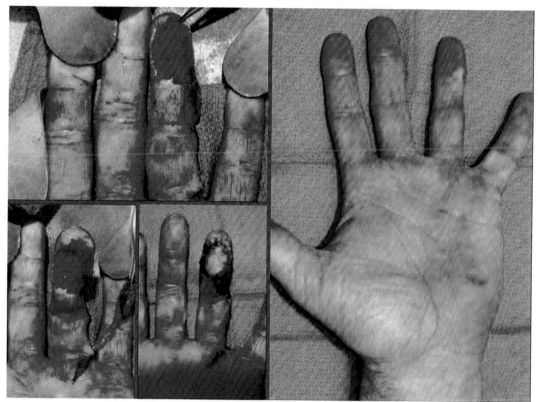

Fig. 9. A case example showing an extensive volar ring finger defect being resurfaced with an anterograde homodigital neurovascular island flap harvested on the ulnar neurovascular bundle. (*Top left*) A clinical photo of a ring finger wound. The defect includes almost the entire pulp of the digit. (*Bottom far left*) A demonstration of the mobility gained by elevating the homodigital island flap. (*Bottom second from left*) An early postoperative photo demonstrating a viable flap that provided complete coverage for this defect. (*Far right panel*) The postoperative result. The flap has incorporated well into the surrounding tissues.

Pearls

1. Perform under tourniquet with loupe magnification[30].
2. Identify the pedicle proximally first.
   a. Do not skeletonize the neurovascular bundle. Sparing the perivascular tissue around the pedicle likely preserves venous outflow.
3. If the pedicle seems to be diminutive or diseased, release the tourniquet and perform a digital Allen test. If the pedicle does not seem to be suitable for perfusing the designed flap, do not elevate the flap.
4. The flap is completely elevated only after ensuring the correct course and adequacy of the pedicle. It is then advanced and inset into the wound in a tension free manner. This is often facilitated by allowing slight flexion.
5. The donor defect should be resurfaced with a hand-harvested FTSG.

   a. The skin graft should not be inset on tension because this maneuver could potentially compromise the flap pedicle
   b. No tie-over bolster should be used on the skin graft because this element could compromise the flap pedicle
6. The hand is protected with a dorsal blocking splint for 1 week followed by a removable dorsal blocking splint for 2 weeks thereafter.
7. Therapy for range of motion can begin at postoperative week 3.

Retrograde Homodigital Island Flap

The retrograde homodigital island flap also offers a reasonably large (up to 4 × 2 cm) vascularized flap of glabrous skin that can be used to cover extensive volar tip wounds.[36] Unlike the antegrade homodigital island flap, which is supplied directly by the digital artery on the same side of the digit as the flap, the retrograde island flap relies on perfusion stemming from the digital artery on the side opposite the proposed flap. The retrograde flap takes advantage of the vascular interconnections between the proper digital arteries of the finger and, specifically, the middle transverse anastomotic arch at the level of the C3 pulley. This flap can be raised with or without sacrifice of the proper digital nerve or dorsal digital nerve branch. Including either in the harvest allows for a distal neurorrhaphy to the contralateral distal nerve stump. Including a nerve for a distal neurorrhaphy has been described as a way to encourage an improved sensory outcome.[37,38] This flap is reliable and offers relatively predictable and favorable outcomes, with a reported 98% survival rate, a near normal interphalangeal joint, range of motion, and an average return to work within 7 weeks.[37] One of the main benefits of the flap is that it does not require interphalangeal joint flexion to facilitate a tension-free inset. When including the digital nerve or the dorsal sensory branch, the flap has reasonable sensory outcomes, with a static 2PD of 4 to 10 mm.[37,38]

Drawbacks

- The flap is retrograde and therefore depends on an intact and healthy contralateral artery and digital vascular arch.[5]
- Harvesting the flap without the digital nerve requires skeletonization of the pedicle, which could harm the perivascular tissues that likely contribute to flap venous drainage.
- Creating a sensate flap requires sectioning the digital nerve proximally and performing a nonanatomic neurorrhaphy distally.
- If the digital nerve or a portion thereof is sacrificed with the flap, there is potential for periscar dysesthesia, numbness, or hypersensitivity.
- A skin graft may be necessary at the donor site.

Pearls

1. Design the flap along the volar–lateral aspect of proximal phalanx, limited to a noncontact area of the digit and avoiding the webspace.
2. Once the pedicle has been identified, trace it proximally to ensure that it runs directly under the premarked skin island.
3. The flap is completely elevated only after ensuring the correct course and adequacy of the pedicle.
4. The digital artery should be ligated proximally. If the digital nerve is to be included in the flap, it should be transected proximally as well.

5. The flap is completely islandized on the pedicle and mobilized up to the level of the PIPJ. The reach is then assessed.
6. If appropriately designed, the flap should be able to reach the distal digit without tension.
7. If needed, the interphalangeal joints may be flexed for tension-free inset
8. If a nerve was included in the flap, the neurorrhaphy should be performed between the elevated digital nerve and the contralateral distal nerve stump.

Dorsal Digital Island Flap

Unlike the antegrade and retrograde homodigital island flaps, which are supplied by the volar digital arteries, the dorsal digital island flap relies on dorsal branches of the proper digital artery. These branches are traced back to the source digital artery, which could be divided proximally to extend flap reach distally.[39,40] When harvested with a dorsal nerve branch, a nerve coaptation can be performed to one of the transected nerve stumps upon inset to encourage a better sensory outcome. When innervated, the static 2PD has been reported to range from 6 to 9 mm.[39,40]

Drawbacks

- Limited reach may necessitate dividing the proper digital artery proximally.
- If the digital nerve or a portion thereof is sacrificed with the flap, there is the potential for periscar dysesthesia, numbness, or hypersensitivity.
- Depending on the size of the flap, a skin graft is often necessary at the donor site.

Pearls

1. The flap is designed on the dorsolateral aspect of the proximal or middle phalanx.
   a. Placing the flap closer to the defect may facilitate reaching the defect without needing to divide the proper digital artery.
   b. The flap is often designed 10% to 15% larger than the defect to accommodate the primary contracture that occurs once the flap is freed from surrounding attachments.
2. The initial incision is made along proximal and central margins of the flap.
3. The flap is then elevated off the underlying tenosynovium.
   a. During this dissection, the dorsal branches of the digital artery may be visible on the underside of the flap.
   b. A cuff of perivascular tissue should be preserved around the dorsal digital artery.

4. If a neurorrhaphy is desired, the dorsal digital nerve should be harvested with the flap.
5. The flap should only be mobilized as much as needed to reach the defect.
   a. The pedicle should not be skeletonized.
   b. If more reach is needed, the proper digital artery can be ligated and transected proximally.
6. The neurorrhaphy is performed between the harvested nerve and the proper digital nerve stump.
7. The flap should be loosely inset.
8. The donor defect will likely need to be covered with FTSG.

Vascularized Heterodigital Island Flap (Without Nerve)

The heterodigital island flap is a neurovascular island flap harvested from an uninjured digit. This is a single-stage flap used to cover large fingertip wounds in which trauma to the injured digit precludes homodigital flaps. With this technique, many patients recover some element of light touch, temperature, and pain discrimination, even though these flaps are not routinely innervated. This flap has the option of including a dorsal branch of the digital nerve for a neurorrhaphy. A static 2PD of 3 to 7 mm has been reported for those flaps with a dorsal nerve branch and distal neurorrhaphy as compared with 10 mm for noninnervated flaps.[41]

Drawbacks

- Involves an uninjured digit.
- Sacrifices an intact digital artery of an uninvolved digit.
- Potential for cold intolerance, hypersensitivity, and hyperesthesia in the reconstructed finger and the donor finger.
- Risk of contour deformity at recipient and/or donor site.
- A skin graft is often necessary at the donor site.

Pearls

1. The flap is designed according to a wound template positioned on the volar-lateral aspect of a finger adjacent to the injured finger.
   a. The template should be placed proximal to the DIP flexion crease to avoid morbidity to donor finger volar pulp.
2. The pedicle should be identified before elevating and islandizing the flap.
3. The flap is completely elevated only after ensuring the correct course and adequacy of the pedicle.

a. The proper digital artery with surrounding perivascular tissue is taken with the flap. The proper digital nerve is left behind.
b. Inclusion of the proper digital nerve creates a neurovascular island flap as described by Littler (discussed elsewhere in this article).
4. The digital artery is ligated and divided distally and then dissected back to the common digital artery bifurcation to allow maximum freedom and reach.
5. The flap should be inset loosely. As the flap is harvested from the middle phalanx level, the recipient digit may need to be slightly flexed to allow for reach past the level of the distal interphalangeal joint.
6. The donor site should be covered with a skin graft.

Littler Neurovascular Island Flap

The Littler neurovascular island flap is a specific heterodigital island flap used primarily to resurface volar thumb defects, although in theory it could be used as a 1-stage flap to reconstruct any volar fingertip injury. Similar to the not-innervated vascularized heterodigital island flap, the Littler flap is designed on the distal volar–lateral aspect of a donor digit using a template of the defect to aid in flap design. Because this flap harvests a proper digital nerve, a noncritical sensory dermatome is selected by the surgeon. This usually corresponds with either the ulnar aspect of the long finger or the radial aspect of the ring finger. If harvested from the ring finger to reconstruct the thumb, the proper ulnar digital artery of the middle finger must be sacrificed to facilitate reach. If harvested from the long finger, the proper radial digital artery of the ring finger must be sacrificed to ensure reach to the thumb. Failure to sacrifice the proper digital artery of the finger adjacent to the donor finger could result in flap tethering and limited reach. Multiple studies demonstrate high rates of flap survival, reasonable range of motion in the donor finger, and a good static 2PD despite the fact that only 60% of patients recognize that the sensation comes from the thumb.[42,43]

Drawbacks

- This flap involves an uninjured finger.
- This flap requires sacrifice of both proper digital arteries off the common and the proper digital nerve of the donor finger for optimal mobilization.
- There is a loss of sensation at the donor site.
- There is need for a skin graft at the donor site.
- There is often dual sensibility at the recipient site.

- There exists the need for cortical reorientation at the recipient site.

Pearls

1. The flap is designed according to wound template positioned on the distal volar–lateral aspect of the donor finger at the level of the middle phalanx.
   a. The donor finger should be selected in advance and the ramifications of harvest, including loss of sensation on this aspect of the donor finger, should be discussed with the patient.
   b. The donor site is most often either the ulnar aspect of the long finger or the radial aspect of the ring finger.
2. A midlateral or Bruner incision is designed to allow for exposure and identification of the underlying neurovascular pedicle.
3. Once the course and adequacy of the pedicle is determined, the flap may be elevated and islandized completely on its neurovascular pedicle.
   a. The pedicle should not be skeletonized.
4. The digital artery is ligated and divided distally, and the digital nerve is transected distally. The freed skin island is then completely islandized on the neurovascular pedicle and dissected back to the common digital artery bifurcation.
   a. For optimal flap mobilization, the second arterial branch off the common is ligated at this point.
   b. If there is any concern about the impact of dividing the proper digital artery to any finger, an off-tourniquet Doppler Allen test may be performed, or perfusion can be assessed off tourniquet after dissection by placing a small, atraumatic vascular clamp on the proper digital artery before division.
5. An intraneural neurolysis of the common digital nerve can be performed to fully mobilize the flap digital nerve and extend reach.
6. The flap is then either tunneled subcutaneously under the skin of the palm or passed through open palmar access incisions and inset into the donor defect.
7. The donor site is covered with a skin graft.
8. The digit is protected with a splint for 2 to 3 weeks, after which time formal therapy may be initiated and the splint discontinued.

First Dorsal Metacarpal Artery Flap

The first dorsal metacarpal artery flap is a pedicled heterodigital island flap from the dorsal index finger that can provide coverage of dorsal or volar thumb defects. This full-thickness flap is elevated off of the dorsal aspect of the index finger proximal phalanx and islandized on an adipofascial leash that includes the fascia of the first dorsal interosseous muscle. Within the leash resides the first dorsal metacarpal artery, which provides arterial inflow to the flap, and multiple subcutaneous veins, which provide venous outflow. The flap contains branches of the dorsal radial sensory nerve, which can provide some sensation. The perfusion of the first dorsal metacarpal artery takes advantage of collateral branches to the dorsal skin, which are located on the radial aspect of the index finger. These branches, critical to flap survival, are located at the proximal radial aspect of the flap approximately at the level of the metacarpophalangeal joint. The versatility of this flap is derived from its large size, proximity to the thumb, and large arc of rotation. This flap is often used to resurface the entire distal volar or dorsal thumb (**Fig. 10**). Because this flap uses dorsal finger skin to cover a volar wound, the sensory outcomes are suboptimal with a static 2PD somewhere in the 7- to 10-mm range.[44–46] Sensation may be improved by including dorsal digital branches from the proper digital nerves that are then coapted to transected digital nerves at the recipient site.

Drawbacks

- This flap is harvested from an uninjured digit.
- The flap donor site requires a skin graft (FTSG preferable).
- The index finger may develop stiffness or pain as a result of flap harvest.
- The flap provides nonglabrous tissue.
- The flap is innervated by branches of the dorsoradial sensory nerve and therefore provides suboptimal and nonanatomic sensory restoration.
- Need for cortical reorientation.
  ○ Only 50% of patients recognize the sensation as coming from their thumb as opposed to the back of their index finger.[44–46]

Pearls

1. The flap is designed on the dorsal aspect of the index finger and is usually proximal to the PIPJ extension creases.
2. The initial incisions are made distally and ulnarly, where there is little risk of injuring the pedicle.
3. The dissection proceeds in an ulnar-to-radial fashion, elevating the skin off of the underlying paratenon while preserving the paratenon to support a later skin graft.

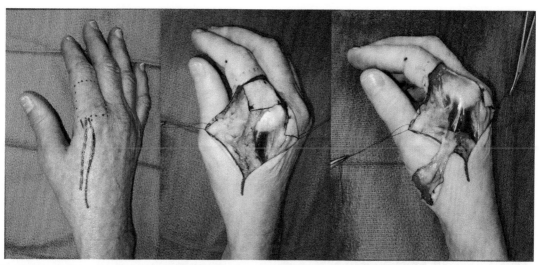

Fig. 10. A clinical series demonstrating the markings and elevation of the first dorsal metacarpal artery flap. (*Left*) The proposed flap markings have been drawn over the dorsal aspect of the index finger. (*Middle*) The flap has been elevated and isolated on its pedicle. (*Right*) The flap has been completely mobilized and is ready for inset. Note the thick adipofascial leash that encompasses the pedicle.

4. At the proximal radial aspect of the flap, the dissection is performed on the sagittal band.
   a. Some surgeons take a portion of the sagittal band to ensure, including the collateral branches perfusing the flap.
5. A longitudinal incision is made over the radial aspect of the index finger metacarpal. The skin is elevated radially and ulnarly in the immediate subdermal plane, preserving the underlying adipofascial layer.
6. The adipofascial layer is incised radially, elevating the fascia of the first dorsal interosseous with the flap, off of the underlying muscle, in a radial-to-ulnar fashion.

7. The adipofascial leash is mobilized by releasing any tethering radial attachments, just enough to ensure the flap will reach the thumb without tension.
   a. A thick adipofascial leash should be preserved.
   b. Overdissection of the adipofascial leash may compromise the flap.
8. The flap may be tunneled subcutaneously under the ulnar aspect of the thumb or positioned through open access incisions.
9. The flap is inset without tension. This can be facilitated by adducting the thumb toward the index finger if needed.

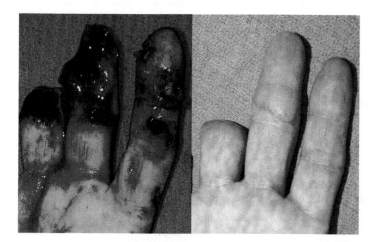

Fig. 11. A clinical series showing the outcome after replantation of amputated middle finger pulp. (*Left*) A photo demonstrating the defect after an amputation of the middle finger at the distal phalanx level that included an extensive amount of volar skin. (*Right*) A photo demonstrating the excellent aesthetic achievable with a replantation.

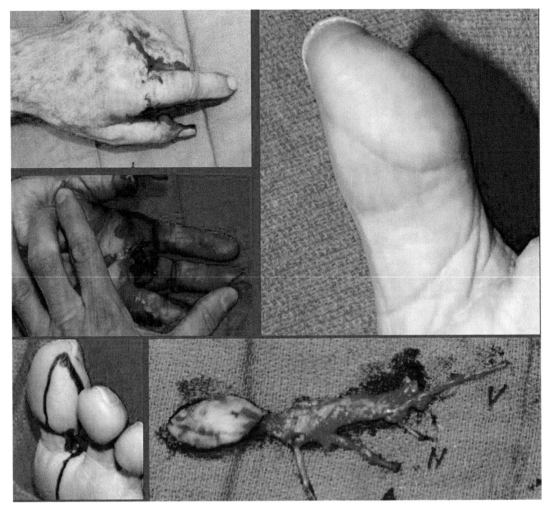

Fig. 12. A clinical series demonstrating microsurgical reconstruction of volar soft tissue defects of the hand. In this series, the critical ulnar thumb pulp has been reconstructed with a free neurovascular toe pulp flap from the great toe. (*Top left*) A sizable defect of the thumb pulp can be appreciated. (*Middle left*) An first dorsal metacarpal artery flap could not be used in this case given extensive volar trauma that involved the index and middle fingers. (*Bottom left*) A free toe pulp flap has been designed along the fibular aspect of the great toe. (*Bottom right*) The free toe pulp after elevation. Vein (V), nerve (N), and artery (A) are isolated and displayed. (*Top right*) Long-term follow-up demonstrates the excellent aesthetic outcome achievable with this method of reconstruction.

10. An FTSG is placed on the donor site with a bolster dressing.
11. Both the thumb and index finger should be temporarily splinted. Therapy is initiated after 1 to 3 weeks.

DISCUSSION

There are a multitude of reconstructive options for volar fingertip injuries (**Figs. 11** & **12**). These options vary in technical ease, number of stages, sensory outcome, involvement of uninjured digits, donor site morbidity, donor tissue quality, and possible complications. It is important to treat each patient and his or her injury on an individualized basis. There is no one best procedure for all distal finger or thumb wounds, and no true infallible algorithm by which to follow. Knowledge of the options available will allow the reconstructive surgeon to select the most appropriate flap for the patient. To facilitate how one approaches volar fingertip injuries, think of the patient's needs as well as the functional and aesthetic considerations of each digit.

CLINICS CARE POINTS

- Fingertip reconstruction should optimize digital motion, sensation, and aesthetics.
- It is important to understand the pros and cons of the multitude of options for fingertip reconstruction.
- The ideal reconstruction produces a sensate, well-padded fingertip.

DISCLOSURE

The authors have nothing to disclose.

ACKNOWLEDGMENTS

Clinical photos provided by Dr. Kevin Chung. Clinical photos courtesy of Dr. Jonas Matzon.

REFERENCES

1. Koh SH, You Y, Kim YW, et al. Long-term outcomes of nail bed reconstruction. Arch Plast Surg 2019;46(6):580–8.
2. de Berker D. Nail anatomy. Clin Dermatol 2013;31(5):509–15.
3. Johansson RS, Vallbo AB. Tactile sensibility in the human hand: relative and absolute densities of four types of mechanoreceptive units in glabrous skin. J Physiol 1979;286:283–300.
4. Chang J, Legrand A, Valero-Cuevas F, et al. "Anatomy and biomechanics of the hand." in Neligan PC, plastic Surgery: hand and upper extremity. 4th edition. New York (NY): Elsevier; 2017.
5. Kim J, Lee YH, Kim MB, et al. Innervated reverse digital artery island flap through bilateral neurorrhaphy using direct small branches of the proper digital nerve. Plast Reconstr Surg 2015;135(6):1643–50.
6. Hustedt JW, Chung A, Bohl DD. Development of a risk stratification scoring system to predict general surgical complications in hand surgery patients. J Hand Surg Am 2018;43(7):641–8.e6.
7. Lipira AB, Sood RF, Tatman PD, et al. Complications within 30 days of hand surgery: an analysis of 10,646 patients. J Hand Surg Am 2015;40(9):1852–9.e3.
8. Goodman AD, Gil JA, Starr AM, et al. Thirty-day reoperation and/or admission after elective hand surgery in adults: a 10-year review. J Hand Surg Am 2018;43(4):383.e1–7.
9. Evans DM, Bernardis C. A new classification for fingertip injuries. J Hand Surg Br 2000;25(1):58–60.
10. Muneuchi G, Tamai M, Igawa K, et al. The PNB classification for treatment of fingertip injuries: the boundary between conservative treatment and surgical treatment. Ann Plast Surg 2005;54(6):604–9.
11. Kumar VP, Satku K. Treatment and prevention of "hook nail" deformity with anatomic correlation. J Hand Surg Am 1993;18(4):617–20.
12. Bubak PJ, Richey MD, Engrav LH. Hook nail deformity repaired using a composite toe graft. Plast Reconstr Surg 1992;90(6):1079–82.
13. Hwang E, Park BH, Song SY, et al. Fingertip reconstruction with simultaneous flaps and nail bed grafts following amputation. J Hand Surg Am 2013;38(7):1307–14.
14. Weichman KE, Wilson SC, Samra F, et al. Treatment and outcomes of fingertip injuries at a large metropolitan public hospital. Plast Reconstr Surg 2013;131(1):107–12.
15. Hoigné D, Hug U, Schürch M, et al. Semi-occlusive dressing for the treatment of fingertip amputations with exposed bone: quantity and quality of soft-tissue regeneration. J Hand Surg Eur 2014;39(5):505–9.
16. Mennen U, Wiese A. Fingertip injuries management with semi-occlusive dressing. J Hand Surg Br 1993;18(4):416–22.
17. Heistein JB, Cook PA. Factors affecting composite graft survival in digital tip amputations. Ann Plast Surg 2003;50(3):299–303.
18. Lee PK, Ahn ST, Lim P. Replantation of fingertip amputation by using the pocket principle in adults. Plast Reconstr Surg 1999;103(5):1428–35.
19. Hong JP, Lee SJ, Lee HB, et al. Reconstruction of fingertip and stump using a composite graft from the hypothenar region. Ann Plast Surg 2003;51(1):57–62.
20. Wang K, Sears ED, Shauver MJ, et al. A systematic review of outcomes of revision amputation treatment for fingertip amputations. Hand (N Y) 2013;8(2):139–45.
21. Tuncali D, Barutcu AY, Gokrem S, et al. The hatchet flap for reconstruction of fingertip amputations. Plast Reconstr Surg 2006;117(6):1933–9.
22. Yam A, Peng YP, Pho RW. "'Palmar pivot flap' for resurfacing palmar lateral defects of the fingers. J Hand Surg Am 2008;33(10):1889–93.
23. Laoulakos DH, Tsetsonis CH, Michail AA, et al. The dorsal reverse adipofascial flap for fingertip reconstruction. Plast Reconstr Surg 2003;112(1):121–5.
24. Lee NH, Pae WS, Roh SG, et al. Innervated cross-finger pulp flap for reconstruction of the fingertip. Arch Plast Surg 2012;39(6):637–42.
25. Nishikawa H, Smith PJ. The recovery of sensation and function after cross-finger flaps for fingertip injury. J Hand Surg Br 1992;17(1):102–7.
26. Paterson P, Titley OG, Nancarrow JD. Donor finger morbidity in cross-finger flaps. Injury 2000;31(4):215–8.
27. Dellon AL. The proximal inset thenar flap for fingertip reconstruction. Plast Reconstr Surg 1983;72(5):698–704.

28. Gatewood MD. A plastic repair of finger defects without hospitalization. JAMA 1926;87:1479.

29. Flatt AE. The thenar flap. J Bone Joint Surg Br 1957; 39:80.

30. Katz RD. The anterograde homodigital neurovascular island flap. J Hand Surg Am 2013;38(6):1226–33.

31. Arsalan-Werner A, Brui N, Mehling I, et al. Long-term outcome of fingertip reconstruction with the homodigital neurovascular island flap. Arch Orthop Trauma Surg 2019;139(8):1171–8.

32. Lok LW, Chan WL, Lau YK. Functional outcomes of antegrade homodigital neurovascular island flaps for fingertip amputation. J Hand Surg Asian Pac Vol 2017;22(1):39–45.

33. Wang B, Chen L, Lu L, et al. The homodigital neurovascular antegrade island flap for fingertip reconstruction in children. Acta Orthop Belg 2011;77(5): 598–602.

34. Varitimidis SE, Dailiana ZH, Zibis AH, et al. Restoration of function and sensitivity utilizing a homodigital neurovascular island flap after amputation injuries of the fingertip. J Hand Surg Br 2005; 30(4):338–42.

35. Venkataswamy R, Subramanian N. Oblique triangular flap: a new method of repair for oblique amputations of the finger-tip and thumb. Plast Reconstr Surg 1980;66:296.

36. Lai CS, Lin SD, Yang CC. The reverse digital artery flap for fingertip reconstruction. Ann Plast Surg 1989;22(6):495–500.

37. Regmi S, Gu JX, Zhang NC, et al. A systematic review of outcomes and complications of primary fingertip reconstruction using reverse-flow homodigital island flaps. Aesthetic Plast Surg 2016;40(2):277–83.

38. Seah BZQ, Sebastin SJ, Chong AKS. Retrograde flow digital artery flaps. Hand Clin 2020;36(1):47–56.

39. Chen C, Tang P, Zhang X. A comparison of the dorsal digital island flap with the dorsal branch of the digital nerve versus the dorsal digital nerve for fingertip and finger pulp reconstruction. Plast Reconstr Surg 2014;133(2):165e–73e.

40. Chen C, Tang P, Zhang X. The dorsal homodigital island flap based on the dorsal branch of the digital artery: a review of 166 cases. Plast Reconstr Surg 2014;133(4):519e–29e.

41. Pham DT, Netscher DT. Vascularized heterodigital Island flap for fingertip and dorsal finger reconstruction. J Hand Surg Am 2015;40(12):2458–64.

42. Oka Y. Sensory function of the neurovascular island flap in thumb reconstruction: comparison of original and modified procedures. J Hand Surg Am 2000; 25(4):637–43.

43. Teoh LC, Tav SC, Yong FC, et al. Heterodigital arterialized flaps for large finger wounds: results and indications. Plast Reconstr Surg 2003;111(6): 1905–13.

44. Chen C, Zhang X, Shao X, et al. Treatment of thumb tip degloving injury using the modified first dorsal metacarpal artery flap. J Hand Surg Am 2010; 35(10):1663–70.

45. Yang JY. The first dorsal metacarpal flap in first web space and thumb reconstruction. Ann Plast Surg 1991;27(3):258–64.

46. Sherif MM. First dorsal metacarpal artery flap in hand reconstruction. II. clinical application. J Hand Surg Am 1994;19(1):32–8.

Management of Tendon and Bony Injuries of the Distal Phalanx

Janice C.Y. Liao, MBBS, MRCS, FAMS[a,b], Soumen Das De, MBBS, FRCS, MPH[b],*

KEYWORDS

- Anatomy • Distal phalanx • Flexor injuries • Extensor injuries • Fractures

KEY POINTS

- Acute tendon and bony injuries of the distal phalanx are challenging injuries because they may result in chronic pain, hypersensitivity, stiffness, and deformity if they are not adequately treated.
- Flexor tendon avulsions require early surgical repair. Conversely, most extensor tendon injuries and fractures heal well with nonoperative treatment.
- In this article, we outline the pertinent clinical anatomy of the distal phalanx, review the current literature regarding treatment options, and highlight key management points to ensure good clinical outcomes while minimizing complications.

INTRODUCTION

The fingertip consists of the distal phalanx, nail complex, and specialized pulp. The distal phalanx has an intricate arrangement of soft tissue attachments that stabilize the distal interphalangeal joint (DIPJ) while allowing a large range of motion. This article begins with a review of the applied anatomy of the distal phalanx and its associated soft tissue attachments. We then discuss the classification, treatment, and rehabilitation of acute zone I flexor and extensor tendon injuries. Finally, we review distal phalangeal fractures and highlight key management points.

PERTINENT ANATOMY

The anatomy of the distal phalanx was described in detail by Shrewsbury and Johnson in 1975.[1] Understanding the osseous, ligamentous, and tendinous anatomy is essential to achieve good treatment outcomes after tendon and bony injuries of the fingertip.

Bony Architecture and Landmarks

The distal phalanx makes up approximately 18% of the fingertip volume.[2] It has a base, shaft, and tuft (**Fig. 1**). The *base* is broad and it narrows distally into the waist of the *shaft* and ends in a bulbous *tuft* with a rough volar surface called the ungual tuberosity.[1] The lateral prominences at the base are called *lateral tubercles,* which are in line with the projections just proximal to the ungual tuberosity called *ungual spines*. On the sagittal projection, the base of the distal phalanx has a dorsal ridge and a flat volar surface (see **Fig. 1**B). The volar cortex slopes dorsally toward the ungual tuberosity and forms a concavity called the *ungual fossa*. The entry point of an axial Kirschner (K-) wire should be just volar to the sterile matrix-hyponychium junction. Starting too volarly would place the wire within the ungual tuberosity but volar to the shaft of the phalanx. The average length of the distal phalanx of the middle finger is 11.2 mm, the coronal width of the tuft is 7.8 mm, and the narrowest width of

Funded by: NA.
[a] Department of Orthopaedic Surgery, Ng Teng Fong General Hospital, Singapore; [b] Department of Hand and Reconstructive Microsurgery, National University Hospital, Singapore
* Corresponding author. Department of Hand and Reconstructive Microsurgery, National University Health System, 1E Kent Ridge Road, Singapore 119228, Singapore.
E-mail address: soumendasde@gmail.com

Hand Clin 37 (2021) 27–42
https://doi.org/10.1016/j.hcl.2020.09.005
0749-0712/21/© 2020 Elsevier Inc. All rights reserved.

hand.theclinics.com

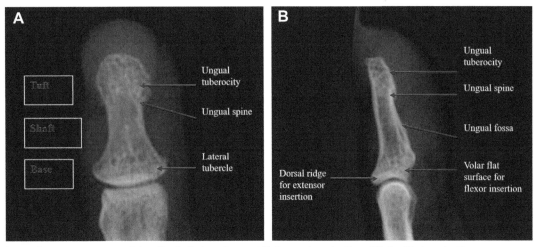

Fig. 1. Osseous anatomy of the distal phalanx bone. (*A*) Coronal projection. (*B*) Sagittal projection.

the shaft (the *isthmus*) is 2.7 mm.[3] In the lateral projection, the average widths of the tuft and isthmus are only 4.0 mm and 3.3 mm, respectively.[3] The surgeon must be mindful of these dimensions when inserting a headless compression screw. A screw that is wider than the isthmus will perforate the dorsal cortex and damage the overlying sterile matrix.

Ligaments

The *lateral interosseous ligaments (LIL)* attach to the lateral tubercles and ungual spines on both sides of the distal phalanx. The *rima ungualum* is the space between the LIL and the bony shaft, and it allows passage of neurovascular branches (**Fig. 2**).[1] The LIL effectively increases the surface area of the fingertip and provides a firm fibrous

attachment for the lateral portions of the nailbed. The proximal margin of the nailbed is loosely attached to the periosteum. The *collateral ligaments* of the DIPJ originate from the head of the middle phalanx, project along the sides of the joint, and insert into the lateral tubercles.

Tendons

The terminal extensor tendon inserts into the dorsal ridge at the base of the distal phalanx, approximately 1.2 mm from the proximal edge of the germinal matrix (**Fig. 3**).[4] The rectangular extensor tendon insertion is free from the dorsal capsule of the joint. The surgeon must take great care to avoid injury to the germinal matrix when mobilizing the terminal extensor tendon or placing a hook plate for fixation of a mallet fracture. The footprint

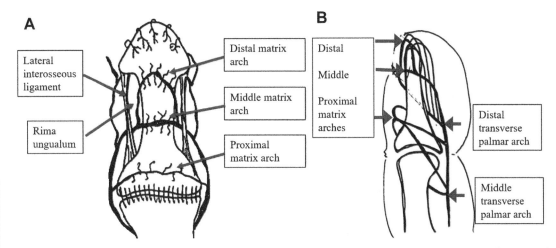

Fig. 2. Illustrations demonstrating the lateral interosseous ligament and passage of arterial branches. (*A*) Coronal view. (*B*) Sagittal view. (*Illustration courtesy of* Dr Sze-Ryn Chung, Singapore General Hospital.)

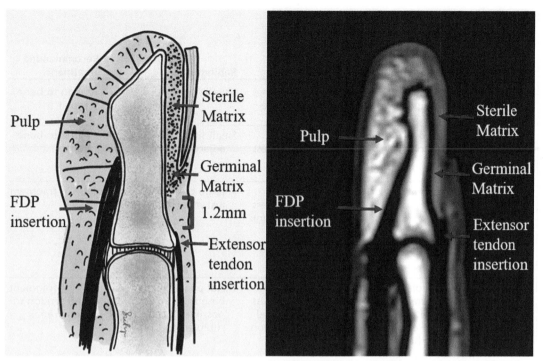

Fig. 3. Illustration and MRI showing the flexor and extensor attachments and their intricate relationship with the germinal matrix. (*Illustration courtesy of* Dr Chung Sze-Ryn, Singapore General Hospital.)

of the flexor digitorum profundus (FDP) insertion is much larger than the extensor tendon, occupying 20% of the distal phalanx surface area with an average insertion length and width of 6.2 mm and 7.9 mm respectively.[5] Unlike the extensor tendon, the FDP tendon has loose areolar connections to the DIPJ via the volar plate and the proximal part of the FDP insertion is approximately 1.2 mm from the articular surface. A surgical incision extending distally to the mid-pulp is required to fully expose the entire FDP insertion and facilitate primary repair.

Blood Supply and Innervation

The finger is predominantly supplied by the palmar digital arteries which lie lateral and deep to the digital nerves at the level of proximal and middle phalanx. At approximately 0.5 cm distal to the distal digital crease, the arteries turn medially, crossing the nerves on their dorsal aspect to anastomose with the contralateral artery. The fingertip has a rich and complex network of blood vessels (see **Fig. 2**).[6,7] However, a dorsal skin incision that is made too close to the lunula may endanger the vascularity of the skin flaps. This may lead to full-thickness skin necrosis and exposure of underlying implants. There is little skin mobility over the dorsum, and

full-thickness defects may require reconstruction with flaps.

ACUTE FLEXOR TENDON INJURIES
Classification

Avulsion of the FDP is a common injury in athletes, with 75% of them occurring in the ring finger.[8] It has been termed the "jersey finger" as it commonly occurs during a tackle in football. The small finger slips away from the pants or jersey as the tackled player moves away, while the longer ring finger gets caught and is forced into hyperextension. The powerful contraction of the FDP leads to an avulsion injury. Leddy and Packer[8] described 3 types of FDP avulsion injuries (**Table 1**). This classification is counterintuitive, because a Type I injury with a small avulsion fragment leads to retraction of the tendon into the palm with complete disruption of its vincular blood supply and delayed repair leads to poor outcomes. Type IV and type V injuries were later added to the classification.[9,10]

The treatment of zone I FDP injuries depends on size of the fracture fragments, extent of tendon retraction, and chronicity. Flexion and stability of the DIPJ against hyperextension forces contribute significantly to grip and pulp pinch, respectively, and early primary repair is generally advocated.

Table 1
Classification of FDP avulsion injuries

Types	Description	Clinical Features	Radiographs	Recommended Treatment
I	FDP retracted into palm (all vinculae disrupted)	Absent DIPJ flexion, tender mass in the palm	Usually normal	Tendon to bone repair
II	FDP retracted to PIPJ (VLP preserved)	Absent DIPJ flexion, swelling, tenderness and some loss of motion at PIPJ	Small fleck of bone adjacent to PIPJ	Tendon to bone repair
III	FDP avulsed with a large bony fragment incarcerated at A4 pulley (vascularity preserved)	No DIPJ flexion, swelling, tenderness over middle phalanx	A large bone fragment just proximal to DIPJ	ORIF of fragment
IV	Fracture of volar base of distal phalanx with separation of FDP from the fracture fragment	No DIPJ flexion, swelling, tenderness depending on level of tendon retraction	Distal phalanx volar base fracture with possible dorsal subluxation of DIPJ	ORIF of fragment and tendon to bone repair
V	Bony avulsion of FDP with distal phalanx fracture	No DIPJ flexion, swelling, tenderness depending on level of tendon retraction	Volar avulsion fragment with distal phalanx fracture	ORIF

Abbreviations: FDP, flexor digitorum profundus; ORIF, open reduction and internal fixation; PIPJ, proximal interphalangeal joint; VLP, vinculum longus profundus.

There is a limited number of large case series to review the outcomes of surgery for FDP avulsion injuries. Early primary repair generally results in satisfactory functional outcome.[11] Patients are expected to regain good flexion and grip strength with 10° to 15° loss of extension.[8]

Isolated Tendon Injuries

In type I and II avulsion injuries, the avulsed tendon must be repaired primarily to bone. Type I injuries must be repaired within 1 to 2 weeks before there is necrosis of the tendon and myostatic contracture sets in. Type II injuries have shown good outcomes even when repaired up to 3 months after injury.[8] However, we recommend that repair be performed as soon as possible because there is a risk of further tendon retraction, converting a type II injury to a type I injury. We use a Bruner incision and open the flexor sheath distal to the A4 pulley. If the proximal tendon end is not retrievable from the wound, we make a transverse incision over the distal palmar crease and open the flexor sheath proximal to the A1 pulley. The proximal

tendon end can be retrieved in the correct orientation with minimal dissection using an infant feeding tube.[12]

The pullout button technique has traditionally been used to repair avulsed tendons directly to bone. It is associated with complications including infection, nail plate deformity and skin necrosis. We prefer primary repair with a suture anchor instead. Several biomechanical studies have shown a superior load to failure of suture anchor repair compared with a 2-strand suture pullout technique.[13] A clinical study has shown comparable DIPJ motion (57° for the pullout vs 56° for the anchor group), but an infection rate of 13% in the pullout group and quicker return to work for the anchor group.[14] The main concerns with suture anchor are inadvertent penetration of the far cortex and impaired pull out strength in osteoporotic bone. We use two 1.3-mm double-loaded suture anchors that provide greater strength than a single 1.8-mm suture anchor and minimizes the risk of cortex penetration. Directing the anchor in a 45° retrograde fashion further reduces the risk and results in significantly less gap formation.[15]

Bony Avulsion Injuries

Avulsion fractures of the FDP (types III, IV, and V) are much less common than pure tendinous avulsions.[8] These injuries are treated with open reduction and internal fixation of the fracture fragment. In type IV injuries, the tendon is then repaired to bone after fixation. We expose the injury site as described for pure tendinous avulsions. Any dorsal subluxation of the DIPJ is reduced and held with a dorsal blocking pin (**Fig. 4**). Various fixation methods including K-wires, interosseous wiring, screws, and small plates can be used for fixation and the exact choice depends on the size of the fracture fragment and surgeon's preference. Type III injuries usually present with a large bony fragment. We fix the fragment with several 1.0-mm screws to achieve rigid fixation and permit early rehabilitation. K-wires are used for preliminary fixation and are sequentially replaced with screws (**Fig. 5**). For small avulsion fragments, a hook plate fashioned from a 1.3-mm plate can be used for fixation.[16] No single technique has been proven to be superior. Most case reports of various techniques have reported satisfactory functional outcome despite reduction in DIPJ range of motion.[16,17] To optimize outcome, we recommend early rigid fixation with correction of dorsal subluxation, independent tendon repair in concomitant tendon avulsions, and early mobilization.

Rehabilitation

The aim of flexor tendon rehabilitation is to allow adequate gliding to prevent adhesions while preventing rupture of the tendon repair. Over the past century, rehabilitation has evolved from static immobilization to early passive mobilization, combined "place-and-hold" regimens, to early active motion protocols. These depend on the strength of repair, patient's ability to participate, and the surgeon's preference. The load to failure in dual micro anchor repair and with the pullout technique (69N and 43N, respectively) are both significantly higher than the baseline forces encountered during active DIPJ flexion (28N).[13] A recent systematic review failed to demonstrate any superiority with a

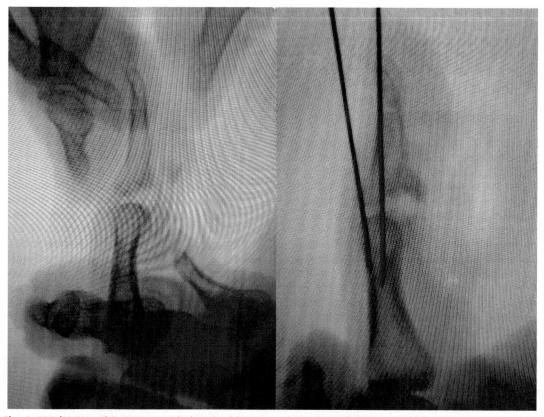

Fig. 4. FDP bony avulsion injury with dorsal subluxation of the joint. (*Left*) Dorsal subluxation reduced. (*Right*) Reduction temporarily held with 2 dorsal blocking pins. (*Case courtesy of* Dr David Tan, Orthopaedic and Hand Surgery Partners).

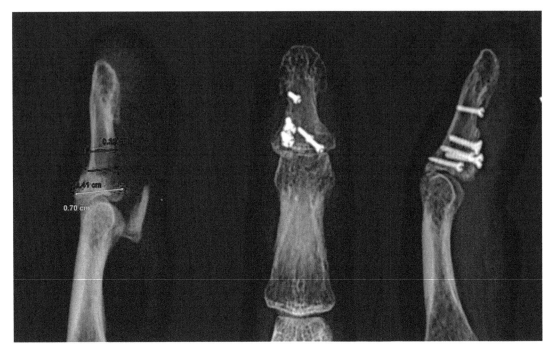

Fig. 5. FDP bony avulsion injury. (*Left*) Preoperative measurements on the plain radiograph to determine the lengths of the screws. This allows preliminary fixation with K-wires which are then replaced with screws. (*Center and Right*) Postoperative radiographs. (*Case courtesy of Dr Ellen Lee, National University Health System.*)

true active mobilization protocol.[18] We prefer to start with early place-and-hold exercises and progress compliant patients to an active motion protocol.

ACUTE EXTENSOR TENDON INJURIES

Disruption of the terminal tendon results in an extension lag of the DIPJ, the so-called "mallet finger." The most common mechanism of injury is an axial load with forced flexion of the DIPJ. Younger individuals tend to be male and have high-energy mechanisms (eg, ball sports) and older patients are more commonly female with low-energy mechanisms (eg, household chores).[19–22] The 2 main patterns of injury are a pure soft tissue disruption ("soft tissue mallet") or a dorsal avulsion fracture ("bony mallet"). A large series indicated that bony mallet injuries comprised slightly more than 25% of mallet finger injuries.[23] The most common classification systems are all radiological and were described by Wehbe and Schneider,[23] Tubiana (1986), and Doyle (1993). Salazar Botero and colleagues[19] contended that the thresholds for fragment size and articular involvement used in these classification systems were arbitrary and did not have a pathophysiological or biomechanical basis. Lange and Engber described a variant of the bony mallet

injury resulting from hyperextension of the DIPJ, the so-called "hyperextension mallet".[24] This injury resulted in volar subluxation of the DIPJ and a large dorsal fragment (usually >50% of the articular surface). They advocated surgery because congruent reduction could rarely be achieved using closed methods.

There is considerable debate about the optimal treatment of mallet injuries. Lin and Samora[25] recently performed a comprehensive systematic review. Of the 1098 cases that were treated nonoperatively, 65% were soft tissue injuries. Conversely, almost 94% of surgically treated cases were bony injuries. The main study outcomes were DIPJ extension lag and the criteria developed by Abouna and Brown,[26] Crawford,[27] and Warren and Norris (1988).[26–28] The average extension lag of the DIPJ was 7.6° with nonoperative treatment and 5.7° with surgery. The most common methods of nonoperative treatment were custom-made thermoplastic splints and padded aluminum splints that were applied volarly, dorsally, or stacked. There was no difference in outcomes between the different types of splints. The average length of immobilization was approximately 7 weeks, with soft tissue mallet injuries having a slightly longer period of immobilization than bony injuries. The complication rate from conservative treatment was about

13% and composed mainly minor skin issues (eg, ulceration, maceration), occasional cold intolerance, and one case of full-thickness skin necrosis. The main indications for surgery were subluxation of the distal phalanx, a sizable fracture fragment, open injuries, and aesthetic reasons. The complication rate after surgery was 14.5% and included nail deformity, infection, redisplacement of the fracture, wound breakdown, resorption of the fracture fragment, and avascular necrosis. Only 5 studies compared surgery (mostly trans-articular K-wire fixation) and conservative treatment and did not show a clear benefit of one modality over the other. None of the studies evaluated long-term issues such as DIPJ osteoarthritis and swan-neck deformity with functional limitation.

It is evident that the literature is equivocal regarding the optimal treatment of mallet finger injuries. There is no consensus on the optimal strategy, choice of splint/implants, or duration of immobilization. One may summarize that nonoperative treatment leads to more transient and manageable adverse events, while surgery provides modest gains in *DIPJ extension* at the risk of more permanent complications. Surgery must be executed skillfully because there is little room for error. We have distilled our treatment philosophy and current practices in the subsequent sections. Our algorithm for treating mallet injuries is shown in **Fig. 6**. We use a simple workflow based on an initial plain radiograph followed by fluoroscopic assessment of bony mallet injuries.[29] We regard any injury with a DIPJ extension lag that is fully correctable as an "acute" injury because of the potential for near-complete recovery, regardless of time since injury.

Soft Tissue Mallet Injuries

We recommend nonoperative treatment for closed soft tissue mallet injuries and use a streamlined protocol that minimizes outpatient visits and health care resources. At the initial office visit, occupational therapists fabricate a custom-made thermoplastic stack splint and provide educational material outlining splint use, personal care, and the rehabilitation process. The proximal interphalangeal joint (PIPJ) is placed in mild (10°–15°) flexion if there is significant volar plate laxity, to prevent a swan-neck deformity. We initiate intermittent, active motion exercises at 6 weeks if there is minimal extension lag at the DIPJ. If there is a persistent lag exceeding 10°, we continue immobilization for a further 2 weeks before commencing motion exercises. The patient continues another 4 to 6 weeks of self-directed

therapy with the aid of printed worksheets and videoconferencing consults, as necessary. This protocol has reduced the number of hospital visits and enhances patient satisfaction without compromising clinical outcomes.

A small group of patients (eg, healthcare workers) do not tolerate a splint and a subcutaneous, trans-articular pin across the DIPJ allows these patients to use the hand for routine tasks without substantial difficulty. We perform thorough debridement, trans-articular pinning, and a tenodermodesis for open soft tissue mallet injuries without skin loss (Doyle type II). A homodigital flap (eg, based on a digital artery perforator) or heterodigital flap (eg, reverse cross finger) may be necessary if there is soft tissue loss (Doyle type III).[30]

Bony Mallet Injuries

We use the algorithm in **Fig. 6** to guide decision-making. The main benefits of surgery for bony mallet injuries are anatomic reduction and reconstitution of the articular surface, earlier joint motion, and a better aesthetic outcome. Surgery for bony mallet injuries is very exacting. Nevertheless, we should not write off surgery because good outcomes are achievable, provided we employ careful preoperative planning and a meticulous technique. The skin incisions must be designed properly to avoid flap necrosis and implant exposure. The surgeon must be fastidious about implant placement, because prominent or inappropriately placed hardware can result in skin ulceration, sensitivity, and permanent injury to the germinal matrix. Finally, the surgeon must scrutinize his/her clinical outcomes, including "minor" issues like a dorsal bump - because the patient who has elected surgical treatment will almost certainly do the same![31]

Several surgical techniques have been described, including extension block pinning, direct fixation with K-wires, screws, and plate/screw constructs. Lucchina and colleagues[32] compared several surgical techniques and did not find significant differences in outcome. However, they reported differences in operative time (pinning was faster), return to work (<3 weeks with screws vs >6 weeks with pins), and higher complications from improper screw placement. We use extension block pinning for dorsal fragments that can be passively reduced with the DIPJ in flexion (**Fig. 7**).[33,34] Fine adjustments to fracture reduction can be made using a hypodermic needle, additional pin, a small burr, and a skin hook.[29] Garg and colleagues[35] reported good outcomes with the "delta wiring" technique

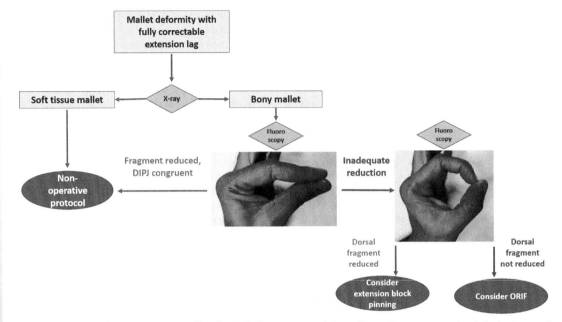

Fig. 6. Algorithm for management of mallet injuries. We use plain radiographs to categorize injuries into soft tissue and bony mallet injuries. Bony mallet injuries are further evaluated using fluoroscopy with the DIPJ in full extension and full flexion. A digital block may be administered if there is significant pain. We recommend nonoperative management if the dorsal bony fragment remains reduced and the DIPJ is congruent with the DIPJ in extension. If the DIPJ remains subluxated, fluoroscopy with the DIPJ in flexion helps to guide the choice of surgery. Extension block pinning may be considered if the dorsal fragment can be reduced by placing the DIPJ in flexion. ORIF should be considered for fragments that do not reduce with DIPJ flexion. (*Acknowledgments*: Dr Sandeep Sebastin, Orthopaedic and Hand Surgery Partners.)

that avoids trans-articular pinning and permits immediate DIPJ motion.

We perform open reduction internal fixation (ORIF) when the dorsal fragment is not reducible with the DIPJ in flexion and prefer to use a hook plate for smaller fragments (**Fig. 8**) and screw fixation for larger fragments (**Fig. 9**).[36–38] Open reduction and extension block pinning is an alternative for irreducible fractures, but we prefer direct fixation methods once the fracture has already been exposed. We initiate immediate PIPJ and DIPJ (for plate and screw fixations) motion and remove K-wires once the fracture has united adequately, usually at 6 weeks.

DISTAL PHALANX FRACTURES

Distal phalanx fractures are the most common type of hand fracture, and the thumb and middle finger are the most affected digits. Most of these injuries arise from occupational accidents. These statistics make sense: the fingertip is the most exposed part of the hand, and the thumb and middle finger project the furthest during manual tasks.[39–41] The most common mechanisms of injury are a blunt, crushing injury (eg, heavy objects

at work), forced loading in various positions of the DIPJ (eg, ball sports), and lacerating injuries from power tools and machinery. Well-taken anteroposterior and lateral radiographs of the affected digit are usually enough to make the diagnosis. Computed tomography scans are sometimes necessary to assess multi-fragmentary fractures, determine the extent of articular involvement, and evaluate bony union when there is persistent pain.

Schneider classified fractures of the distal phalanx by location and the relative frequency of each type is shown in **Fig. 10**.[41] We have added "comminuted/pilon-type injury" as an additional category for proximal (articular) injuries because these injuries are usually associated with poor outcomes and arthrodesis is often indicated (**Box 1**). An unstable injury is one in which the soft tissues have been disrupted to the extent that the fracture will displace under physiologic loads. A seemingly innocuous injury is the transverse mid-shaft fracture, which occurs at the "hard-soft" junction between the nail plate and its eponychial recess (**Fig. 11**).

The treatment, and eventual clinical outcomes, of most of these fractures centers more around

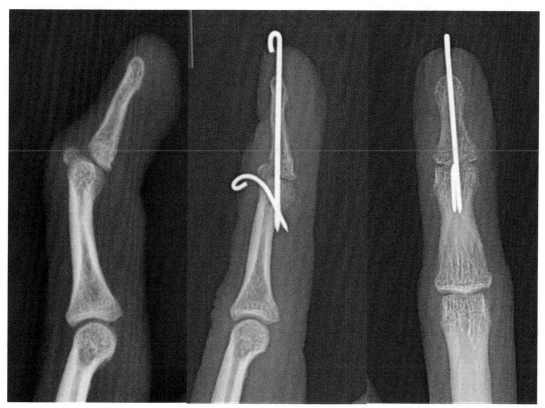

Fig. 7. We insert the central (axial) wire midway into the distal phalanx first. The dorsal fragment is then brought into its anatomic position by placing the DIPJ in flexion and the dorsal blocking wire is inserted. The DIPJ is then extended, thus reducing the fracture, and the axial wire is advanced across the DIPJ. A subtle point is that this trans-articular wire should be placed slightly volar so that it does not block reduction of the dorsal fragment. An alternative method is inserting this wire obliquely across the DIPJ.

the associated soft tissue injuries rather than the bone injury. Most distal phalangeal fractures can be treated nonoperatively because they are either inherently stable and/or some degree of malunion has little consequence. The fibrous septa of the pulp and dorsal nail complex provide intrinsic support and, apart from the flexor and extensor insertions, there are no major deforming forces.[42] Therefore, meticulous soft tissue repair and a well-padded protective splint that spares the PIPJ is often all that is needed. Prophylactic antibiotics do not seem to reduce the incidence of infection.[43] Internal fixation is reserved for unstable fractures and displaced fractures where malunion will lead to functional and aesthetic consequences such as visible fingertip and nail deformity (eg, ridging, nonadherence).

hypersensitivity can last for several weeks after injury and splinting provides adequate pain relief during this period. Undisplaced nailbed injuries, as suggested by a minimally displaced fracture and an intact nail plate, do not require nail avulsion. A tense, painful subungual hematoma can be drained using simple trephination in both adults and children.[44] An axial K-wire sparing the DIPJ may be necessary for *soft tissue support* if there is extensive soft tissue injury. Finally, a large proportion of these injuries heal with a stable fibrous union and further radiographs are not necessary once fingertip pain has subsided. Malunion of a tuft fracture can produce a prominent, painful "bump" under the pulp. Excision of the offending fragment with revision of any soft tissue scarring is occasionally necessary.

Tuft Fractures

Tuft fractures are inherently stable and anatomic repair of a displaced nailbed injury is usually enough to reduce the fracture. Pain and

Shaft Fractures

The most common patterns of diaphyseal fractures are transverse, longitudinal (split), oblique, and segmental fractures. Minimally displaced,

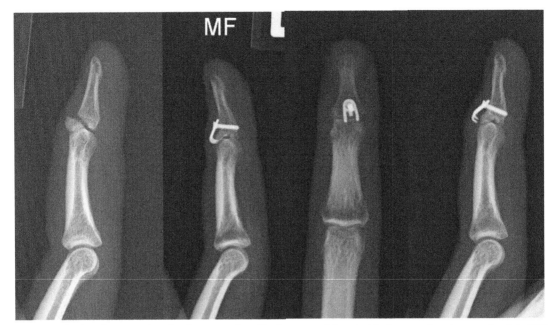

Fig. 8. Hook plate fixation of mallet fractures. A mallet fracture with a sizable fragment and approximately 50% articular involvement (*left*) was treated with open reduction and internal fixation using a pre-contoured hook plate (*middle*). Excellent articular reduction was achieved, and the fracture healed within 10 weeks. However, radiographs taken at about 4 months indicated that the proximal hooks of the implant had backed out (*right*). It is possible that the screw was directed too proximally and created a clockwise moment that caused the hooks to back out. The patient had excellent motion at the joint with no nail deformity and the implant did not irritate the soft tissue. The hardware was left in place.

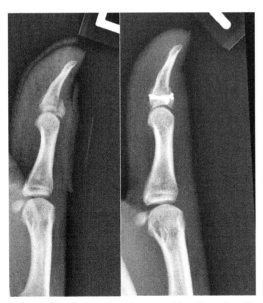

Fig. 9. Open reduction and internal fixation of mallet fracture using screws. There is excellent articular reduction and the low-profile screws do not irritate the overlying soft tissues. The risk of injury to the germinal matrix is also low.

stable fractures can be managed nonoperatively because of the robust soft tissue envelope (**Fig. 12**). Fractures with substantial angular displacement and unstable fractures (eg, metaphyseal comminution; extensive soft tissue injury) should be treated surgically because of the consequences of malunion on nail growth. We prefer to use K-wires because the technique is straight-forward, reproducible, and is unlikely to damage the articular cartilage and nail complex if done properly. We initially hand-drill the phalanx using an 18-G hypodermic needle mounted on a 5-cc syringe and then insert the K-wire through the track thus created. This technique minimizes heat and damage to the bone and articular cartilage. If the fracture is open, the K-wire can be inserted in a distal direction through the fracture site, brought out through the pulp and then re-directed proximally into the base of the distal phalanx. Once adequate placement is confirmed, the wire is cut flush with the skin so that it does not interfere with hand function. A single wire is usually sufficient, and it is removed under local anesthesia once union is confirmed clinically and radiologically, usually after 5 to 6 weeks.

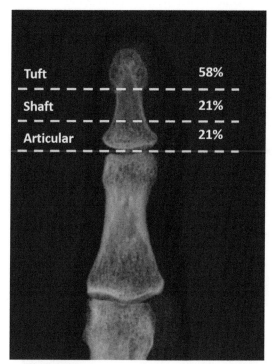

Fig. 10. Classification and relative frequency of distal phalangeal fractures by location (based on data from our institution).

Various other methods of internal fixation have been described, including axial variable pitch compression screws, cerclage wires, and plate and screws.[45–47] The advantages of using an axial compression screw are a minimally invasive

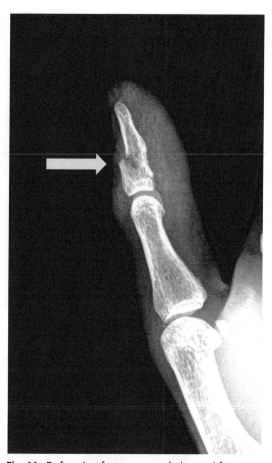

Fig. 11. Deforming forces across phalangeal fractures. This transverse fracture is at the "hard-soft" junction at the root of the nail (*arrow*). The resultant deforming forces generated around this fulcrum by repeated pulp and lateral pinching can displace the fracture, resulting in residual dorsal angulation. Nonoperative treatment requires offloading the fracture with a well molded protective splint until union is evident.

Box 1
Classification of distal phalangeal fractures

Distal (tuft) fractures

- Simple
- Comminuted

Central (shaft) fractures

- Stable
- Unstable

Proximal (articular) fractures

- Volar (flexor digitorum profundus avulsion)
- Dorsal (extensor avulsion)
- Epiphyseal separation
- Comminuted/pilon

Adapted from Schneider LH. Fractures of the distal phalanx. Hand Clin. 1988;4(3):537-547; with permission.

---

technique and the increased rigidity. However, there is a risk of dorsal screw penetration which can result in disturbance of the nail bed, particularly in smaller individuals and in the ring and small fingers. A simple and effective method of reducing small, displaced fragments is using a Prolene tie-over suture that can be easily removed (**Fig. 13**).

A special situation worth highlighting is an unstable fracture with a segmental bone defect. These injuries have a higher propensity to develop painful nonunion, pulp instability, and nail deformity. We prefer to reconstruct these defects immediately using cortico-cancellous bone graft from either the olecranon or distal radius and stabilize it using a single K-wire (**Fig. 14**). Established nonunion can be treated using bone grafting and fixation with axial screws.[48,49] Shinomiya and

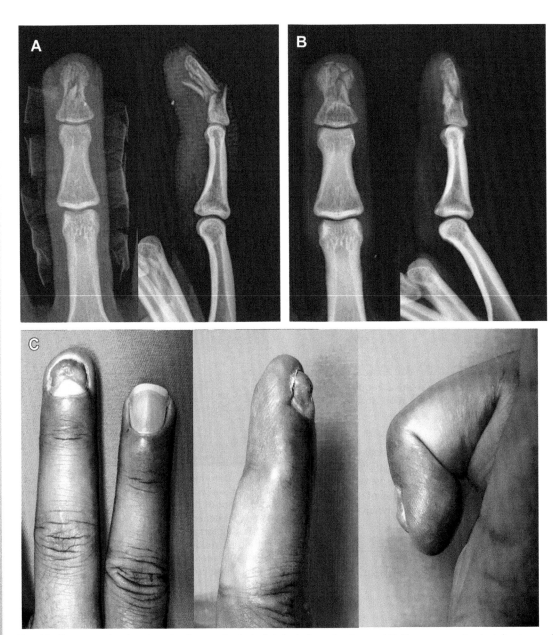

Fig. 12. Nonoperative treatment of comminuted distal phalanx fractures. (*A*) Open, comminuted fracture of distal phalanx shaft with seawater contamination. The wound was thoroughly debrided, and a nailbed repair was performed at a second operation. (*B*) The fracture was well reduced and internal fixation was not required. It healed within 10 weeks with areas of fibrous union. (*C*) There was excellent motion at the DIPJ with no residual hypersensitivity and minimal nail deformity at 3 months.

colleagues[50] have also described good results with the "bone peg fixation" method.

Articular Fractures

Articular fractures are commonly due to axial loading injuries. This results in impaction and fragmentation of the articular surface, akin to pilon fractures of the middle phalanx. Avulsion fractures of the FDP and extensor mechanism have already been covered earlier. Physeal (Seymour) fractures and epiphyseal injuries in children are covered in a separate article, elsewhere in this issue. Fractures with extensive articular comminution pose a challenging problem. The fragments are usually too small to permit accurate

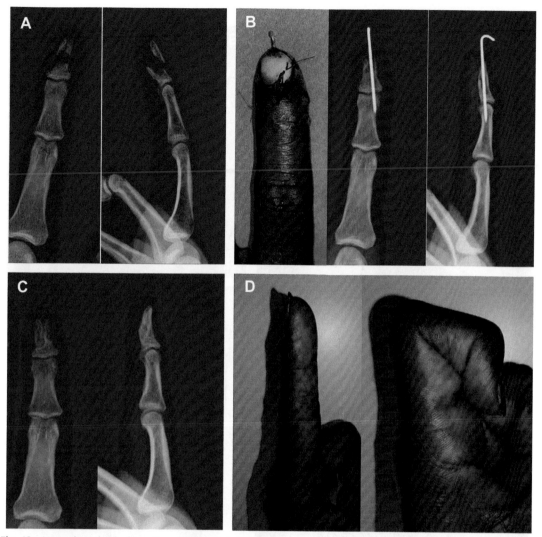

Fig. 13. A novel method of treating displaced shaft fractures. (*A*) A comminuted distal phalanx fracture with displaced volar segment. (*B*) This segment was reduced using Prolene sutures that were brought out dorsally and tied over the nail plate. The fracture was stabilized using an axial, trans-articular K-wire. (*C, D*) The fracture healed well with excellent function and no nail deformity. (*Case courtesy of* Dr Lim Jin Xi, National University Health System.)

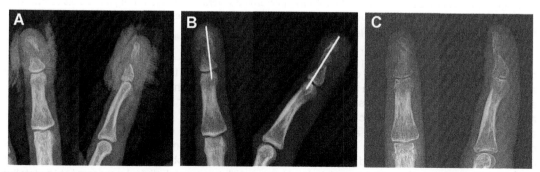

Fig. 14. Distal phalanx shaft fractures with segmental bone loss. (*A, B*) An intercalary cortico-cancellous bone graft was harvested from the dorsal part of the distal radius and inserted into the defect. An axial K-wire was used to provide stability. (*C*) The fracture healed well with no residual tenderness, hypersensitivity or donor site complications.

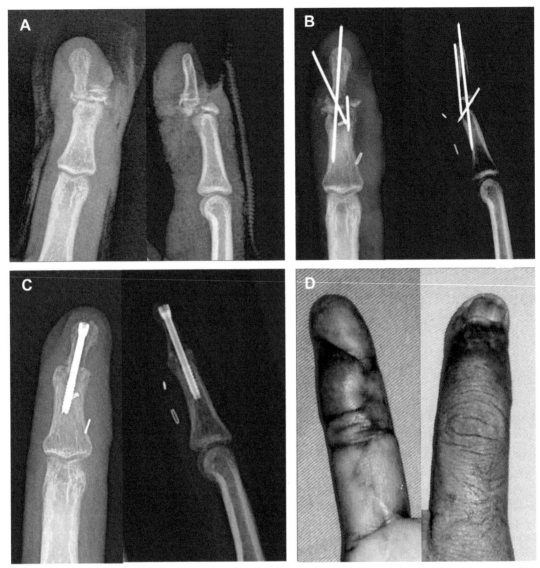

Fig. 15. DIPJ arthrodesis for comminuted articular fractures. (*A*) A comminuted, intra-articular fracture of the distal phalanx with extensive soft tissue injury. (*B*) Initial debridement and trans-articular pinning was performed to maintain length and bone stock. A heterodigital vascular island flap was also necessary for soft tissue coverage. (*C*) A definitive arthrodesis of the DIPJ was performed several weeks later using a headless compression screw. There is an area of screw extrusion under the sterile matrix. (*D*) However, there was no nail deformity and the patient regained good functional use of the finger.

placement of implants. Excessive dissection may also cause avascular necrosis. On the other hand, excision of all bone fragments and primary arthrodesis can result in significant bone loss and shortening. An intermediate approach is to obtain initial stabilization using K-wires. This method preserves bone stock and provides sufficient stability to allow the soft tissue injuries to heal. A formal arthrodesis can subsequently be performed if there is symptomatic nonunion and/or deformity (**Fig. 15**). Unlike the PIPJ,

arthrodesis of the DIPJ is well tolerated and is compatible with good hand function.

SUMMARY

Tendon and bony injuries of the distal phalanx are challenging problems and treating them properly mandates careful clinical assessment, a detailed knowledge of anatomy, and judicious decision-making. Flexor tendon avulsions warrant early surgical repair. Conversely, most extensor tendon injuries and fractures heal well with nonoperative treatment. However, surgery is indicated in selected patients, and a meticulous technique and attention to detail is required to achieve good postoperative outcomes.

CLINICS CARE POINTS

- A thorough understanding of the anatomy of the distal phalanx is essential for accurate implant placement and tendon repair.
- Zone I flexor tendon injuries should be repaired early to avoid postoperative problems such as stiffness and finger flexion contracture.
- The results of nonoperative treatment of mallet injuries are universally favorable. A comprehensive treatment protocol must streamline the use of resources and optimize patient comfort. Conversely, surgery for these injuries is exacting but can provide improved outcomes in selected patients.
- Most distal phalangeal fractures heal well with nonoperative treatment. However, it is crucial to identify specific fracture configurations where operative treatment will lead to better outcomes.

DISCLOSURE

The authors have no conflicts of interest to declare. There was no funding received for this work.

REFERENCES

1. Shrewsbury M, Johnson RK. The fascia of the distal phalanx. J Bone Joint Surg Am 1975;57(6):784–8.
2. Murai M, Lau HK, Pereira BP, et al. A cadaver study on volume and surface area of the fingertip. J Hand Surg Am 1997;22(5):935–41.
3. Mintalucci D, Lutsky KF, Matzon JL, et al. Distal interphalangeal joint bony dimensions related to headless compression screw sizes. J Hand Surg Am 2014;39(6):1068–74.e1.
4. Shum C, Bruno RJ, Ristic S, et al. Examination of the anatomic relationship of the proximal germinal nail matrix to the extensor tendon insertion. J Hand Surg Am 2000;25(6):1114–7.
5. Chepla KJ, Goitz RJ, Fowler JR. Anatomy of the flexor digitorum profundus insertion. J Hand Surg Am 2015;40(2):240–4.
6. Brunelli F, Brunelli G. Vascular anatomy of the distal phalanx. The hand and upper limb 7, vol. 17. Edinburgh (United Kingdom): Churchill Livingstone; 1991.
7. Strauch B, de Moura W. Arterial system of the fingers. J Hand Surg Am 1990;15(1):148–54.
8. Leddy JP, Packer JW. Avulsion of the profundus tendon insertion in athletes. J Hand Surg Am 1977;2(1):66–9.
9. Smith JH Jr. Avulsion of a profundus tendon with simultaneous intraarticular fracture of the distal phalanx–case report. J Hand Surg Am 1981;6(6):600–1.
10. Al-Qattan MM. Extra-articular transverse fractures of the base of the distal phalanx (Seymour's fracture) in children and adults. J Hand Surg Br 2001;26(3):201–6.
11. Tuttle HG, Olvey SP, Stern PJ. Tendon avulsion injuries of the distal phalanx. Clin Orthop Relat Res 2006;445:157–68.
12. Wong J, McGrouther DA. Minimizing trauma over 'no man's land' with flexor tendon retrieval. J Hand Surg Eur Vol 2014;39(9):1004–6.
13. Huq S, George S, Boyce DE. Zone 1 flexor tendon injuries: a review of the current treatment options for acute injuries. J Plast Reconstr Aesthet Surg 2013;66(8):1023–31.
14. McCallister WV, Ambrose HC, Katolik LI, et al. Comparison of pullout button versus suture anchor for zone I flexor tendon repair. J Hand Surg Am 2006;31(2):246–51.
15. Schreuder FB, Scougall PJ, Puchert E, et al. The effect of mitek anchor insertion angle to attachment of FDP avulsion injuries. J Hand Surg Br 2006;31(3):292–5.
16. Kang GC, Yam A, Phoon ES, et al. The hook plate technique for fixation of phalangeal avulsion fractures. J Bone Joint Surg Am 2012;94(11):e72.
17. Henry SL, Katz MA, Green DP. Type IV FDP avulsion: lessons learned clinically and through review of the literature. Hand (N Y) 2009;4(4):357–61.
18. Neiduski RL, Powell RK. Flexor tendon rehabilitation in the 21st century: A systematic review. J Hand Ther 2019;32(2):165–74.
19. Salazar Botero S, Hidalgo Diaz JJ, Benaida A, et al. Review of acute traumatic closed mallet finger injuries in adults. Arch Plast Surg 2016;43(2):134–44.
20. Moss JG, Steingold RF. The long term results of mallet finger injury. A retrospective study of one hundred cases. Hand 1983;15(2):151–4.
21. Handoll HH, Vaghela MV. Interventions for treating mallet finger injuries. Cochrane Database Syst Rev 2004;(3):CD004574.
22. Yeh PC, Shin SS. Tendon ruptures: mallet, flexor digitorum profundus. Hand Clin 2012;28(3):425–30, xi.
23. Wehbe MA, Schneider LH. Mallet fractures. J Bone Joint Surg Am 1984;66(5):658–69.
24. Lange RH, Engber WD. Hyperextension mallet finger. Orthopedics 1983;6(11):1426–31.
25. Lin JS, Samora JB. Surgical and nonsurgical management of mallet finger: a systematic review. J Hand Surg Am 2018;43(2):146–63.e2.
26. Abouna JM, Brown H. The treatment of mallet finger. The results in a series of 148 consecutive cases and

a review of the literature. Br J Surg 1968;55(9): 653–67.

27. Crawford GP. The molded polythene splint for mallet finger deformities. J Hand Surg Am 1984;9(2): 231–7.

28. Warren RA, Norris SH, Ferguson DG. Mallet finger: a trial of two splints. J Hand Surg Br 1988;13(2):151–3.

29. Chin YC, Foo TL. Tips and tricks in mallet fracture fixation. J Hand Surg Asian Pac Vol 2016;21(3):432–5.

30. Das De S, Sebastin SJ. Soft tissue coverage of the digits and hand. Hand Clin 2020;36(1):97–105.

31. Lubahn JD. Mallet finger fractures: a comparison of open and closed technique. J Hand Surg Am 1989; 14(2 Pt 2):394–6.

32. Lucchina S, Badia A, Dornean V, et al. Unstable mallet fractures: a comparison between three different techniques in a multicenter study. Chin J Traumatol 2010;13(4):195–200.

33. Ishiguro T, Itoh Y, Yabe Y, et al. Extension block with Kirschner wire for fracture dislocation of the distal interphalangeal joint. Tech Hand Up Extrem Surg 1997;1(2):95–102.

34. Hofmeister EP, Mazurek MT, Shin AY, et al. Extension block pinning for large mallet fractures. J Hand Surg Am 2003;28(3):453–9.

35. Garg BK, Rajput SS, Purushottam GI, et al. Delta wiring technique to treat bony mallet finger: no need of transfixation pin. Tech Hand Up Extrem Surg 2020; 24(3):131–4.

36. Teoh LC, Lee JY. Mallet fractures: a novel approach to internal fixation using a hook plate. J Hand Surg Eur Vol 2007;32(1):24–30.

37. Theivendran K, Mahon A, Rajaratnam V. A novel hook plate fixation technique for the treatment of mallet fractures. Ann Plast Surg 2007;58(1):112–5.

38. Tie J, Hsieh MKH, Tay SC. Outcome of hook plate fixation of mallet fractures. J Hand Surg Asian Pac Vol 2017;22(4):416–22.

39. Absoud EM, Harrop SN. Hand injuries at work. J Hand Surg Br 1984;9(2):211–5.

40. Butt WD. Fractures of the hand. I. Description. Can Med Assoc J 1962;86:731–5.

41. Schneider LH. Fractures of the distal phalanx. Hand Clin 1988;4(3):537–47.

42. Gaston RG, Chadderdon C. Phalangeal fractures: displaced/nondisplaced. Hand Clin 2012;28(3): 395–401, x.

43. Metcalfe D, Aquilina AL, Hedley HM. Prophylactic antibiotics in open distal phalanx fractures: systematic review and meta-analysis. J Hand Surg Eur Vol 2016;41(4):423–30.

44. Roser SE, Gellman H. Comparison of nail bed repair versus nail trephination for subungual hematomas in children. J Hand Surg Am 1999;24(6):1166–70.

45. Richards RR, Khoury G, Young MC. Internal fixation of an unstable open fracture of a distal phalanx with a Herbert screw. J Hand Surg Am 1988;13(3): 428–32.

46. Shim WC, Yang JW, Roh SY, et al. Percutaneous cerclage wiring technique for phalangeal fractures. Tech Hand Up Extrem Surg 2014;18(1):36–40.

47. Bhatt RA, Schmidt S, Stang F. Methods and pitfalls in treatment of fractures in the digits. Clin Plast Surg 2014;41(3):429–50.

48. Henry M. Variable pitch headless compression screw treatment of distal phalangeal nonunions. Tech Hand Up Extrem Surg 2010;14(4):230–3.

49. Chim H, Teoh LC, Yong FC. Open reduction and interfragmentary screw fixation for symptomatic nonunion of distal phalangeal fractures. J Hand Surg Eur Vol 2008;33(1):71–6.

50. Shinomiya R, Sunagawa T, Ochi M. Bone peg fixation for the treatment of nonunion of the shaft of the distal phalanx. J Hand Surg Eur Vol 2010; 35(9):769–71.

Non-microsurgical Composite Grafting for Acute Management of Fingertip Amputation

Kate Elzinga, MD[a], Kevin C. Chung, MD, MS[b]

KEYWORDS

- Composite grafting • Fingertip amputation • Microvascular replantation • Tissue cooling

KEY POINTS

- Following a fingertip amputation, if vessels are present and of adequate condition and size, microsurgical replantation is the preferred technique for management. However, the technical demands of distal, small-vessel replantation limit the availability of replantation.
- Composite grafting has a limited role in the management of fingertip amputations due to its unreliable nature but can be an option when an amputated fingertip is not replantable and the patient (in particular a child) needs and desires restoration of fingertip length and aesthetics.
- When composite grafting is selected as the treatment of choice for a particular patient, there are methods of optimizing the chances of graft revascularization and survival, including early grafting, graft cooling, and a moist wound healing environment.

INTRODUCTION

Fingertip injuries are the most common injury to the hand.[1,2] Children 4 years of age and younger and adults 55 years of age and older are most commonly injured, by doors and power tools, respectively.[3] When a fingertip amputation occurs, there are 4 main options available to the patient:

- Secondary intention healing
- Revision amputation
- Microsurgical replantation
- Composite grafting

SECONDARY INTENTION HEALING

Permitting a fingertip amputation to heal by secondary intention preserves the remaining digital length, permits the ingrowth of durable and sensate soft tissue coverage, prevents the need for surgery and hospitalization, and results in excellent functional and aesthetic outcomes.[4,5] Even in cases with exposed bone, secondary intention healing has been shown to result in regeneration of the soft tissue thickness to 90% of its former extent with reformation of dermal ridges.[6]

Krauss and Lalonde[7] advocate for secondary intention healing for open wounds, including those with exposed tendon and bone. They reviewed more than 1592 fingertip injuries treated without surgery. Wounds smaller than 1 cm healed within 2 weeks on average. The mean time to healing for all wounds was 4 weeks. A daily shower is recommended, followed by a simple dressing such as Vaseline and Coban wrap (**Fig. 1**).

[a] Section of Plastic Surgery, University of Calgary, South Health Campus, 4448 Front Street Southeast, Calgary, Alberta T3M 1M4, Canada; [b] Section of Plastic Surgery, The University of Michigan Medical School, The University of Michigan Health System, 1500 East Medical Center Drive, 2130 Taubman Center, SPC 5340, Ann Arbor, MI 48109-0340, USA
E-mail address: kecchung@med.umich.edu

Hand Clin 37 (2021) 43–51
https://doi.org/10.1016/j.hcl.2020.09.007
0749-0712/21/© 2020 Elsevier Inc. All rights reserved.

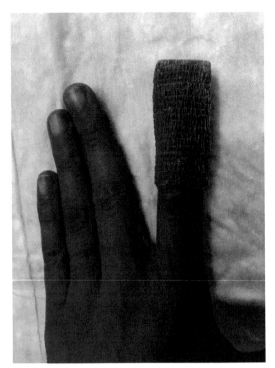

Fig. 1. Vaseline is applied to open fingertip wound and covered by flexible Coban wrap. The dressing provides a moist wound healing environment, protection, and does not restrict the ability to perform range of motion exercises.

Hoigné and colleagues[6] treated 19 fingertip amputations with exposed bone using a semi-occlusive dressing (OpSite Flexifix, Smith and Nephew, London, UK) and secondary intention healing. Lee and colleagues[5] reported good outcomes using an occlusive fingertip cap dressing (Hyphecan) for management of 156 fingertip injuries, including those with exposed distal phalanx bone (63% of cases). Early return to work was possible and a low occurrence of nail deformity was observed as no distal phalanx shortening was performed.

REVISION AMPUTATION

Revision amputation procedures are straightforward and permit early return to work.[8] The primary disadvantage is the need for bone shortening to permit soft tissue coverage. If a fingertip replantation or grafting procedure fails, revision amputation can be performed secondarily.

MICROSURGICAL REPLANTATION

Microsurgical replantation results in excellent functional outcomes and appearance but is technically challenging. At the fingertip level, extensive microsurgical skill is required to repair 0.3 to 0.5 mm arteries and veins to permit successful outcomes.[9,10] A systematic review of 30 studies and 2273 distal fingertip replantations noted a mean survival rate of 86%.[11] Arterial repair is mandatory. Venous repair improves survival rates.[11] The digital nerves regenerate well without repair.[12] For patients with strong beliefs regarding the restoration of wholeness, microvascular replantation provides a reliable means of restoring native anatomy.

Venous outflow can be very difficult to establish at the fingertip level. Delayed venous anastomosis can be attempted once the veins have dilated due to congestion.[13] Vein grafts or venous flow-through flaps can be beneficial if there is a distal vein available.[14] If there is no adequate distal vein for anastomosis, controlled external bleeding can prevent venous congestion of a replanted fingertip while new venous channels are established. External bleeding can be achieved using topical and systemic heparin, medicinal leeches, and/or a fingertip pulp or paraungual incision.[15] Techniques that rely on spontaneous venous connection require at least 72 hours of venous egress, necessitating a prolonged hospital stay, and may be unreliable in achieving revascularization of the reattached fingertip.

COMPOSITE GRAFTING

In situations in which the amputated fingertip is not replantable (very distal amputation, inadequate vessels, severe crush, lack of microsurgical equipment or surgeon expertise), nonvascularized composite grafting can be undertaken in the hopes of restoring digital length and aesthetics for patients who are opposed to healing by secondary intention. Maintenance of body integrity and physical appearance is more important in certain cultures than others, in particular those with Confucian moral values.[16]

The main disadvantage of composite grafting is its unpredictable nature. Success rates are highly variable, less than 50% unless specific interventions are used that require hospitalization and prolonged treatment time, in particular, cooling of the graft. Patients must be counseled preoperatively on the risk of partial or complete graft necrosis and thus the potential need for secondary procedures.[17]

Composite grafting of an amputated fingertip is indicated primarily for the management of patients younger than 4 years with clean, sharp, distal amputations. Beyond these narrow indications, grafting generally has a low success rate. In young children with small digits, replantation is rarely technically possible.

Better results are reported for composite grafting in children compared with adults and those with smaller grafts. Composite grafts with dimensions smaller than 1 cm³ have higher success rates than larger grafts because no area of the graft is further than 1 cm from the underlying vascularized wound bed to permit revascularization. Bone should be removed from the graft to improve the chances of graft survival. If necrosis of the bone within a composite graft occurs, the entire graft will likely fail.

Grafting is not recommended in smokers, diabetic individuals, and patients with vascular disease and poor peripheral arterial flow due to high failure rates.[18,19] The mechanism of injury is an important predictor of outcome for composite grafting. Sharp injuries can be considered for grafting. Crush injuries have poor outcomes and other treatment options should be discussed with the patient, in particular, healing by secondary intention should be considered.

In many cases, composite grafting is performed and patients are discharged home on the day of surgery or the following day. However, better outcomes have been reported by centers that admit patients for close postoperative monitoring and ongoing management after surgery. Experimental studies have shown that 3 to 5 days are required for tissue neovascularization.[20–23] During this time, the graft must be supported with adjunct techniques until reperfusion occurs. Most notably, cooling has shown promising results.[24]

ANATOMY

Fingertip injuries are defined as injuries distal to the tendinous insertions of the flexor digitorum profundus and the extensor tendon on the distal phalanx.[25] Composite grafting involves more than one type of tissue (eg, skin, nail, bone) with no microvascular anastomoses.

The Ishikawa classification of fingertip injuries has 4 zones, starting from distal and moving proximally (**Fig. 2**):[26–28]

1. Injuries from the mid-nail to the fingertip
2. Injuries from the eponychium (base of the nail, proximal nailfold) to the mid-nail
3. Injuries from midway between the eponychium and the distal interphalangeal joint (DIPJ) to the eponychium
4. Injuries from the DIPJ to midway between the eponychium and the DIPJ

Using the Ishikawa classification of fingertip injuries, Kiuchi and colleagues[29] recommended

that all zone I injuries are candidates for composite grafting. In zone II, only clean-cut injuries should be grafted; blunt-cut and crush-avulsion injuries were unlikely to survive. Zone III and IV injuries do poorly with grafting and microsurgery anastomosis is preferred. With larger volumes of tissue and greater hyponychium and bone involvement, the metabolic demands of the grafted tissues increase, resulting in higher graft failure rates.[30]

TECHNIQUES TO IMPROVE COMPOSITE GRAFT SURVIVAL

Composite graft survival depends on the ability of the surrounding tissues to provide plasmatic imbibition, inosculation, and neovascularization. During this multiday process, prevention of tissue death in the graft is paramount. Techniques recommended to improve graft viability include the following:

- Early grafting
- Debulking of the amputated fingertip
- Maintenance of a moist healing environment
- Support for arterial ingrowth
- Cooling of the amputated fingertip

Clinical data are lacking to support the use of hyperbaric oxygen following composite grafting.[31]

Early Grafting

Early grafting of amputated fingertips is recommended. Eo and colleagues[24] had improved graft

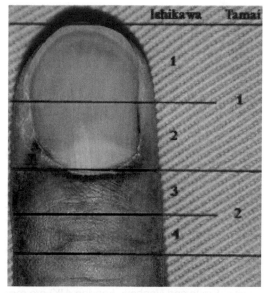

Fig. 2. The Ishikawa classification of fingertip injuries has 4 zones, as illustrated here. (*From* Hattori Y, Doi K, Sakamoto S, et al. Fingertip replantation. *J Hand Surg Am.* 2007 Apr;32(4):548-55; with permission.)

survival when repair was performed within 4 hours of the amputation. Similarly, Moiemen and Elliot[32] found a significant improvement in survival for grafting performed within 5 hours of injury. Butler and colleagues[33] found that no grafts survived if replanted 10 hours after amputation. Cooling may improve the viability of grafts. The amputated fingertip should be kept cool before grafting, using an ice-water bath or a refrigerator.[34]

Debulking of the Amputated Fingertip

If there is bone in the amputated fingertip, the bone can be included in the graft in patients younger than 4 years, if the bone appears viable. The bone is reduced and can be held in position with a K-wire or hypodermic needle. However, if the bone fails to revascularize, it can lead to complete graft necrosis. Removal of the bone from composite grafts may improve graft take.[19,35] Bone removal is performed gently using a scalpel or rongeur, to minimize trauma to the surrounding soft tissues of the amputated fingertip. Removal of bone will result in a loss of distal nail support, and the distal nail bed may need to be ablated. We prefer a shorter distal phalanx and a shorter nail than risking complete loss of the composite graft and therefore typically remove bone in the amputated part in Ishikawa zone 1 amputations. In more proximal amputations, microvascular replantation is preferred, but if composite grafting is pursued, the amputated bone is stabilized with 1 to 2 K-wires for 4 to 6 weeks.

Chen and colleagues[36] removed the bone from the amputated fingertip and defatted half of the pulp fat to decrease the graft thickness. For 31 amputated fingertips, they had complete graft survival in 94% of cases. Lai and colleagues[37] described a pulp adipofascial advancement flap from the intact proximal finger to create distal bulk for the fingertip while improving graft success rates by defatting the graft, removing any bone, and trimming the proximal aspect of the amputated part circumferentially (**Fig. 3**). All of their grafts (n = 16) took with 75% to 100% (average 89%) survival.

Maintenance of a Moist Healing Environment

Prevention of tissue desiccation and dermal necrosis is critical to survival of a grafted fingertip. If the tissues are exposed to the air and become too dry, they will no longer be viable. Antibiotic ointment and occlusive dressings (eg, OpSite Flexifix; Smith and Nephew, London, UK) are recommended.[5,38] A study of 60 composite grafts had a 70% survival rate when ofloxacin ophthalmic antibiotic ointment (Ocuflox) was applied once or twice hourly to maintain a moist healing environment.[39] This ointment is translucent, permitting monitoring of the graft.

A moist environment supports reepithelization of open wounds, keeps small vessels open until inosculation and neovascularization occur, prevents eschar formation, supports endothelial cells, reduces inflammation, and shortens the inflammatory phase of wound healing.[39]

Support for Arterial Ingrowth

The amputated fingertip is debrided; removal of unhealthy tissue and any foreign debris is performed. Bleeding is controlled at the finger recipient wound bed, ideally with pressure or sparingly with bipolar cautery, to avoid a hematoma which will impair graft take. The skin surrounding the proximal fingertip wound is deepithelialized circumferentially by 2 to -3 mm to increase the surface area available for contact with the amputated part to improve graft take. A hole can be made in the central aspect of the amputated part to permit fluid outflow.

The recipient wound bed must be clean and well-vascularized to optimize survival of the composite graft through plasmatic imbibition, capillary inosculation, and neoangiogenesis. The diffuse tissue damage caused by crush injuries limits plasmatic imbibition and graft success rates. Initially the graft will survive on nutrient diffusion. A large surface area of contact is important between the graft and the amputation site to permit adequate fluid uptake into the graft. Elevation of the hand is recommended postoperatively for 7 days to be helpful in limiting edema that could hinder vascular ingrowth.[29]

All forms of nicotine should be avoided postoperatively. Vasospasm and vasoconstriction induced by nicotine will impair revascularization.[40] Composite grafting should be avoided in smokers.[41] If composite grafting is performed and is successful in a patient who smokes, a higher rate of postoperative wound contraction is expected compared to a non-smoker.[42]

Cooling of the Amputated Fingertip

Cooling decreases the biological activity demands of tissue. Decreasing the tissue's metabolic demand and preventing cellular death are important while neovascularization occurs. Plasmatic imbibition supports the graft for the first 48 hours; the graft obtains nutrients and dissolved oxygen from the fluid exuded from the recipient finger bed.[43] The cuts ends of the vessels in the recipient bed and in the graft can reconnect 2 to 5 days after grafting. Capillary budding follows and typically

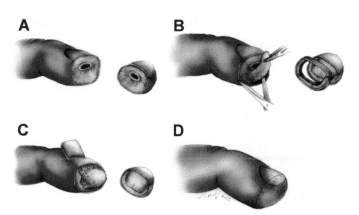

Fig. 3. After a distal fingertip amputation (*A*), bone and fat are removed from the composite graft and the proximal graft is trimmed (*B*) and a pulp adipofascial advancement flap (*C*) is used from the intact proximal finger to create distal bulk for the fingertip while improving graft take rates (*D*). (*Adapted from* Lai HT, Wu SH, Lai YW, et al. Composite grafting with pulp adipofascial advancement flaps for treating non-replantable fingertip amputations. *Microsurgery.* 2016 Nov;36(8):651-657; with permission.)

occurs 5 days after grafting.[44] Vascularization can be seen in skin grafts 3 to 4 days after graft placement with anastomosis between the recipient bed and the graft vessels on stereomicroscopy.[43]

Cooling of the composite graft is started immediately after grafting, ideally under nursing supervision in a hospital. Patients with financial or other constraints can be discharged home if requested, after reviewing how to apply a bag of crushed ice and water to the graft. Cooling is performed continuously for 3 days after grafting; compliance can be difficult for patients, especially for young children, and during sleep. Hospital admission is preferred rather than outpatient care to facilitate graft monitoring and adequate cooling. Anticoagulation is not used in cases of composite grafting.

The use of prostaglandin E1 (ie, Alprostadil) as a vasodilator can be discussed with the patient. Hospitalization is required to administer the medication as a continuous intravenous infusion, which may be cost prohibitive in some situations. Prostaglandin E1 encourages angiogenesis and vasodilation and decreases platelet aggregation and superoxide formation from neutrophils.[45] It increases wound bed microcirculation blood flow and modulates inflammation.[46,47] It is readily available as it is commonly used intravenously to maintain a patent ductus arteriosus in neonates with ductus-dependant cardiac lesions.[48] It is also used for peripheral vascular disease (including Raynaud disease, Buerger disease, scleroderma, and cutaneous ulcers), erectile dysfunction, pulmonary hypertension, and diabetic angiopathy.[49–51] Lipo-prostaglandin E1 infusions at 0.4 µg/h have been noted to significantly increase the maximal blood flow velocity intra-operatively and postoperatively for free flap reconstructions.[52] Fever is the most common adverse effect, occurring in greater than 10% of patients.[51] Other adverse effects include hypotension, flushing, and bradycardia

due to effects of prostaglandin E1 on vascular smooth muscle and the heart.[52,53]

Hirase[54] described keeping a composite graft cool for 3 days continuously after grafting to prevent cellular degeneration until neovascularization. The graft was wrapped in aluminum foil and then a vinyl bag filled with crushed ice and water was applied to the foil. The foil maintains a moist wound healing environment by preventing evaporation.[39] After 3 days, prostaglandin E1 was administered intravenously at 40 to 60 µg/d for 3 days to enhance angiogenesis and to promote vasodilation. Graft survival of 86% (n = 14) was achieved using cooling, compared with a survival rate of 24% (n = 21) without cooling. In more recent publications, Hirase[55,56] described using prostaglandin E1 for 7 days at 60 to 120 µg/d intravenously after cooling for 3 days with a composite graft survival rate of 92% (n = 11).

Eo and colleagues[24,44] recommended cooling of the amputated part for 2 weeks and starting intravenous (IV) lipo-prostaglandin E1 immediately after composite graft surgery. The fingertip was covered with a vinyl bag and balls of ice were applied to the graft. The ice-cooling decreased the skin temperature from 36° Celsius to 26° Celsius. The prostaglandin E1 infusion was used with a rate of 0.167 µg/kg/d for a mean of 12 days postoperatively. The resulting graft survival rate was 89% for 94 patients.

To cool a composite fingertip graft, we wrap the graft with a single layer of Xeroform (Covidien, Minneapolis, MN) then cover it with a layer of aluminum foil. We use a reusable, resealable plastic bag (ie, Ziploc; SC Johnson, Racine, WI) to continuously apply a slush of ice and water to the finger (**Fig. 4**). The bag is changed when the ice melts, approximately every 4 hours, maintaining a slush temperature of 4° Celsius. In young children, we splint the hand and put copious impermeable padding between the affected finger

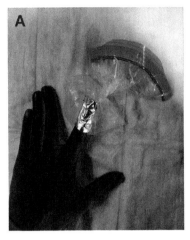
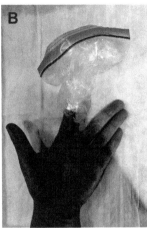

Fig. 4. Following composite grafting, the fingertip is covered with Xeroform and foil and then a bag containing a slush of ice and water is applied (*A*) and wrapped around the fingertip (*B*) for uniform continuous cooling for 3 to 7 days while graft revascularization occurs.

and the other digits to exclude the uninjured digits from cooling. Given the expense and hospital resources required for prolonged hospitalization, we typically admit patients for 24 hours following composite grafting to teach the patient (and their parents when applicable) the cooling protocol and then we discharge them home to continue cooling for a minimum of 3 days, but preferably for up to 7 days while revascularization occurs.

The subdermal pocket procedure has been used as an adjunct for composite grafting and replantation. To prevent composite graft necrosis,

prevention of bone necrosis is essential. This is achieved by removal of the bone from the amputated fingertip or by exposing the bone in the graft directly to the subdermal flap by removal of the soft tissues over the dorsal bone in the amputated fingertip. An abdominal pocket is most commonly used.[41,57–61] The fingertip is deepithelialized and grafted onto the finger and then placed under 2 skin flaps. The pocket skin flaps are sutured to the paraungual area of the fingertip. Lin and colleagues[41] treated 11 fingertips with an abdominal subdermal pocket: 7 had complete survival, 3

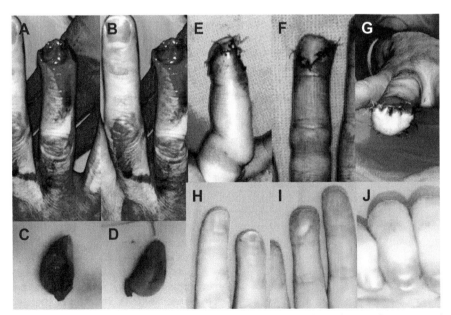

Fig. 5. The injured finger (*A*, *B*) and the amputated fingertip (*C*, *D*) are debrided. Immediate composite grafting restores the fingertip length and contour (*E–G*). Three months after composite grafting, the fingertip is well vascularized and fully healed (*H–J*). Mild pulp atrophy is common (*H*). Full extension (*I*) and flexion (*J*) of the DIPJ has been regained.

had partial survival, and 1 did not survive. Jung and colleagues[61] treated 10 patients with palmar subdermal pocketing for composite grafts: 9 grafts survived completely and one graft survived with 20% partial necrosis. Cross-finger subdermal pockets have been used to salvage fingertip replantations.[58,62] Venous outflow was maintained by venous blood egress from the surgical incision to the dressings and plasmatic exchange between the deepithelialized composite graft and the cross-finger dermal flap. Patient acceptance is greater for the cooling technique compared with the pocket procedures.

CLINICS CARE POINTS

- Postoperative cooling of composite grafts has shown promising results with improved graft survival rates.
- Early grafting and a moist wound healing environment will also support graft take.
- Outcomes for composite grafting are better in younger patients, in more distal amputations, and with a sharp mechanism of injury (**Fig. 5**).
- If the bone in the composite graft undergoes necrosis, typically the entire composite graft will fail. The benefit of retaining bone in the amputated part to maintain digital length and nail support must be weighed against the risk of graft failure.

ACKNOWLEDGMENTS

Dr K.C. Chung receives funding from the National Institutes of Health and book royalties from Wolters Kluwer and Elsevier. He has received financial support from Axogen as a consultant.

DISCLOSURE

The authors have nothing to disclose.

REFERENCES

1. Venkatramani H, Sabapathy SR. Fingertip replantation: technical considerations and outcome analysis of 24 consecutive fingertip replantations. Indian J Plast Surg 2011;44(2):237–45.
2. Peterson SL, Peterson EL, Wheatley MJ. Management of fingertip amputations. J Hand Surg Am 2014;39(10):2093–101.
3. Conn JM, Annest JL, Ryan GW, et al. Non-work-related finger amputations in the United States, 2001-2002. Ann Emerg Med 2005;45(6):630–5.
4. Champagne L, Hustedt JW, Walker R, et al. Digital Tip Amputations from the Perspective of the Nail. Adv Orthop 2016;2016:1967192.
5. Lee LP, Lau PY, Chan CW. A simple and efficient treatment for fingertip injuries. J Hand Surg Br 1995;20(1):63–71.
6. Hoigné D, Hug U, Schürch M, et al. Semi-occlusive dressing for the treatment of fingertip amputations with exposed bone: quantity and quality of soft-tissue regeneration. J Hand Surg Eur Vol 2014;39(5):505–9.
7. Krauss EM, Lalonde DH. Secondary healing of fingertip amputations: a review. Hand (N Y) 2014;9(3):282–8.
8. Wang K, Sears ED, Shauver MJ, et al. A systematic review of outcomes of revision amputation treatment for fingertip amputations. Hand (N Y) 2013;8(2):139–45.
9. Hattori Y, Doi K, Ikeda K, et al. A retrospective study of functional outcomes after successful replantation versus amputation closure for single fingertip amputations. J Hand Surg Am 2006;31(5):811–8.
10. Brown M, Lu Y, Chung KC, et al. Annual hospital volume and success of digital replantation. Plast Reconstr Surg 2017;139(3):672–80.
11. Sebastin SJ, Chung KC. A systematic review of the outcomes of replantation of distal digital amputation. Plast Reconstr Surg 2011;128(3):723–37.
12. Zhu ZW, Zou XY, Huang YJ, et al. Evaluation of sensory function and recovery after replantation of fingertips at Zone I in children. Neural Regen Res 2017;12(11):1911–7.
13. Koshima I, Yamashita S, Sugiyama N, et al. Successful delayed venous drainage in 16 consecutive distal phalangeal replantations. Plast Reconstr Surg 2005;115(1):149–54.
14. Zheng D, Li Z, Xu L, et al. Application of venous flow-through flap in finger replantation with circularity soft tissue defect. Zhongguo Xiu Fu Chong Jian Wai Ke Za Zhi 2014;28(8):977–80 [in Chinese].
15. Lafosse T, Jehanno P, Fitoussi F. Complications and pitfalls after finger replantation in young children. J Hand Microsurg 2018;10(2):74–8.
16. Chen NC, Srinivasan RC, Shauver MJ, et al. A systematic review of outcomes of fasciotomy, aponeurotomy, and collagenase treatments for Dupuytren's contracture. Hand (N Y) 2011;6(3):250–5.
17. Heistein JB, Cook PA. Factors affecting composite graft survival in digital tip amputations. Ann Plast Surg 2003;50(3):299–303.
18. Lemmon JA, Janis JE, Rohrich RJ. Soft-tissue injuries of the fingertip: methods of evaluation and treatment. An algorithmic approach. Plast Reconstr Surg 2008;122(3):105e–17e.
19. Uysal A, Kankaya Y, Ulusoy MG, et al. An alternative technique for microsurgically unreplantable fingertip amputations. Ann Plast Surg 2006;57(5):545–51.
20. Hirase Y, Valauri FA, Buncke HJ. Prefabricated sensate myocutaneous and osteomyocutaneous

free flaps: an experimental model. Preliminary report. Plast Reconstr Surg 1988;82(3):440–6.

21. Hirase Y, Valauri FA, Buncke HJ, et al. Customized prefabricated neovascularized free flaps. Microsurgery 1987;8(4):218–24.

22. Converse JM, Rapaport FT. The vascularization of skin autografts and homografts; an experimental study in man. Ann Surg 1956;143(3):306–15.

23. Young DM, Greulich KM, Weier HG. Species-specific in situ hybridization with fluorochrome-labeled DNA probes to study vascularization of human skin grafts on athymic mice. J Burn Care Rehabil 1996; 17(4):305–10.

24. Eo S, Doh G, Lim S, et al. Analysis of the risk factors that determine composite graft survival for fingertip amputation. J Hand Surg Eur Vol 2018;43(10): 1030–5.

25. Fassler PR. Fingertip injuries: evaluation and treatment. J Am Acad Orthop Surg 1996;4(1):84–92.

26. Ishikawa K, Ogawa Y, Soeda H, et al. A new classification of the amputation level for the distal part of the fingers. J Jpn Soc Microsurg 1990; 3:54–62.

27. Borrelli MR, Dupré S, Mediratta S, et al. Composite grafts for pediatric fingertip amputations: a retrospective case series of 100 patients. Plast Reconstr Surg Glob Open 2018;6(6):e1843.

28. Hattori Y, Doi K, Sakamoto S, et al. Fingertip replantation. J Hand Surg Am 2007;32(4):548–55.

29. Kiuchi T, Shimizu Y, Nagasao T, et al. Composite grafting for distal digital amputation with respect to injury type and amputation level. J Plast Surg Hand Surg 2015;49(4):224–8.

30. Henderson JT, Schulz SA, Swiergosz AM, et al. Preservation of the sterile matrix, hyponychium, and fingertip pad in fingertip reconstruction with composite fingertip and nail bed graft and volar V-Y advancement flap. Eplasty 2017;17:e28.

31. Alper N, Sood A, Granick MS. Composite graft repair for distal fingertip amputation. Eplasty 2013; 13:ic32.

32. Moiemen NS, Elliot D. Composite graft replacement of digital tips. 2. A study in children. J Hand Surg Br 1997;22(3):346–52.

33. Butler DP, Murugesan L, Ruston J, et al. The outcomes of digital tip amputation replacement as a composite graft in a paediatric population. J Hand Surg Eur Vol 2016;41(2):164–70.

34. Elsahy NI. When to replant a fingertip after its complete amputation. Plast Reconstr Surg 1977;60(1): 14–21.

35. Rose EH, Norris MS, Kowalski TA, et al. The "cap" technique: nonmicrosurgical reattachment of fingertip amputations. J Hand Surg Am 1989;14(3): 513–8.

36. Chen SY, Wang CH, Fu JP, et al. Composite grafting for traumatic fingertip amputation in adults: technique reinforcement and experience in 31 digits. J Trauma 2011;70(1):148–53.

37. Lai HT, Wu SH, Lai YW, et al. Composite grafting with pulp adipofascial advancement flaps for treating non-replantable fingertip amputations. Microsurgery 2016;36(8):651–7.

38. Lalonde D, Joukhadar N, Janis J. Simple effective ways to care for skin wounds and incisions. Plast Reconstr Surg Glob Open 2019;7(10):e2471.

39. Son D, Han K, Chang DW. Extending the limits of fingertip composite grafting with moist-exposed dressing. Int Wound J 2005;2(4):315–21.

40. Black CE, Huang N, Neligan PC, et al. Effect of nicotine on vasoconstrictor and vasodilator responses in human skin vasculature. Am J Physiol Regul Integr Comp Physiol 2001;281(4):R1097–104.

41. Lin TS, Jeng SF, Chiang YC. Fingertip replantation using the subdermal pocket procedure. Plast Reconstr Surg 2004;113(1):247–53.

42. Hong JP, Lee SJ, Lee HB, et al. Reconstruction of fingertip and stump using a composite graft from the hypothenar region. Ann Plast Surg 2003;51(1): 57–62.

43. Greenwood J, Amjadi M, Dearman B, et al. Real-time demonstration of split skin graft inosculation and integra dermal matrix neovascularization using confocal laser scanning microscopy. Eplasty 2009; 9:e33.

44. Eo S, Hur G, Cho S, et al. Successful composite graft for fingertip amputations using ice-cooling and lipo-prostaglandin E1. J Plast Reconstr Aesthet Surg 2009;62(6):764–70.

45. Simmet T, Peskar BA. Prostaglandin E1 and arterial occlusive disease: pharmacological considerations. Eur J Clin Invest 1988;18(6):549–54.

46. Greaves MW, McDonald-Gibson W. Itch: role of prostaglandins. Br Med J 1973;3(5881):608–9.

47. Hasegawa H, Ichioka S. Effects of lipo-prostaglandin E1 on wound bed microcirculation. J Wound Care 2015;24(7):293–4, 296, 298-299.

48. Akkinapally S, Hundalani SG, Kulkarni M, et al. Prostaglandin E1 for maintaining ductal patency in neonates with ductal-dependent cardiac lesions. Cochrane Database Syst Rev 2018;(2): CD011417.

49. Mizushima Y, Yanagawa A, Hoshi K. Prostaglandin E1 is more effective, when incorporated in lipid microspheres, for treatment of peripheral vascular diseases in man. J Pharm Pharmacol 1983;35(10): 666–7.

50. Collantes-Rodríguez C, Jiménez-Gallo D, Arjona-Aguilera C, et al. Treatment of skin ulcers secondary to Sneddon syndrome with alprostadil (prostaglandin E1). JAMA Dermatol 2016;152(6):726–7.

51. Hew MR, Gerriets V. Prostaglandin E1. Treasure Island (FL): StatPearls Publishing; 2020. Available at: https://www.ncbi.nlm.nih.gov/pubmed/31536236.

52. Jin SJ, Suh HP, Lee J, et al. Lipo-prostaglandin E1 increases immediate arterial maximal flow velocity of free flap in patients undergoing reconstructive surgery. Acta Anaesthesiol Scand 2019; 63(1):40–5.

53. Gul M, Serefoglu EC. An update on the drug safety of treating erectile dysfunction. Expert Opin Drug Saf 2019;18(10):965–75.

54. Hirasé Y. Postoperative cooling enhances composite graft survival in nasal-alar and fingertip reconstruction. Br J Plast Surg 1993;46(8):707–11.

55. Hirase Y. Salvage of fingertip amputated at nail level: new surgical principles and treatments. Ann Plast Surg 1997;38(2):151–7.

56. Hirasé Y. Free composite graft to claw nail deformity using the ice water cooling method. Tech Hand Up Extrem Surg 1998;2(1):47–9.

57. Tsai PL, Scaglioni MF, Lin TS, et al. Combined subdermal pocket procedure and abdominal flap for distal finger amputations in a toddler. Plast Reconstr Surg Glob Open 2015;3(5):e386.

58. Li YS, Chen CY, Yang SW, et al. Cross-finger subdermal pocketplasty as a salvage procedure for thumb tip replantation without vascular anastomosis: a case report. J Int Med Res 2018;46(9): 3717–23.

59. Arata J, Ishikawa K, Soeda H, et al. Replantation of multi-level fingertip amputation using the pocket principle (palmar pocket method). Br J Plast Surg 2003;56(5):504–8.

60. Shim HS, Kim DH, Kwon H, et al. Contralateral abdominal pocketing in salvation of replanted fingertips with compromised circulation. ScientificWorldJournal 2014;2014:548687.

61. Jung MS, Lim YK, Hong YT, et al. Treatment of fingertip amputation in adults by palmar pocketing of the amputated part. Arch Plast Surg 2012;39(4):404–10.

62. Tan VH, Murugan A, Foo TL, et al. Cross-finger dermal pocketing to augment venous outflow for distal fingertip replantation. Tech Hand Up Extrem Surg 2014;18(3):131–4.

Fingertip Replantation
Technique Details and Review of the Evidence

Amelia C. Van Handel, MD, Mitchell A. Pet, MD*

KEYWORDS

• Fingertip • Replantation • Amputation

KEY POINTS

• Fingertip replantation is technically challenging, but in a motivated patient excellent aesthetic and functional outcomes can be achieved.
• Careful preoperative patient selection and a deliberate process of informed consent are necessary.
• A detailed understanding of fingertip microanatomy by zone is critical to inform an orderly replantation plan that minimizes soft tissue dissection.
• Several authors advocate for venous anastomosis to improve success rates, shorten hospital time, and decrease blood loss from external bleeding; however, similar rates of success are reported with alternative methods of venous egress.
• Patient-reported outcomes of pain and satisfaction have been studied only in a limited capacity.

INTRODUCTION

Because the world is quite literally "at our fingertips," the fingertip is particularly vulnerable to harm. Although replantable fingertip amputations constitute only a small portion of fingertip injuries, they represent a substantial challenge. In this article, we outline our preferred techniques for fingertip replantation and review the current body of evidence surrounding indications and outcomes. Opportunities for future investigations are highlighted in the context of existing evidence.

ANATOMY

The nail protects the dorsal surface of the phalanx, facilitates sensory function, and enables stable pinch.[1] The nail complex is made up of the nail plate, nail bed, eponychium (cuticle), perionychium, and hyponychium. Within the nail bed, the germinal matrix produces the nail plate and the sterile matrix adheres the nail plate to the fingertip. The volar pulp skin is glabrous, stable, resistant to injury, and critical for optimal grip.

The fingertip is dense with sensory receptors, which help to fulfill its exploratory role in hand function. Each digit has 2 proper digital nerves, one each on the ulnar and radial borders of the digit. These nerves are located volar to the digital arteries along the respective border of the finger before branching distally. In the thumb, 60% of digital nerves branch distal to the interphalangeal joint (IPJ) crease. In the remaining digits, 78% of terminal branching is distal to the distal IPJ (DIPJ) crease, 18% at the DIPJ crease, and only 4% of digital nerves branch proximal to the DIPJ crease. Most digital nerves have a terminal trifurcation, though the number of branches ranges from 2 to 7.[2]

Each digit has 2 proper digital arteries paired with its radial and ulnar digital nerves. These arteries join distally at the level of the nail base to form the distal transverse palmar arch (DTPA). The arterial diameter at this level is 0.85 ± 0.10 mm.[3] The DTPA gives off 1 or more dominant central arteries distally. This pattern of central artery branching was described by Nam

Division of Plastic & Reconstructive Surgery, Washington University in St. Louis, 660 South Euclid Avenue, Suite 1150, St Louis, MO 63110, USA
* Corresponding author.
E-mail address: mpet@wustl.edu

Hand Clin 37 (2021) 53–65
https://doi.org/10.1016/j.hcl.2020.09.006
0749-0712/21/© 2020 Elsevier Inc. All rights reserved.

and colleagues in a 2017 anatomic study in which they described 3 branching types:

Type I: Only 1 dominant artery branching off the DTPA

Type II: Two dominant branching arteries off the DTPA

Type III: Three or more dominant branching arteries off the DTPA

The incidence of types I, II, and III was 27%, 28%, and 45%, respectively. The largest central artery branches typically run close to the midline and just volar to the distal phalanx, with a diameter range of 0.58 ± 0.10 mm.[3]

Venous drainage of the fingertip occurs through dorsal and volar venous systems, but the dorsal system is more robust and predictable.[4] At the level of the DIPJ, there is a terminal dorsal vein that subsequently drains into both the radial and ulnar longitudinal dorsal veins.[5] This terminal dorsal vein is present in the central one-third of the dorsal digit 68% of the time and is reliably greater than 0.5 mm.[4] There exists a volar equivalent of this terminal dorsal vein, but it can be difficult to dissect owing to its intimate relationship with the glabrous skin at the DIPJ flexion crease.[4] Additional reliable venous structures at the DIPJ level are the commissural veins, which are lateral conduits that connect the volar and dorsal systems.[4] These commissural veins are also present more distally, usually in the 3 to 5 o'clock and 7 to 9 o'clock positions (where 12 o'clock corresponds with the dorsal distal midline).[6]

HISTORY

Kleinert and colleagues[7] were the first to report success in revascularization of a digit in 1965, and 3 years later Komatsu and Tamai[8] reported replantation of an amputated thumb. Shortly thereafter, Serafin and colleagues[9] and Snyder and associates[10] reported the first "artery only" replants. The 1970s saw advances in microinstruments, sutures, and microscopes, and by the end of the decade, Buncke and associates[11] were publishing microsurgical techniques including methods of progressively distal replantation. Early adopters of the techniques pushed the boundaries of replantation[12–14] and ushered in the era of routine replantation. Currently, capabilities for very distal replantation continue to evolve,[15] and indications are becoming more evidence based.[16]

DEFINITIONS

In this review, distal fingertip amputation will be defined as occurring at or distal to the flexor digitorum superficialis insertion. The majority of classification systems separate injuries by proximodistal level[12,17–21] (**Fig. 1**). Other investigators delineate zones and treatment recommendations based on injury geometry.[22,23] We find the Sebastin and Chung[20] classification system to be most useful because the boundaries are easily defined by external inspection and each zone is associated with distinct surgical considerations.

INDICATIONS

Early indications for replantation were for injuries threatening a catastrophic functional deficit (hands, thumbs, multiple digits, pediatric).[16,24–26] However, in the era of routine microsurgery, increased surgical capabilities and patient expectations have necessitated a more nuanced discussion. A modern approach to indications for distal fingertip replantation must include evaluation of patient, injury, and circumstance factors which have been recently outlined by the senior author (**Table 1**).[16]

Contraindications to fingertip replantation are consistent with those for amputation at any level and include:

- Severely crushed or mangled parts
- Multilevel injury to the same digit
- Comorbid or otherwise injured patients
- Severe atherosclerotic disease
- Mental illness

A prolonged warm ischemia time is also a traditional contraindication to replant, but the absence of ischemia-sensitive muscle at the fingertip level make these amputations less time-sensitive. The traditional limit of warm ischemia for a digit replantation is 6 to 12 hours,[27] but even in excess of 12 hours, success rates of more than 90% have been reported.[28]

PATIENT MANAGEMENT

Fingertip replantation requires specialized skill and equipment and should be performed at referral centers.[29] The referring hospital should be given specific instructions on how to handle the patient and part before transfer. The amputated part should be rinsed with normal saline to remove gross contamination and then wrapped in moist gauze. The wrapped part should be placed in a waterproof bag and placed in a container of ice water. The part should not be placed directly on ice, because this contact risks causing tissue damage.[30] Radiographs should be taken of the part and hand to identify injuries in other digits and to facilitate surgical planning for the amputated digit. Antibiotics and

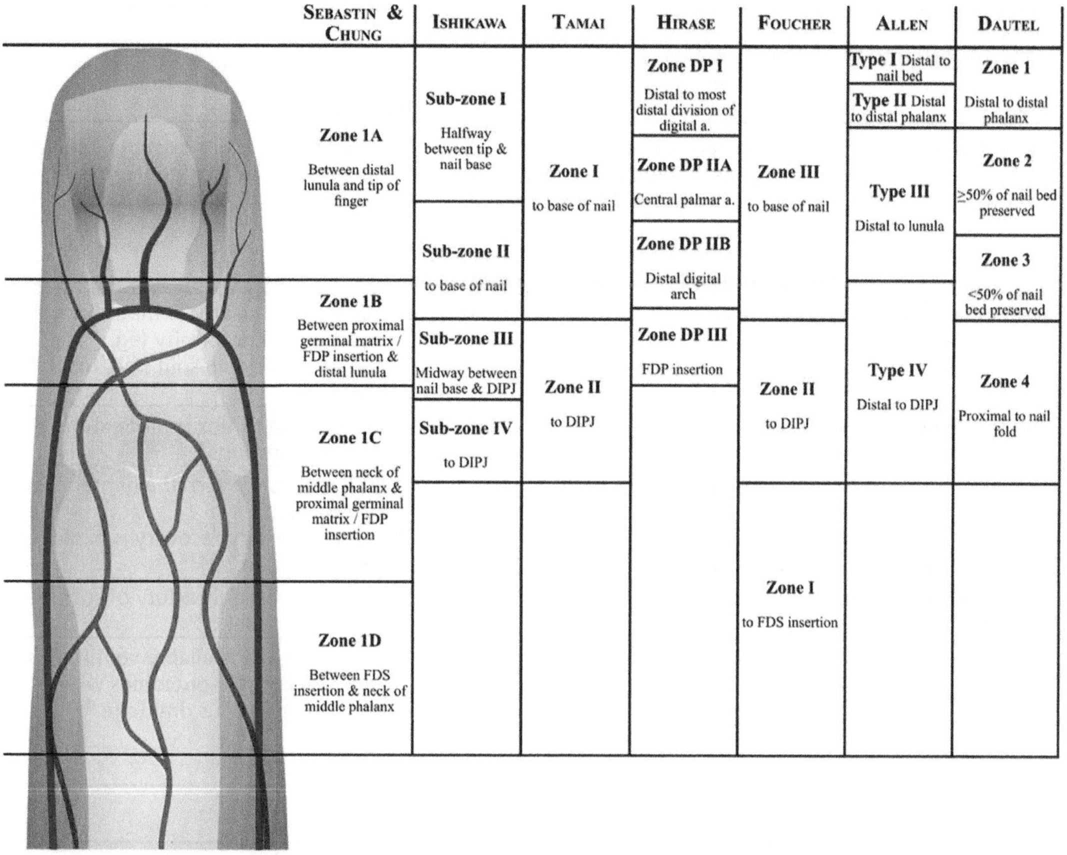

Sebastin & Chung	Ishikawa	Tamai	Hirase	Foucher	Allen	Dautel
Zone 1A Between distal lunula and tip of finger	**Sub-zone I** Halfway between tip & nail base	**Zone I** to base of nail	**Zone DP I** Distal to most distal division of digital a.	**Zone III** to base of nail	**Type I** Distal to nail bed **Type II** Distal to distal phalanx	**Zone 1** Distal to distal phalanx
			Zone DP IIA Central palmar a.		**Type III** Distal to lunula	**Zone 2** ≥50% of nail bed preserved
Zone 1B Between proximal germinal matrix / FDP insertion & distal lunula	**Sub-zone II** to base of nail		**Zone DP IIB** Distal digital arch			**Zone 3** <50% of nail bed preserved
	Sub-zone III Midway between nail base & DIPJ	**Zone II** to DIPJ	**Zone DP III** FDP insertion	**Zone II** to DIPJ	**Type IV** Distal to DIPJ	**Zone 4** Proximal to nail fold
Zone 1C Between neck of middle phalanx & proximal germinal matrix / FDP insertion	**Sub-zone IV** to DIPJ					
Zone 1D Between FDS insertion & neck of middle phalanx					**Zone I** to FDS insertion	

Fig. 1. Classification systems of distal fingertip amputations. The Sebastin and Chung classification system is referenced in this article. DIPJ, distal interphalangeal joint; FDP, flexor digitorum profundus; FDS, flexor digitorum superficialis. (Figure acknowledgement: Kevin Shim, MD, PhD.)

tetanus vaccination should be administered as appropriate. Procedural consent should cover all possibilities including replantation, vein graft, nerve allograft or autograft, skin graft, arthrodesis, and revision amputation.

AUTHORS' PREFERRED SURGICAL TECHNIQUES

Fingertip replantation is similar to replantation at any level, with some specialized techniques and considerations given the diminutive size, fragility, and anatomic variability present at this level. Our general approach is reviewed here, and zone-specific considerations are outlined in **Tables 2–5**.

Anesthesia

Our preference is for general anesthesia with brachial plexus regional anesthetic. We believe that an indwelling regional block catheter

Table 1		
Factors for consideration when deciding whether replantation/revascularization should be offered		
Patient Factors	**Injury Factors**	**Circumstantial Factors**
Medical comorbidity Age Physical and occupational demands Social factors Cultural and personal values Psychiatric disease	Level of injury Digits involved Mechanism Injury to adjacent fingers Incomplete or complete amputation	Time to presentation Availability of postreplantation care

From Pet MA, Ko JH. Indications for Replantation and Revascularization in the Hand. *Hand Clin.* 2019;35(2):119-130; with permission.

Table 2
Zone 1A: distal to the lunula (see Fig. 2)

Step	Technique	Rationale
Bony fixation	If bone fragment of sufficient size present, one or 2 longitudinal K-wires extending across the DIPJ into the P2 base. In the absence of a bone fragment, use lateral sutures for tissue stabilization.	If bony fixation is not possible, repair of the lateral skin and sterile matrix will stabilize the part during microsurgery.[69]
Nail apparatus	Remove the nail plate and repair sterile matrix with 5-0 fast gut.	Disruption of the sterile matrix can result in nail deformity (eg, nonadherent nail, split nail, irregular contour).
Tendon repair	No flexor or extensor tendon repair is performed.	Injury is distal to flexor and extensor tendon insertions.
Nerve repair	No nerve repair is performed.	Digital nerves are terminally branched at this level.[2] Adequate sensory recovery is expected without repair.[6,20,34,35]
Artery repair	Repair of central artery.	Central artery is only artery of sufficient size at this level.[3,70]
Vein repair	No vein repair is performed. Fish mouth incision in the fingertip with intermittent heparin scrubs.[14] Immediate leeching is an alternative[56]	Unlikely to have available vein in this zone, acceptable outcomes with alternative venous drainage.[42]

Data from Refs.[2,3,6,14,20,34,35,42,56,69,70]

Table 3
Zone 1B: root of germinal matrix/FDP insertion to distal lunula (see Fig. 3)

Step	Technique	Rationale
Bony fixation	Two longitudinal 0.035 K-wires inserted anterograde into the part, then driven proximally across the DIPJ into the P2 base.	Two small wires confer some rotational stability. A single 0.045 K-wire may be better suited to small distal bone fragments, with rotational stability offered by skin closure.
Nail apparatus	Remove nail plate and repair germinal matrix with 5-0 fast gut.	Failure to repair germinal matrix can result in nail plate absence or deformity.
Tendon repair	Same as zone 1A.	Same as zone 1A.
Nerve repair	Explore proximal nerve first. If injury is proximal to trifurcation, microsurgical repair is performed. If injury is beyond trifurcation, no repair is performed.	Terminal branches of nerves sometimes visible and repairable at this level.[2] Adequate sensory recovery is expected without repair.[6,20,34,35]
Artery repair	Repair of central artery. If necessary, divide DTPA on one side and mobilize for additional length.	Central artery and DTPA both available at this level; DTPA has larger diameter for easier anastomosis, but can result in size mismatch with distal target.[3,70]
Vein repair	Anastomosis of one or more dorsal veins is often possible. If suitable veins cannot be found, fishmouth incision and heparin scrubs or leeching[14,56]	Suitable caliber dorsal veins (>0.3 mm) are present at this level. Smaller volar veins are variable.[6]

Data from Refs.[2,3,6,14,20,34,35,56,70]

Table 4
Zone 1C: middle phalangeal neck to base of germinal matrix (see Fig. 4)

Step	Technique	Rationale
Bony fixation	Most cases include DIPJ articular injury. Perform DIPJ arthrodesis using K-wire fixation.	DIPJ unlikely to recover significant motion, arthrodesis unlikely to compromise overall hand function.
Nail apparatus	No nail bed repair.	Proximal to nail plate.
Tendon repair	No FDP repair performed after DIP arthrodesis. In cases of DIP preservation, FDP is reinserted using suture anchors. Repair terminal extensor with a 4-0 braided nonabsorbable suture.	Flexor tendon repair not required in the setting of arthrodesis. Suture anchor technique is preferable to suture button, as pressure on the nail may impair circulation. Extensor digitorum communis repair may prevent swan neck deformity that can occur even in the setting of DIPJ arthrodesis.[33]
Nerve repair	Repair digital nerves if injured proximal to the trifurcation.	Proper digital nerves do not branch until distal to DIPJ in 78% of digits.[2]
Artery repair	Anastomosis of a single proper digital artery on the dominant border.	Proper digital arteries present at level of DIPJ.[3]
Vein repair	Anastomosis of one or more veins.	Volar and dorsal veins available at this level.[4]

Data from Refs.[2–4,33]

functions both to enhance patient comfort and reduce vasospasm in the postoperative period.

Preparation of the Amputated Part

As soon as the decision is made to pursue replantation, the amputated part can be taken to the operating room ahead of the patient to expedite the procedure. The part is cleansed with betadine and a sterile back table can be used to prepare the part. A plan for skeletal shortening should be developed early. In general, shortening is done proximally to preserve the small volume of bone in the amputated part. However, proximal shortening should not violate intact tendon insertions

Table 5
Zone 1D: flexor digitorum superficialis insertion to middle phalangeal neck (see Fig. 5)

Step	Technique	Rationale
Bony fixation	90–90 wire fixation of the middle phalanx fracture is preferable when possible. Crossed or parallel K-wire fixation is an acceptable alternative.	90–90 wiring is preferable when possible because fixation is rigid and does not cross the DIPJ. This facilitates early motion.[71] K-wires are preferable when soft tissues are unfavorable.
Nail apparatus	Same as zone 1C.	Same as zone 1C.
Tendon repair	A4 and A5 pulleys should be divided. Four to 8 core strand locking cruciate repair is performed with 4-0 looped braided nonabsorbable suture. This is supplemented with a 5-0 monofilament epitendinous stitch.	Robust flexor tendon repair allows early rehabilitation.
Nerve repair	Repair both the radial and ulnar digital nerves.	Injury is expected to be proximal to the trifurcation at this level.[2]
Artery repair	Same as zone 1C.	Same as zone 1C.
Vein repair	Same as zone 1C.	Same as zone 1C.

Data from Refs.[2,71]

or exceed that which would be necessary for a revision amputation in the case of an unsuccessful replantation. Retrograde K-wire(s) are inserted into the distal bone fragment if one is present.

Although some authors[31–33] advocate using the operating microscope at this stage to identify and mark vascular and nervous structures in the part, it is our practice to use the back table only for the preparation of bony fixation. We forego dissection of vascular and nervous structures until the bony fixation has been accomplished, because the cues of normal anatomy in the context of a whole finger are helpful during structure identification. Additionally, the structures are larger and easier to identify proximally, and, once identified, can guide dissection of the distal structures in the part. Dissecting these structures immediately before repair also avoids desiccation and inadvertent injury during bony fixation and tendon repair.

Bone

Bony fixation in the fingertip is accomplished before raising the tourniquet, usually using 1 or 2 longitudinal K-wires previously placed into the amputated part. After appropriate shortening, the fracture is reduced and the K-wires are driven retrograde into the proximal fragment, crossing the DIPJ and terminating in the subchondral bone of the middle phalanx. If the amputation occurs through the DIPJ, the opposing cartilaginous surfaces are formally prepared during shortening and arthrodesis is performed. After fixation is completed and confirmed using fluoroscopy, the tourniquet is raised.

Tendon

Extensor tendon injury should be repaired in all cases to prevent both mallet and swan-neck deformities. To facilitate tendon repair, the dorsal skin is lifted off of the underlying extensor tendon using a double skin hook both proximally and distally. The skin and adipofascial tissues are separated from the tendon using a blade without making an additional incision, and the extensor tendon is repaired in the usual fashion. It is important that the soft tissues overlying the extensor tendon be carefully protected during the placement and tying of these sutures, because this tissue may contain venous structures that can be unintentionally entrapped or injured.

Flexor tendon injury may occur by transection or disinsertion from the distal phalangeal base. Repair is only pertinent if a functional DIPJ is expected. Repair may be accomplished using a core and epitendinous suture when a suitable distal stump is present or using suture anchors in the absence of a distal tendon.

Neurovascular structures

Microsurgery commences on the volar side. It is sometimes necessary to make an additional incision to provide adequate exposure, and it should be customized to the injury pattern such that there will be adequate soft tissue to cover the anastomosis, even if skin closure is not possible.

The target for arterial repair is chosen based on the expected dominant side for that finger and the geometry of the laceration. The proximal artery is identified first, using a small mid lateral incision. The termination of the proximal artery points the surgeon to the cut distal arterial end, which can be difficult to identify without this guide. Each cut end is tagged with a microclip once identified. These markers are limited to the zone of injury that will be excised before repair.

In our practice, nerve repair is infrequently performed during distal fingertip replantation. Beyond zone 1D, the nerve has usually trifurcated,[2] and we believe that the additional dissection to isolate and repair these terminal nerve branches is not justified by the amount of trauma it can cause to the diminutive fingertip.[6,20,34,35] If the injury is proximal to the trifurcation and primary repair is possible, the nerve ends are dissected and tagged for repair after arterial anastomosis.

Both ends of the chosen artery are trimmed until a healthy appearing lumen is visualized and can be irrigated with heparinized saline using a small anterior chamber ophthalmic syringe. Arterial anastomosis is then performed using 10-0 or 11-0 nylon microsuture. Because of the diminutive size of these vessels and the restricted operative field, this repair is generally done using a back-wall technique without the use of Acland clamps. Four to 6 sutures are usually required.

The tourniquet is then released and the arterial anastomosis is examined under the microscope, bathed with papaverine, and repair stitches are added if necessary. Once patency is confirmed, the volar skin is loosely closed with 4-0 nylon suture. We do not routinely administer intravenous heparin to avoid excessive oozing, but heparin is used if there is an instance of intraoperative anastomotic thrombosis. The finger is then warmed with saline and allowed to reperfuse for 10 minutes.

After this reperfusion period, the fingertip should show visible signs of blood flow, including color, turgor, and venous egress. If these signs are absent, the arterial anastomosis should be interrogated. If perfusion is evident, attention can be turned to venous outflow. In zone 1A replantation, we do not seek veins, and recommend drainage using a fish-mouth incision with intermittent heparin scrubs.[14,36] In more proximal amputations, we examine the dorsal and lateral aspects of the distal part for points of bleeding or engorged veins. These veins are exposed through small dorsal incisions and the corresponding proximal veins are similarly isolated. After minimal trimming, venous anastomoses are performed using 10-0 or 11-0 nylon microsuture using a back-wall technique. Usually, only 4 sutures are needed. This anastomosis is made quite difficult by ongoing venous bleeding, but this bleeding can be mitigated by slow continuous irrigation of heparinized saline via an anterior chamber ophthalmic syringe. It is our preference to repair at least 2 veins if possible.[37]

Nerve and Vascular Gaps

In cases of an arterial gap, we use a small caliber reversed vein graft from the volar aspect of the distal forearm. This graft can be taken as a venous flow through flap if there is both a vascular and soft tissue deficit.[38] In cases of a nerve gap, we have used nerve allograft in zone 1D, but recommend foregoing nerve gap repair distal to this level.[6,20,34,35]

Zone-Specific Considerations

In addition to general principles of fingertip replantation, there are specific considerations and technical nuances to achieve success in each zone. (**Tables 2-5**; **Figs. 2-5**).

POSTOPERATIVE CARE

Postoperatively, patients are admitted for monitoring and support of the replantation. The operative arm is warmed using a forced air blanket. The patient is kept on 81 mg of oral aspirin and routine deep vein thrombosis prophylaxis during hospitalization. Systemic therapeutic heparinization is avoided. Patients are permitted to eat and postoperative monitoring is used only for decision making regarding external measures to promote venous drainage. Ambulation is encouraged after 48 hours. We do not routinely offer reoperation for salvage of a failing fingertip replantation, and patients are counseled as such preoperatively. In cases of arterial insufficiency, we advocate watchful waiting until the replant has clearly failed. In cases of venous insufficiency, the wide range of supportive measures are discussed elsewhere in this article.

The block catheter is discontinued after 72 to 96 hours, and discharge occurs between the third and fifth days. The postoperative dressing is left in place if it is clean and changed if heavily soiled in

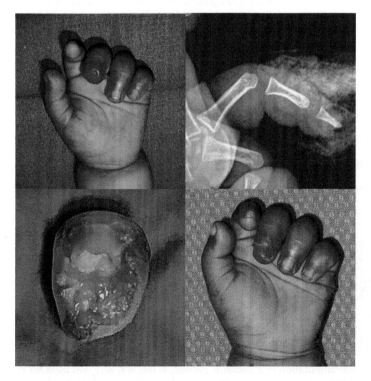

Fig. 2. Replantation of zone 1A long finger amputation in a pediatric patient. No bone or tendon repair was indicated. (Photo Credit: Brinkley Sandvall, MD.)

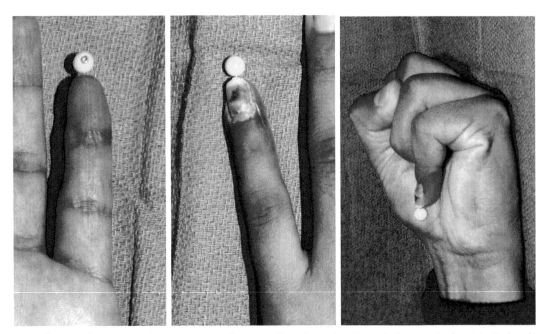

Fig. 3. The 6-week postoperative appearance after zone 1B replantation through the germinal matrix. Early rehabilitation has led to excellent PIPJ motion. (Photo credit: Ryan Katz, MD.)

blood. Two weeks postoperatively, all wounds are assessed, and if deemed stable the patient commences hand therapy beginning with active motion, progressing to passive motion and desensitization over the next several weeks.

VENOUS CONGESTION

One of the greatest challenges and most impactful factors in successful fingertip replantation is achieving adequate venous outflow. When possible, most authors advocate for vein repair. Hahn and Jung[37] reported on outcomes of 510 fingertip replants, 25 of which were performed without venous anastomosis; in this group, the success rate was 68%, significantly lower than their average success rate of 92%, and they found that each additional venous anastomosis improved their success rate. In 1996, Kim and

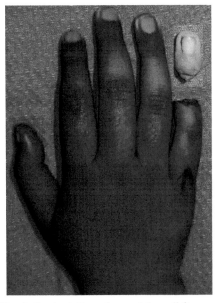
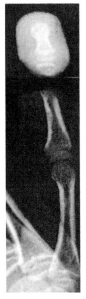
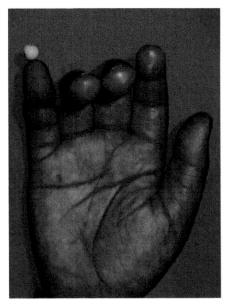

Fig. 4. Replantation of zone 1C small finger amputation in a pediatric patient. A single K-wire was used for P2 fixation, the DIPJ was preserved and both tendons were repaired. (Photo Credit: Brinkley Sandvall, MD.)

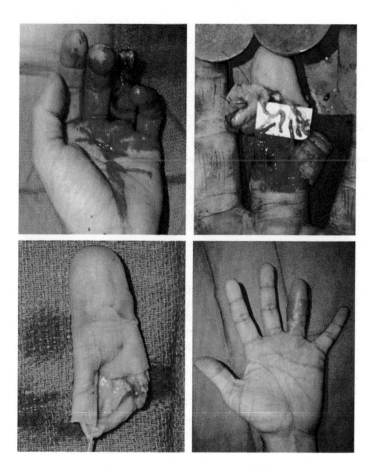

Fig. 5. In this avulsive injury, the bony injury was at the level of the DIPJ (1C), while the arterial and venous injuries were within zone 1D. DIPJ arthrodesis was achieved with 2 K-wires. A single arterial and 2 venous anastomoses were possible.

colleagues[39] reported on 135 fingertip replants with a 70% success rate in Tamai zone I and an 86% success rate in zone II, a difference they attributed to the ability to perform venous anastomosis in progressively proximal zones. This result was replicated by Hattori and colleagues[40] in 2003, who had an 84% success rate in Tamai zone I and 90% success in zone II. The systematic review by Sebastin and Chung[20] found no statistically significant difference in survival between Tamai zones I and II, but did find that venous anastomosis significantly improved survival in all zones. Aksoy and colleagues[41] also demonstrated significantly improved survival in replants with venous anastomosis over those without, 92.6% and 77.3% respectively. Their data did not support significant improvement in venous congestion postoperatively, but those replants with vein anastomosis did require less postoperative intervention for external bleeding and thus shorter hospital stays.

Not all data support the absolute necessity of venous anastomosis. The success rate of artery-only replantation has been reported at 64% to 100%, which is very similar to the 70% to 92% success rate with venous repair.[42] Li and colleagues[43] evaluated 211 fingertip replants and found no difference in survival between 0 and 2 veins repaired. In a 2010 study, Ito and colleagues[44] aimed to determine the limitations of artery-only replant by Ishikawa zone. Their success rate was 87% overall and they found no statistically significant difference between artery-only and artery with vein replant distal to zone IV. A more recent study by Ryu and colleagues[45] specifically aimed to evaluate the importance of venous anastomosis and failed to find a correlation between the number of veins anastomosed and replant survival, although they did note that more anastomoses were correlated with a decreased need for external bleeding.

In cases where arterial anastomosis is successful but venous anastomosis cannot be performed, several surgical techniques for alternative venous outflow have been proposed. Venocutaneous fistula, first proposed by Kamei and colleagues,[46] involves using a vein graft to temporarily connect a vein from the stump to a punch wound in the replanted fingertip. Koshima and colleagues[47] first proposed arteriovenous fistula creation with 91% success, and a recent study by Wu and colleagues[35] replicated this survival rate using the technique. The same authors also proposed a method of delayed venous repair in which artery-only replant is performed and the patient subsequently returns to the operating room a second time after venous congestion develops and veins are dilated, allowing easier anastomosis and survival of 83.5% of replanted digits.[48] Subdermal pocketing was first suggested by Lin and colleagues,[49] and subsequent studies of dermal pocketing in the hand or adjacent digit have demonstrated 68.0% to 85.7% survival.[50,51] Nakajima and colleagues[52] recently published a novel pulp tissue reduction method in which pulp tissue is removed to the level of the fingerprint core to decrease tissue burden for drainage. Their technique demonstrated an 89% success rate in replants as proximal as Ishikawa zone IV.

Critics of these alternative surgical techniques cite the prolonged operative time and specific technical expertise required. Additionally, the delayed venous repair[48] and dermal pocketing[49] techniques require a second procedure. The various surgical techniques have never been rigorously compared, and it is unknown if they offer an advantage over simpler, nonsurgical methods.

Fortunately, relatively high rates of success[53] have been demonstrated for several simple and inexpensive methods of nonsurgical external venous drainage. Venous outflow has been established through a fishmouth incision,[14] nail plate removal,[54] paraungual stab incision,[55] and leech application.[56,57] Owing to inconsistent availability, infection risk, and patient objection, alternatives to medical leeches have been described. In particular, the "chemical leech" was first described by Barnett and associates in 1989[58] and consists of subcutaneous injection of heparin calcium into the replanted finger. This modality has been proposed as a useful means of maintaining external bleeding in patients who cannot receive systemic anticoagulation,[59] and several authors have reported survival rates ranging from 83.3% to 100.0%.[59–61]

The variety of methods described for nonsurgical venous drainage reflects the lack of evidence demonstrating any superior method. Kayalar and colleagues[53] performed a retrospective review of 228 artery-only fingertip replants and compared nail matrix bleeding with pulp skin area bleeding (the "crater" method). They reported a high incidence of venous insufficiency at 86.8%, but an overall survival of 79.8% with no difference between methods of bleeding. Comparison of other methods of external bleeding is absent in the literature, as are data to compare external bleeding with the surgical methods of creating alternative venous outflow.

The perceived necessity and methods of systemic anticoagulation are similarly variable and poorly studied, such that surveyed surgeons reported using 21 different chemical agents, independent of the variable dosages and durations.[62] One study by Lee and colleagues[63] showed a survival benefit to continuous heparin drip as compared with intermittent bolus heparin, 91.2% and 59.3%, respectively, but data regarding other agents, durations, or combinations of anticoagulants for fingertip replantation are lacking.

One notable concern with any method of external bleeding is the blood transfusion requirement, which may be required in up to 88% of patients.[55] However, some authors have been able to use external bleeding without transfusion.[44,59,61] Additionally, external bleeding commits the patient to a long hospitalization of 7 to 15 days.[34,42,55,60,64] This is in part owing to the time required for neovascularization of the replanted part, which takes approximately 7 to 8 days.[65] At a minimum, when discussing the possibility of distal fingertip replantation with a patient, the potential need for prolonged hospitalization and/or blood transfusion should be disclosed during the decision-making process.

Outcomes

Survival of replanted digit
Referral centers with large volumes of distal replantation cases report success rates commensurate with more proximal replantation.[20,35,65,66] A systematic review of distal digital replantation found a mean survival rate of 86% and demonstrated no difference between amputations in Tamai zone I versus zone II.[20] However, it is important to understand that the success rate of fingertip replantation depends heavily on a surgeon's indications for replantation in addition to his or her experience and technical expertise.

Motion and strength
Urbaniak and colleagues[67] demonstrated 82° of proximal interphalangeal joint (PIPJ) motion for replantation distal to the flexor digitorum superficialis insertion, compared with 35° for replantation proximal to this level. Sebastin and Chung's systematic review found that range of motion at the DIPJ ranged from 60° to 90°,[20] and subsequently published outcomes have reinforced these findings.[34,35] An article by Hattori and colleagues[68]

comparing distal replant with revision amputation found no difference in grip strength and superior active flexion at the PIPJ in replanted fingers. This outcome was attributed to increased use of replanted digits as compared with those digits which underwent revision amputation.[68]

Sensation

Sensory recovery is favorable in fingertip replantation because of the proximity to the sensory end-organs of the fingertip. Although direct neurorrhaphy has been shown to improve 2-point discrimination,[35] this is not always possible distal to the DIPJ where the digital nerves have terminally branched. Even in the absence of direct nerve repair, however, reported outcomes in average 2-point discrimination range from 4.2 to 12.0 mm.[6,20,34,35] This result suggests that, even in amputations too distal to accommodate nerve repair, protective sensation or better often returns. Patient-specific analyses have suggested that crush injury and older patient age contribute to poor sensory recovery.[36]

Pain

There has been limited study of pain outcomes for patients with fingertip amputations. In the single published series comparing replantation with revision amputation, Hattori and colleagues[68] reported significantly decreased pain in patients undergoing replant. However, prior publications of replantation series have not evaluated pain, indicating a gap in our understanding of patient outcomes after replantation.

Aesthetic

Many patients pursue replantation to avoid the cosmetic deformity and social stigma they anticipate after digital loss. Although the aesthetic outcomes of replantation are difficult to quantify, a 2013 study by Cheng and colleagues[6] reported digital length, width, and thickness were greater than 90% of the contralateral digit. Despite this finding, replantation does not ensure a perfect aesthetic outcome, and pulp atrophy and nail deformity have been reported in 35% and 38% of cases, respectively.[20] These imperfections notwithstanding, reports of patient satisfaction with the appearance of their replanted digits exceeds 90%.[6,35]

Satisfaction

When reported, patient satisfaction is consistently high in the replant literature, ranging from 68% to 100%.[35,60,64] Hattori's study comparing revision amputation to replantation found that all patients undergoing replant were highly or fairly satisfied, whereas only 61% of revision amputations reported that level of satisfaction.[68] The current literature lacks direct comparison of patient satisfaction using the various replantation techniques and is not granular enough to draw conclusions about which aspects of function or appearance contribute most to patient satisfaction.

SUMMARY

Distal fingertip replantation is a technically challenging operation; but, in a motivated patient, excellent aesthetic and functional outcomes can be achieved. Although the literature is replete with series documenting replant survival using a variety of techniques, comparative studies aimed at identifying best practices are lacking. More research is required to determine the functional, cosmetic, and survival benefits conferred by various techniques, especially those related to venous drainage and patient-reported outcomes of pain and satisfaction.

CLINICS CARE POINTS

- Fingertip replantation is technically challenging; however, in a motivated patient, excellent aesthetic and functional outcomes can be achieved.
- Careful preoperative patient selection and a deliberate process of informed consent are necessary.
- A detailed understanding of fingertip microanatomy by zone is critical to inform an orderly plan for replantation that minimizes soft tissue dissection.
- Several authors advocate for venous anastomosis to improve success rates, shorten hospital time, and decrease blood loss from external bleeding; however, similar rates of success are reported with alternative methods of venous egress. Evidence-based comparison of these alternative methods is lacking.
- Patient-reported outcomes of pain and satisfaction have been studied only in a limited capacity and represent a gap in our understanding of patient outcomes after replantation.

DISCLOSURE

The authors have no commercial or financial conflicts of interest. This work was completed without funding sources.

REFERENCES

1. Tos P, Titolo P, Chirila NL, et al. Surgical treatment of acute fingernail injuries. J Orthop Traumatol 2012; 13(2):57–62.

2. Zenn MR, Hoffman L, Latrenta G, et al. Variations in digital nerve anatomy. J Hand Surg Am 1992;17(6): 1033–6.

3. Strauch B, de Moura W. Arterial system of the fingers. J Hand Surg Am 1990;15(1):148–54.

4. Smith DO, Oura C, Kimura C, et al. The distal venous anatomy of the finger. J Hand Surg Am 1991;16(2):303–7.

5. Lucas GL. The pattern of venous drainage of the digits. J Hand Surg Am 1984;9(3):448–50.

6. Cheng L, Chen K, Chai YM, et al. Fingertip replantation at the eponychial level with venous anastomosis: an anatomic study and clinical application. J Hand Surg Eur Vol 2013;38(9):959–63.

7. Kleinert HE, Kasdan ML, Romero JL. Small blood-vessel anastomosis for salvage of severely injured upper extremity. J Bone Joint Surg Am 1963;45-A:788–96.

8. Komatsu S, Tamai S. Successful replantation of a completely cut-off thumb. Plast Reconstr Surg 1968;42(4):374–7.

9. Serafin D, Kutz JE, Kleinert HE. Replantation of a completely amputated distal thumb without venous anastomosis. Case report. Plast Reconstr Surg 1973;52(5):579–82.

10. Snyder CC, Stevenson RM, Browne EZ Jr. Successful replantation of a totally severed thumb. Plast Reconstr Surg 1972;50(6):553–9.

11. Buncke HJ, Alpert BS, RJohnson-Giebink R. Digital Replantation. Surg Clin North Am 1981;61(2): 383–94.

12. Foucher G, Norris RW. Distal and very distal digital replantations. Br J Plast Surg 1992;45(3):199–203.

13. Goldner RD, Stevanovic MV, Nunley JA, et al. Digital replantation at the level of the distal interphalangeal joint and the distal phalanx. J Hand Surg Am 1989; 14(2 Pt 1):214–20.

14. Yamano Y. Replantation of the amputated distal part of the fingers. J Hand Surg Am 1985;10(2):211–8.

15. Tang JB, Wang ZT, Chen J, et al. A Global View of Digital Replantation and Revascularization. Clin Plast Surg 2017;44(2):189–209.

16. Pet MA, Ko JH. Indications for replantation and revascularization in the hand. Hand Clin 2019; 35(2):119–30.

17. Allen MJ. Conservative management of finger tip injuries in adults. Hand 1980;12(3):257–65.

18. Hirase Y. Salvage of fingertip amputated at nail level: new surgical principles and treatments. Ann Plast Surg 1997;38(2):151–7.

19. Ishikawa K, Ogawa Y, Soeda H, et al. A new classification of the amputation level for the distal part of the finger. JJSRM 1990;3:54–62.

20. Sebastin SJ, Chung KC. A systematic review of the outcomes of replantation of distal digital amputation. Plast Reconstr Surg 2011;128(3):723–37.

21. Tamai S. Twenty years' experience of limb replantation–review of 293 upper extremity replants. J Hand Surg Am 1982;7(6):549–56.

22. Evans DM, Bernardis C. A new classification for fingertip injuries. J Hand Surg Br 2000;25(1): 58–60.

23. Fassler PR. Fingertip injuries: evaluation and treatment. J Am Acad Orthop Surg 1996;4(1):84–92.

24. Frykman GK, Wood VE. Saving amputated digits. Current status of replantation of fingers and hands. West J Med 1974;121(4):265–9.

25. Manktelow RT. What are the indications for digital replantation? Ann Plast Surg 1978;1(3):336–7.

26. O'Brien BM, MacLeod AM, Miller GD, et al. Clinical replantation of digits. Plast Reconstr Surg 1973; 52(5):490–502.

27. Lin CH, Aydyn N, Lin YT, et al. Hand and finger replantation after protracted ischemia (more than 24 hours). Ann Plast Surg 2010;64(3):286–90.

28. Waikakul S, Sakkarnkosol S, Vanadurongwan V, et al. Results of 1018 digital replantations in 552 patients. Injury 2000;31(1):33–40.

29. Hustedt JW, Bohl DD, Champagne L. The detrimental effect of decentralization in digital replantation in the United States: 15 years of evidence from the National Inpatient Sample. J Hand Surg Am 2016;41(5):593–601.

30. VanGiesen PJ, Seaber AV, Urbaniak JR. Storage of amputated parts prior to replantation–an experimental study with rabbit ears. J Hand Surg Am 1983;8(1):60–5.

31. Dautel G, Barbary S. Mini replants: fingertip replant distal to the IP or DIP joint. J Plast Reconstr Aesthet Surg 2007;60(7):811–5.

32. Hattori Y, Doi K, Sakamoto S, et al. Fingertip replantation. J Hand Surg Am 2007;32(4):548–55.

33. Jazayeri L, Klausner JQ, Chang J. Distal digital replantation. Plast Reconstr Surg 2013;132(5):1207–17.

34. Huan AS, Regmi S, Gu JX, et al. Fingertip replantation (zone I) without venous anastomosis: clinical experience and outcome analysis. Springerplus 2016;5(1):1835.

35. Wu F, Shen X, Eberlin KR, et al. The use of arteriovenous anastomosis for venous drainage during Tamai zone I fingertip replantation. Injury 2018;49(6): 1113–8.

36. Matsuzaki H, Yoshizu T, Maki Y, et al. Functional and cosmetic results of fingertip replantation: anastomosing only the digital artery. Ann Plast Surg 2004; 53(4):353–9.

37. Hahn HO, Jung SG. Results of replantation of amputated fingertips in 450 patients. J Reconstr Microsurg 2006;22(6):407–13.

38. Roberts JM, Carr LW, Haley CT, et al. Venous flaps for revascularization and soft-tissue coverage in traumatic hand injuries: a systematic review of the literature. J Reconstr Microsurg 2020;36(2):104–9.

39. Kim WK, Lim JH, Han SK. Fingertip replantations: clinical evaluation of 135 digits. Plast Reconstr Surg 1996;98(3):470–6.

40. Hattori Y, Doi K, Ikeda K, et al. Significance of venous anastomosis in fingertip replantation. Plast Reconstr Surg 2003;111(3):1151–8.
41. Aksoy A, Gungor M, Sir E, et al. Replantation without and with palmar venous anastomosis: analysis of the survival rates and vein distribution. Ann Plast Surg 2017;78(1):62–6.
42. Buntic RF, Brooks D. Standardized protocol for artery-only fingertip replantation. J Hand Surg Am 2010;35(9):1491–6.
43. Li J, Guo Z, Zhu Q, et al. Fingertip replantation: determinants of survival. Plast Reconstr Surg 2008;122(3):833–9.
44. Ito H, Sasaki K, Morioka K, et al. Fingertip amputation salvage on arterial anastomosis alone: an investigation of its limitations. Ann Plast Surg 2010;65(3):302–5.
45. Ryu DH, Roh SY, Kim JS, et al. Multiple venous anastomoses decrease the need for intensive postoperative management in Tamai zone I replantations. Arch Plast Surg 2018;45(1):58–61.
46. Kamei K, Sinokawa Y, Kishibe M. The venocutaneous fistula: a new technique for reducing venous congestion in replanted fingertips. Plast Reconstr Surg 1997;99(6):1771–4.
47. Koshima I, Soeda S, Moriguchi T, et al. The use of arteriovenous anastomosis for replantation of the distal phalanx of the fingers. Plast Reconstr Surg 1992;89(4):710–4.
48. Koshima I, Yamashita S, Sugiyama N, et al. Successful delayed venous drainage in 16 consecutive distal phalangeal replantations. Plast Reconstr Surg 2005;115(1):149–54.
49. Lin TS, Jeng SF, Chiang YC. Fingertip replantation using the subdermal pocket procedure. Plast Reconstr Surg 2004;113(1):247–53.
50. Lim R, Lee E, Lim J Jr, et al. External bleeding versus dermal pocketing for distal digital replantation without venous anastomosis. J Hand Surg Eur Vol 2019;44(2):181–6.
51. Puhaindran ME, Paavilainen P, Tan DM, et al. Dermal pocketing following distal finger replantation. J Plast Reconstr Aesthet Surg 2010;63(8):1318–22.
52. Nakajima Y, Iwasawa M, Mishima Y, et al. Fingertip Replantation Using Artery-Only Anastomosis With a Pulp Tissue Reduction Method. Ann Plast Surg 2020.
53. Kayalar M, Gunturk OB, Gurbuz Y, et al. Survival and Comparison of External Bleeding Methods in Artery-Only Distal Finger Replantations. J Hand Surg Am 2020;45(3):256.e1-6.
54. Gordon L, Leitner DW, Buncke HJ, et al. Partial nail plate removal after digital replantation as an alternative method of venous drainage. J Hand Surg Am 1985;10(3):360–4.
55. Han SK, Lee BI, Kim WK. Topical and systemic anticoagulation in the treatment of absent or compromised venous outflow in replanted fingertips. J Hand Surg Am 2000;25(4):659–67.
56. Baudet J. The use of leeches in distal digital replantation. Blood Coagul Fibrinolysis 1991;2(1):193–6.
57. Golden MA, Quinn JJ, Partington MT. Leech therapy in digital replantation. AORN J 1995;62(3):364–6, 369, 371-362, passim.
58. Barnett GR, Taylor GI, Mutimer KL. The "chemical leech": intra-replant subcutaneous heparin as an alternative to venous anastomosis. Report of three cases. Br J Plast Surg 1989;42(5):556–8.
59. Yokoyama T, Hosaka Y, Takagi S. The place of chemical leeching with heparin in digital replantation: subcutaneous calcium heparin for patients not treatable with systemic heparin. Plast Reconstr Surg 2007;119(4):1284–93.
60. Chen YC, Chan FC, Hsu CC, et al. Fingertip replantation without venous anastomosis. Ann Plast Surg 2013;70(3):284–8.
61. Kadota H, Imaizumi A, Ishida K, et al. Successful local use of heparin calcium for congested fingertip replants. Arch Plast Surg 2020;47(1):54–61.
62. Davies DM. A world survey of anticoagulation practice in clinical microvascular surgery. Br J Plast Surg 1982;35(1):96–9.
63. Lee JY, Kim HS, Heo ST, et al. Controlled continuous systemic heparinization increases success rate of artery-only anastomosis replantation in single distal digit amputation: a retrospective cohort study. Medicine (Baltimore) 2016;95(26):e3979.
64. Erken HY, Takka S, Akmaz I. Artery-only fingertip replantations using a controlled nailbed bleeding protocol. J Hand Surg Am 2013;38(11):2173–9.
65. Han SK, Chung HS, Kim WK. The timing of neovascularization in fingertip replantation by external bleeding. Plast Reconstr Surg 2002;110(4):1042–6.
66. Venkatramani H, Sabapathy SR. Fingertip replantation: technical considerations and outcome analysis of 24 consecutive fingertip replantations. Indian J Plast Surg 2011;44(2):237–45.
67. Urbaniak JR, Roth JH, Nunley JA, et al. The results of replantation after amputation of a single finger. J Bone Joint Surg Am 1985;67(4):611–9.
68. Hattori Y, Doi K, Ikeda K, et al. A retrospective study of functional outcomes after successful replantation versus amputation closure for single fingertip amputations. J Hand Surg Am 2006;31(5):811–8.
69. Shim HS, Kwon BY, Seo BF, et al. A prospective randomised comparison of fixation methods in Tamai's zone I amputation. J Plast Reconstr Aesthet Surg 2018;71(7):997–1003.
70. Nam YS, Jun YJ, Kim IB, et al. Reply to a Letter to the Editor: anatomical study of the fingertip artery in Tamai zone I: clinical significance in fingertip replantation. J Reconstr Microsurg 2017;33(1):e5.
71. Whitney TM, Lineaweaver WC, Buncke HJ, et al. Clinical results of bony fixation methods in digital replantation. J Hand Surg Am 1990;15(2):328–34.

Grafting and Other Reconstructive Options for Nail Deformities
Indications, Techniques, and Outcomes

Michael W. Neumeister, MD, FRCSC[a],*, James N. Winters, MD[b]

KEYWORDS

• Nail deformity • Split nail graft • Full nail graft

KEY POINTS

• A breadth of knowledge on nail anatomy, physiologic growth, and appropriate acute injury management helps prevent chronic nail bed deformities.
• Multiple nail growth cycles should be allowed to define the final deformity prior to reconstruction.
• Split or full-thickness nailbed grafts and skin grafts represent viable treatment options to correct such deformities, obtain a good cosmetic outcome, and support a flat adherent nail.

 Video content accompanies this article at http://www.hand.theclinics.com.

INTRODUCTION/HISTORY/DEFINITIONS/BACKGROUND

The nail represents a unique structure in the human body providing sensory feedback in fine pinch, stability and protection, the ability to scratch, and many other functions. Fingertip and associated nailbed injuries are common hand injuries. The anatomic structure injured and quality of acute repair dictate the outcomes. Improper repair leads to aesthetic and functional nail deformities. This article aims to provide technical insight into repair of resulting secondary nail defects.

ANATOMY AND PHYSIOLOGY

A basic understanding of the nomenclature, anatomy, and physiology of the perionychium is necessary to treat these injuries. The anatomic study by Zook and colleagues[1] helped standardize the terminology for discussion within the literature. The perionychium can be divided into paronychium and the nail (**Fig. 1**A, B). The paronychium includes the soft tissue around the nail: proximal eponychium, lateral nail folds, and distal hyponychium. The nail encompasses the germinal matrix, sterile matrix, proximal nail fold, and the nail plate (hard shiny portion). The germinal matrix represents the proximal growth center of the nail and originates 1 to 2 mm distal to the terminal extensor tendon.[2] The dorsal nail fold guides cell growth in a horizontal and distal direction.[3] Distally the nail is composed of sterile matrix cells, which act like glue to adhere the nail plate to the distal phalanx. Multiple studies evaluated the rate of complete nail regeneration ranging from 0.1 mm per day to 3 to 5 months for total regeneration.[4–6] Sensation and vascularity of the nail arises from dorsal branches of the digital nerves and arteries respectively.[1,7]

[a] Department of Surgery, Institute for Plastic Surgery, Southern Illinois University School of Medicine, 747 North Rutledge Street #3, Springfield, IL 62702, USA; [b] Institute for Plastic Surgery, Southern Illinois University School of Medicine, 747 North Rutledge Street #3, Springfield, IL 62702, USA
* Corresponding author.
E-mail address: mneumeister@siumed.edu

Hand Clin 37 (2021) 67–76
https://doi.org/10.1016/j.hcl.2020.09.003
0749-0712/21/© 2020 Elsevier Inc. All rights reserved.

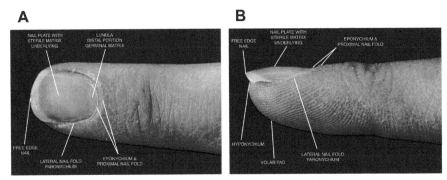

Fig. 1. (*A*) Dorsal view of the perionychium anatomy. (*B*). Lateral view of the perionychium anatomy. The hard nail plate protects the underlying nail bed composed of sterile matrix distally and germinal matrix proximally.

NATURE OF THE PROBLEM: NAIL DEFORMITIES

Nail deformities result from a myriad of etiologies, including traumatic injuries, loss of bony and soft tissue support, congenital absence, subungual masses, and iatrogenic. A thorough history, examination of the fingertip, and basic imaging help guide appropriate treatment algorithms for each individual problem. Restoration of a smooth nail bed is essential to normal nail growth and appearance.[8] Reconstructive options for each deformity are discussed. Free nail transfer and composite nail graft options are discussed elsewhere.

Traumatic Nail Injuries and Resulting Scars

Acute traumatic injuries to the fingertip can result in damage to the nailbed, distal phalanx, paronychium, or a combination of these structures. Comprehensive knowledge of acute nailbed and paronychium treatment options can avoid missed reconstructive opportunities and help prevent chronic nail deformities. Meticulous repair is critically important, as the nail appears to have a greater recovery potential in the acute setting.[9]

Following a traumatic injury, remodeling of the nail requires 3 or 4 growth cycles to determine the final appearance and deformity.[10] Crush and avulsion injuries lead to poorer cosmetic outcomes, with distal phalanx fractures contributing to irregular nail plate characteristics.[11] The amount, direction, and structural location of scarring determines the resulting nail deformity.

Scarring of the sterile matrix produces areas of onycholysis (nonadherence) (**Fig. 2**). The nonadherence is due to a lack of gluelike cell production and replacement with keratinized cells lifting the nail plate. A narrow or very distal area of nonadherence may not be problematic; however, larger scars often require intervention. Treatment involves removal of the nail plate and full-thickness

excision of the scar to the level of periosteum. Small defects may be repaired primarily. A template should be designed for larger defects. Prior treatment attempts used split-thickness skin grafts, dermal and reverse dermal grafts, but these resulted in continued nonadherence.[12–15] Split-thickness sterile matrix grafts from the same digit, adjacent digits, or toes later became the standard of care.[16–18] This technique results in good cosmetic outcomes, adherence, and minimal donor site morbidity.

Split nails result from injury to the germinal matrix, leading to loss of nail production at this level and distally. Synechia, scarring of the eponychial fold to the underlying matrix, can also result in this deformity. To prevent this, the traditional teaching is that a stent should be placed between these 2 structures at the time of initial repair to prevent deformity. Longitudinal split nails and horizontal double nails have been described in the literature depending on the germinal matrix scarring pattern[19] (**Fig. 3**). Removal of the nail plate and exposure of the full germinal matrix via relaxing incisions of the eponychial fold is critical to proper treatment. Thin longitudinal splits may be

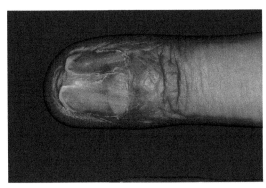

Fig. 2. Onycholysis (nonadherence) of distal nail bed in wedge shaped pattern due to scarring of sterile matrix.

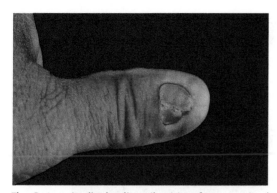

Fig. 3. Longitudinal split nail arising from proximal nail fold due to old injury of germinal matrix.

excised and repaired primarily or with Z-plasties following mobilization of the lateral matrix. Wider splits of the germinal matrix require a full-thickness germinal matrix nail graft as split thickness grafts do not produce nail.[20] The full-thickness graft should be taken from a toe as this results in donor site morbidity and loss of nail. Double nail deformity requires assessment of the thickness and durability of dorsal and ventral nail components. The thinner of the 2 components should be excised with the scar to allow for a uniform singular nail.[19]

Complete absence of the nail can result from avulsion injury or as a congenital anomaly. Microsurgical vascularized nail transfer and composite nail grafts have been described in the literature and are discussed in separate sections.[21–24] Buncke and Gonzales[25] advocated for recreation of an eponychium with folded skin grafts to house a prosthetic nail. Today more elegant prosthetics and methods of attachment are available. A simple alternative to provide the illusion of a nail is to de-epithelialize and skin graft the dorsal fingertip in the shape of a nail.[10]

Hook Nail

A "hook" or "claw" nail deformity results from distal fingertip amputation with loss of bony and soft tissue support causing the redundant distal nailbed to curve volarly[26] (**Fig. 4**A–D). Hook nail is best avoided at the time of initial injury by removing the portion of sterile matrix that extends past the remaining distal phalanx support. However, this deformity often goes unrecognized for many months, until full nail regrowth has occurred. Conservative management involves keeping the nail trimmed proximal to the curvature. Surgical intervention is often necessary due to pain, functional deficits, and a cosmetically unappealing short nail. Surgical treatments involve one or more of the following:

1. Restoration of bony or soft tissue support without excision of the distal nailbed
2. Removal of the curved portion of nailbed and providing soft tissue coverage to any resulting defect
3. Eponychial flaps to give the appearance of a lengthened nail

Atasoy and colleagues[27] described one of the earliest treatments known as the "Antenna procedure," which involves elevation of the hyponychium and curved nailbed, splinting with K-wires for support, and reconstruction of the distal hyponychium defect with a cross-finger flap. Homodigital flaps, osteocutaneous flaps, composite toe grafts, and distraction osteogenesis of the distal phalanx have all been proposed treatment options to provide support without shortening the distal nailbed.[28–31] Kumar and Satku[26] suggested treatment with excision of the distal 2 mm of nailbed hooking, followed by V-Y advancement flaps for coverage. Distal excision is simple, but results in a shorter appearing nail. The average length of nail beneath the eponychial fold is ~40% of the visible nail length.[32] Bakhach and others[33–35] have described eponychial flaps transposed proximally over a deepithelialized area, exposing more of the nail typically covered by the eponychial soft tissue to give the appearance of increased nail length. One modification of this technique utilizes the proximal deepithelialized eponychium to skin graft the defect site at the hyponychium after excision of the curved sterile matrix.[36]

Pincer Nail

The pincer nail deformity was first described by Cornelius and Shelley in 1968.[37] This deformity results from a transverse curvature of the nail that increases distally, "pinching" the soft tissue and often causing pain (**Fig. 5**A, B). The etiology of pincer nails has been proposed as hereditary and acquired factors: trauma, psoriasis, medications, allergic reactions, subungual mass effect, osteoarthritis, and ill-fitting shoes.[38–44] Conservative treatment options have ranged from topical therapies, external shaping devices, sutures, or removal of the nail plate.[37,44–48] These methods often result in recurrence after cessation of treatment. Nail bed ablation and partial excision with skin grafting have also been described, but result in a narrowed, nonadherent, or absent nail.[38,41,43,49,50] More recent methods describe elevating the nailbed off of the distal phalanx and placement of de-epithelialized lateral fold flaps between the distal phalanx and nailbed for prevention of curvature.[51–53] Brown and

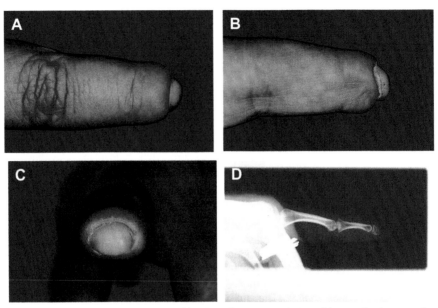

Fig. 4. (*A, B, C*) Dorsal, volar, and end-on view of hook nail. Note proximity of free nail edge to volar DIP crease. (*D*) Lateral radiograph showing loss of distal phalanx bony support for nail bed and plate resulting in volar curvature.

colleagues[54] and Zook and colleagues[55] elevated the curved lateral sterile and germinal matrix off the distal phalanx and tunneled dermal grafts underneath this area to allow flattening of the nail bed and plate. Addition of lateral support beneath the curved nailbed via dermal grafts or local flaps appear to give the best long-term outcomes and minimize recurrence.

Mass Effect and Subungual Tumors

The differential diagnosis for subungual tumors and a recommended treatment algorithm have previously been reviewed by Willard and colleagues[56] and Hinchcliff and Pereira.[57] A detailed history, physical examination, plain films, and sometimes additional imaging are typically sufficient for diagnosis. Treatment with conservative measures should not delay treatment for more than 8 weeks. Excisional biopsy is often diagnostic and therapeutic in most cases. These subungual tumors may be accessed after nail plate removal via direct longitudinal incision of the nail bed, proximally based U-shaped flap, or lateral subperiosteal approaches. This section reviews the more common pathologies and repair of the resulting defects.

Bony irregularities resulting in nail deformity are common following displaced distal phalanx fractures. Bony tumors such as exostosis and osteochondroma are rarer causes of nail deformity.[58] Surgical treatment consists of excision with rongeur and curettage of the lesion.[59] A burr can be used after excision to ensure a smooth distal phalanx is providing support of the nail bed. Bone grafting can be done if there is a resulting depression within the distal phalanx to provide smooth contour.

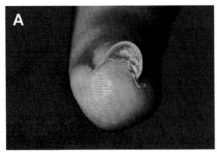
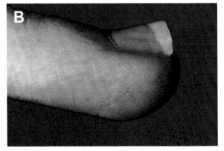

Fig. 5. (*A*) Distal end-on view of pincer nail. Note the U-shaped curvature of the distal nail plate. Pinched hyponychium and nailbed soft tissue distally. (*B*) Lateral view of pincer nail with distal elevation of nail plate.

Glomus tumors, hemangiomas, and pyogenic granulomas represent the more common subungual vascular lesions with clinical history helping to differentiate the diagnosis. Glomus tumors can be bluish in color, sensitive to touch, and painful in cold temperatures.[60] Treatment involves surgical excision with some advocating for Mohs surgery.[61] Hemangiomas can present with pseudoclubbing, red or blue hues, and more superficial location on imaging than glomus tumors.[56,58] No consensus exists for treatment, but surgical excision is recommended if symptomatic. Pyogenic granuloma typically presents as rapidly growing with the tendency to bleed. Recommended treatment involves surgical excision for symptomatic purposes and to ensure no malignancy on pathology.[62]

The most common cystic lesions are epidermal inclusion and myxoid cysts. Epidermal inclusion cysts develop secondary to trauma with retained epidermal tissue beneath the skin. Simple excision is recommended with repair of any bony and nail disruption. Myxoid cysts result from distal interphalangeal joint osteophytes allowing a weak point for joint fluid to escape. Nail plate and eponychial fold disruption are often the first signs. Plain films can help identify osteophytes and help guide surgical excision. Brown and colleagues[63] reported good aesthetic outcomes without recurrence by using a T-shaped or H-shaped incision to expose the distal interphalangeal joint (DIP) to rongeur the osteophyte and excise the cyst. Care must be taken in this operation to avoid damaging the terminal extensor tendon or the germinal matrix. Some advocate DIP fusion for cases of more extensive joint involvement/arthritis to more reliably prevent recurrence.

Solid malignancies including basal cell carcinoma, squamous cell carcinoma, and melanoma are rare. Basal cell carcinoma should be resected to negative margins and has an excellent 5-year cure rate.[64] Squamous cell represents the most common primary malignancy of the subungual space and wide local excision is recommended.[65,66] Melanoma is discussed in the next section. The resulting nail defects can be treated with split or full-thickness nail grafts or split thickness skin grafts depending on the size and location.

Melanonychia

Pigmentation within the nailbed is defined as melanonychia. This broad term encompasses multiple differential diagnoses: subungual hematoma, onychomycosis (fungal infection), striate melanonychia, subungual melanoma, and others.[67,68]

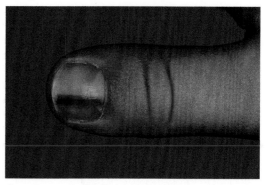

Fig. 6. Longitudinal melanonychia involving the nailbed, which could represent benign (striate melanonychia) versus malignant (subungual melanoma) etiology.

(**Fig. 6**) Differentiation of benign versus malignant lesions is often difficult based on clinical history alone. If there is a history of infection or trauma, then treatment with antifungals or scoring of the nail plate to assess distal movement of the lesion may be appropriate for a few weeks. Clinical features concerning for subungual melanoma include: patient age 50 to 70 years, single digit (thumb), longitudinal band >3 mm, irregular borders, change in size or color, ulceration, destruction of the nail apparatus, or extension of pigmentation onto paronychium (Hutchinson sign).[69,70] Unfortunately, delay in diagnosis and treatment are common for subungual melanoma.[71] Biopsy technique includes full-thickness longitudinal excision of the sterile and germinal matrix, including any surrounding pigmented skin.[72,73] Slight undermining and mobilization of the lateral borders allows for closure of the biopsy site. For benign subungual lesions biopsy is both diagnostic and therapeutic. Diagnosis of a malignant subungual melanoma leads to debate in management and associated reconstruction.

The first described case of malignant subungual melanoma was by Boyer[74] in 1854 and later expanded on by Hutchinson[75] in 1886. The acral lentiginous subtype is the most common and subungual melanoma represents 0.7% to 3.5% of all melanoma subtypes.[76,77] Historically, amputation of the involved digit at the level of the interphalangeal joint represented the treatment of choice.[78] It was initially thought that more proximal amputations yielded better outcomes.[79] Heaton and colleagues[80] later concluded that metacarpophalangeal joint versus proximal interphalangeal joint amputation did not significantly impact overall survival or recurrence. In 1992, Park and colleagues[81] presented the first study treating subungual melanoma with wide local excision (WLE) to preserve length and function of the digit. This practice was supported by Clarkson and colleagues[82] who formally advocated for WLE for subungual melanoma in situ. A systematic review of current management strategies showed poor level of evidence to suggest superiority of amputation versus WLE.[83] This review supported WLE for melanoma in situ and sentinel node biopsy based off cutaneous melanoma guidelines. Reconstruction after WLE can be treated with skin grafting or heterodigital flaps.

PREOPERATIVE/PREPROCEDURE PLANNING

- Determine goals of treatment with patient: aesthetic and functional
- Determine need for split-thickness versus full-thickness nail graft or skin graft
- Review donor side morbidity at great or second toe
- Discuss expected outcomes and timeline for nail regrowth

PREPARATION AND PATIENT POSITIONING

- Patient positioned supine with arm abducted 90° on hand table
- Sterile arm/leg tourniquet or digital tourniquet may be used for finger/toe
- Digital block performed to assist in hemostasis and postoperative pain control at donor and recipient site
- If split-thickness skin graft is needed, shave and prep out the respective donor thigh

PROCEDURAL APPROACHES
Exposure of Nail Bed

- Digital block anesthesia and tourniquet used
- Freer elevator, tip pointed dorsally, to elevate nail plate from sterile matrix
  - Gently sweep with freer underneath lateral nail folds and eponychial fold. Small scissors may also be used.
  - Grasp distal tip of nail plate with mosquito clamp for stability and apply gentle distal traction until nail plate releases
  - Nail plate should be cleansed and trimmed of sharp edges to be replaced later to stent open the eponychial fold
- #15-blade is used to make longitudinal relaxing incisions at the lateral borders of the eponychial fold
  - Incision made over a freer elevator placed under the fold to prevent unintentional damage to the germinal matrix below

oSuture the eponychial fold proximally with 2 stay stitches to fully expose the germinal matrix

Split Sterile Matrix Nail Grafts for Nonadherence

- Expose the nail bed as listed previously. Relaxing incisions are not required (Video 1).
- Mark the area of scar to be excised
- Use #15 blade scalpel or beaver blade to sharply excise the entire scar to the level of the periosteum
- Glove paper or suture foil may be used to make a template of the resulting defect
- Template transposed onto the donor digit sterile matrix, outlined with marking pen
- #15 or Beaver blade used to harvest a split thickness sterile matrix graft
  - As a guide of ideal graft thickness, the blade should be visible beneath the graft during harvest
- Secure the split thickness sterile graft using 6 to 0 chromic suture to the surrounding nail bed for smooth approximation
- The nail plate is then replaced under the proximal eponychial fold and a bulky dressing is applied distally

Full-Thickness Germinal Matrix Nail Graft for Split Nail

- Expose the nail as listed previously for both the donor toe and recipient digit
- Mark the area of scar to be excised on the germinal and sterile matrix
- #15 blade scalpel used to sharply excise the entire area of scar down to the level of the periosteum
- Care is taken to avoid injury to the terminal extensor tendon located 1 to 2 mm proximal to the germinal matrix
- A template and measurements are taken of the defect to determine donor graft size
- The lateral aspect of the great toe is the preferred option for larger defects.
- The full-thickness graft includes the proximal most germinal matrix and distal sterile matrix to the level of the periosteum.
- The donor site can be skin grafted as detailed later in this article. The lateral nail fold can also be advanced to minimize defect size.
- The full-thickness graft is placed into the recipient site and secured with 6 to 0 chromic sutures.
- Nail plate or bolster is then used to secure the graft

Skin Graft Absent Nail

- Marking pen used to outline shape of nail on dorsal distal phalanx
- Template then deepithelialized to accept graft
- Split-thickness or full-thickness skin graft may be harvested and trimmed to fit the nail template
- Secure the graft with 6 to 0 chromic sutures
- Bolster dressing placed with xeroform, cotton balls, and nylon sutures

Hook Nail (Postoperative Result)

- Expose the distal nail bed as described previously (**Fig. 7**A, B).
- Use #15 blade scalpel to excise and elevate the hook portion of the nail bed off of the distal phalanx
- Volar soft tissue elevated off the distal phalanx to expose the bone
- Sagittal saw used to make stair step cut in distal phalanx to allow for lengthening and distal support of the nailbed.
- Secure distal phalanx with K-wires
- Digit flexed and cross-finger flap used for distal and volar fingertip coverage given additional defect with added fingertip length.
- Template designed for remaining distal nailbed defect.
- Beaver blade used to harvest split thickness sterile nail bed graft from adjacent finger or toe.
- Graft secured with 6 to 0 chromic suture and bolster dressing.

Pincer Nail

- Expose the nail bed as described previously.
- Oblique incisions made distal to the hyponychium and proximal to the eponychial fold at the most lateral aspects of the nail bed bilaterally.

- Freer elevator of small scissors used to elevate deformed paronychium off the distal phalanx.
- Tunnel created between the proximal and distal incisions, elevating the lateral sterile and germinal matrix with a freer.
- Thin strips of dermal graft are harvested from the forearm or groin under local anesthesia. Allograft may also be used. Size is roughly 5 to 10 mm × 15 mm.
- Bunnell needle placed eye-first from proximal to distal through tunnels.
- 5 to 0 nylon passed through graft and eye of needle. Grafts then passed through tunnel to elevate the lateral nailbed and paronychial fold.
- Graft secured to proximal skin over a bolster with 5 to 0 nylon and distal incisions closed with 5 to 0 nylon.
- Suture foil or silicone sheeting placed underneath eponychial fold to protect nail and prevent synechia.

RECOVERY AND REHABILITATION

- Occlusive bolster dressing typically left in place for 5 to 7 days and removed at first clinic visit
- Gently wash with warm soapy water daily after bolster removal
- Bacitracin and xeroform dressing/band aid placed over graft and donor site
- Cap splint used for protection and patient comfort
- Active range of motion resumed early postoperatively to prevent stiffness

OUTCOMES AND MANAGEMENT

- Nailbed grafting requires multiple growth cycles to reach maturity
- Final outcome is expected at ~1 year

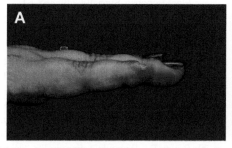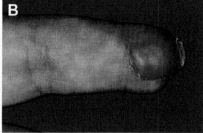

Fig. 7. (*A*) Lateral view of hook nail correction with thenar crease flap for improved soft tissue coverage and distal support. (*B*) Volar view of hook nail correction. Note typical squared off appearance of small local flap for digital reconstruction.

SUMMARY

Meticulous repair of acute nailbed injuries remains the best prevention for chronic deformities. Recognizing these deformities and the etiology is key to secondary repair. Split and full-thickness nailbed grafts remain viable options to correct chronic nailbed deformities with the end goal of a flat adherent nail.

CLINICS CARE POINTS

- A breadth of knowledge on nail anatomy, physiologic growth, and appropriate acute injury management helps prevent chronic nail bed deformities.
- Multiple nail growth cycles should be allowed to define the final deformity prior to reconstruction.
- Reconstruction should be aimed at restoration of function, a flat adherent nail, normal cosmesis, and elimination of pain.
- Split-thickness or full-thickness nailbed grafts and skin grafts represent viable treatment options to correct such deformities and obtain good cosmetic outcomes.

DISCLOSURE

The authors have nothing to disclose.

SUPPLEMENTARY DATA

Supplementary data related to this article can be found online at https://doi.org/10.1016/j.hcl.2020.09.003.

REFERENCES

1. Zook EG, Van Beek AL, Russell RC. Anatomy and physiology of the perionychium: a review of the literature and anatomic study. J Hand Surg 1980;5A:528–36.
2. Shum C, Bruno RJ, Ristic S, et al. Examination of the anatomic relationship of the proximal germinal nail matrix to the extensor tendon insertion. J Hand Surg 2000;25A:1114–7.
3. Kligman AM. Why do nails grow out instead of up? Arch Dermatol 1961;84:313–5.
4. Baden HP. Regeneration of the nail. Arch Dermatol 1964;91:619–20.
5. Pardo-Castello V. Diseases of the nail. 2nd edition. Springfield (IL): Charles C Thomas; 1941. p. 1–9.
6. Jones FW. The principles of anatomy as seen in the hand. 2nd edition. London (United Kingdom): Bailliere Tindall Cox; 1942.
7. Wilgis EFS, Maxwell GP. Distal digital nerve graft clinical and anatomical studies. J Hand Surg 1979;4:439–43.
8. Hashimoto R. Experimental study on histogenesis of the nail and its surrounding tissues. Niigata Med J 1971;85:254.
9. Brucker MJ, Edstrom L. The use of grafts in acute and chronic fingernail deformities. J Hand Surg Am 2002;2:14–20.
10. Zook EG. Reconstruction of a functional and aesthetic nail. Hand Clin 2002;18:577–94.
11. Zook EG, Guy RJ, Russell RC. A study of nail bed injuries: causes, treatment, and prognos is. J Hand Surg Am 1984;9:247–52.
12. Flat AE. Nail-bed injuries. Br J Plast Surg 1956;8:34–7.
13. Hanrahan EM. The split thickness skin graft as a covering following removal of a fingernail. Surgery 1946;20:398–400.
14. Kleinert HK, Purcha S, Ashbell TS, et al. The deformed fingernail, a frequent result of failure to repair nail bed injuries. J Trauma 1967;7:177–90.
15. Clayburgh RH, Wood MB, Cooney WP 3rd. Nail bed repair and reconstruction by reverse dermal grafts. J Hand Surg Am 1983;8:594–8.
16. Shepard GH. Nail graft for reconstruction. Hand Clin 1990;6:79–102.
17. Yong FC, Teoh LC. Nail bed reconstruction with split thickness nail bed grafts. J Hand Surg 1992;17:193–7.
18. Pessa JE, Tsai T-M, Li Y, et al. The repair of nail deformities with the nonvascularized nail bed graft: indications and results. J Hand Surg 1990;15:466–70.
19. Ogo K. Split nails. Plast Reconstr Surg 1990;86:1190–3.
20. Shepard GH. Management of acute nail bed avulsions. Hand Clin 1990;6:39–56.
21. Koshima I, Soeda S, Takase T, et al. Free vascularized nail grafts. J Hand Surg 1988;13:29–32.
22. Morrison WA. Microvascular nail transfer. Hand Clin 1990;6:69–76.
23. Lille S, Brown RE, Zook EG, et al. Free nonvascularized composite nail grafts: an institutional experience. Plast Reconstr Surg 2000;105:2412–5. 7.
24. Endo T, Nakayama Y, Soeda S. Nail transfer: evolution of the reconstructive procedure. Plast Reconstr Surg 1997;100:907913.
25. Buncke HJ, Gonzales RI. Fingernail reconstruction. Plast Reconstr Surg 1962;30:452–61.
26. Kumar VP, Satku K. Treatment and prevention of "hook nail" deformity with anatomic correlation. J Hand Surg 1993;18(4):617–20.
27. Atasoy E, Godfrey A, Kalisman M. The "antenna" procedure for the "hook-nail" deformity. J Hand Surg 1983;8:55–8.
28. Dumontier C, Gilbert A, Tubiana R. Hook-nail deformity: Surgical treatment with a homodigital advancement flap. J Hand Surg Br 1995;20(6):830–5.
29. Bubak PJ, RicheyMD, Engrav LH. Hook nail deformity repaired using a composite toe graft. Plast Reconstr Surg 1992;90(6):1079–82.

30. Kim JY, Kwon ST. Correction of contracted nail deformity by distraction lengthening. Ann Plast Surg 2008;61(2):153–6.
31. Garcıa-Lopez A, Laredo C, Rojas A. Oblique triangular neurovascular osteocutaneous flap for hook nail deformity correction. J Hand Surg Am 2014;39(7):1415–8.
32. Bakhach J. Le lambeau d'eponychium. Ann Chir Plast Esthet 1998;43(3):259–63.
33. Bakhach J, Demiri E, Guimberteau JC. Use of the eponychial flap to restore length of a short nail: a review of 30 cases. Plast Reconstr Surg 2005;116:478–83.
34. Dufourmentel C. Problemes esthetiques dans la reconstruction des moignons digitaux. Ann Chir 1971;25:995.
35. Foucher G, Lenoble E, Goffin D, et al. Le lanbeau "escalator" dans le traitement de l'ongle en griffe. Ann Chir Plast Esthet 1991;36:51.
36. Cambon-Binder A, Le Hanneur M, Doursounian L, et al. Eponychial flap refinement for the treatment of "hook-nail" deformity. J Hand Surg Br 1995;(6):830–5.
37. Cornelius CE 3rd, Shelly WB. Pincer nail syndrome. Arch Surg 1968;96:321–2.
38. Baran R. Pincer and trumpet nails [letter]. Arch Dermatol 1974;110:639–40.
39. Baran R, Broutart JC. Epidermoid cyst of the thumb presenting as pincer nail. J Am Acad Dermatol 1988;19:143–4.
40. Chapman RS. Overcurvature of the nails: an inherited disorder (letter). Br J Dermatol 1973;89:317–8.
41. Baran R, Haneke E, Richert B. Pincer nails: definition and surgical treatment. Dermatol Surg 2001;27:261–6.
42. el-Gammal S, Altmeyer P. Successful conservative therapy of pincer nail syndrome. Hautarzt 1993;44:535–7.
43. Suzuki K, Yagi I, Kondo M. Surgical treatment of pincer nail syndrome. Plast Reconstr Surg 1979;63:570–3.
44. Effendy I, Ossowski B, Happle R. Pincer nail: conservative correction by attachment of a plastic brace. Hautarzt 1993;44:800–2.
45. Sorg M, Kruger K, Schattenkirchner M. Das pincernail syndrome: eine seltene differentiale diagnose des fingerendgelenk/nagelbefalls. Z Rheumatol 1989;48:204.
46. Kim KD, Sim WY. Surgical pearl: nail plate separation and splint fixation–a new noninvasive treatment for pincer nails. J Am Acad Dermatol 2003;48:791–2.
47. Tseng JTP, Ho WT, Hsu CH, et al. A simple therapeutic approach to pincer nail deformity using a memory alloy: measurement of response. Dermatol Surg 2013;39:398–405.
48. Dikmen A, Ozer K, Ulusoy M, et al. Triple combination therapy for pincer nail deformity: surgical matricectomy, thioglycolic acid, and anticonvex sutures. Dermatol Surg 2017;43:1474–82.
49. Aksakal AB, Akar A, Erbil H, et al. A new surgical therapeutic approach to pincer nail deformity. Dermatol Surg 2001;27:55–7.
50. Kosaka M, Kamiishi H. New strategy for the treatment and assessment of pincer nail. Plast Reconstr Surg 2003;111:2014–9.
51. Son E, Tak M, Song W. Correction of pincer nail deformity: using a vertical Z-plasty. Plast Reconstr Surg 2013;132:158.
52. Jung DJ, Kim JH, Lee HY, et al. Anatomical characteristics and surgical treatments of pincer nail deformity. Arch Plas Surg 2015;42:207–13.
53. Shin WJ, Change BK, Shim JW, et al. Nail plate and bed reconstruction for pincer nail deformity. Clin Orthop Surg 2018;10:385–8.
54. Brown RE, Zook EG, Williams J. Correction of pincer-nail deformity using dermal grafting. Plast Reconstr Surg 2000;105:1658–61.
55. Zook EG, Chalekson CP, Brown RE, et al. Correction of pincer-nail deformities with autograft or homograft dermis: modified surgical technique. J Hand Surg 2005;30A:400–3.
56. Willard KJ, Cappel MA, Kozin SH, et al. Benign subungual tumors. J Hand Surg Am 2012;37(6):1276e1286.
57. Hinchcliff KM, Pereira C. Subungual tumors: an algorithmic approach. J Hand Surg Am 2019;44:588–98.
58. Baek HJ, Lee SJ, Cho KH, et al. Subungual tumors: clinicopathologic correlation with US and MR imaging findings. Radiographics 2010;30(6):1621–36.
59. Göktay F, Atıs G, Günes P, et al. Subungual exostosis and subungual osteochondromas: a description of 25 cases. Int J Dermatol 2018;57(7):872–81.
60. Netscher DT, Aburto J, Koepplinger M. Subungual glomus tumor. J Hand Surg Am 2012;37(4):821–3.
61. Lambertini M, Piraccini BM, Fanti PA, et al. Mohs micrographic surgery for nail unit tumors: an update and a critical review of the literature. J Eur Acad Dermatol Venereol 2018;32(10):1638–44.
62. Piraccini BM, Bellavista S, Misciali C, et al. Periungual and subungual pyogenic granuloma. Br J Dermatol 2010;163(5):941–53.
63. Brown RE, Zook EG, Russell RC, et al. Fingernail deformities secondary to ganglions of the distal interphalangeal joint (Mucous Cysts). Plast Reconstr Surg 1991;87:718–25.
64. Ilyas EN, Leinberry CF, Ilyas AM. Skin cancers of the hand and upper extremity. J Hand Surg Am 2012;37(1):171–8.
65. Dijksterhuis A, Friedeman E, van der Heijden B. Squamous cell carcinoma of the nail unit: review

of the literature. J Hand Surg Am 2018;43(4): 374–9.e2.

66. Topin-Ruiz S, Surinach C, Dalle S, et al. Surgical treatment of subungual squamous cell carcinoma by wide excision of the nail unit and skin graft reconstruction: an evaluation of treatment efficiency and outcomes. JAMA Dermatol 2017; 153(5):442–8.

67. Andre J, Lateur N. Pigmented nail disorders. Dermatol Clin 2006;24:329–39.

68. Braun RP, Baran R, LeGal FA, et al. Diagnosis and management of nail pigmentations. J Am Acad Dermatol 2007;56:835–47.

69. Levit EK, Kagen MH, Scher RK, et al. The ABC rule for clinical detection of subungual melanoma. J Am Acad Dermatol 2000;42:269–74.

70. Quinn MJ, Thompson JE, Crotty K, et al. Subungual melanoma of the hand. J Hand Surg Am 1996;21: 506–11.

71. Machol JA, Dzwierzynski WW. Subungual melanoma: a systematic review. Suppl Plas Reconstr Surg 2013;132:635–41.

72. O'Connor EA, Dzwierzynski W. Longitudinal melonychia: clinical evaluation and biopsy technique. J Hand Surg Am 2011;36:1852–4.

73. Tran KT, Wright NA, Cockerell CJ. Biopsy of the pigmented lesion—when and how. J Am Acad Dermatol 2008;59:852–71.

74. Boyer. Cited by: Patterson RYH, Helwig EB. Quoted by Hertzler AE. Gaz Med de Paris. 1854. P 212.

75. Hutchinson JT. Morale in mental handicap hospitals. Br Med J 1978;1:362–3.

76. Feibleman CE, Stoll H, Maize JC. Melanomas of the palm, sole, and nailbed: a clinicopathologic study. Cancer 1980;46:2492–504.

77. Brodland DG. The treatment of nail apparatus melanoma with Mohs micrographic surgery. Dermatol Surg 2001;27:269–73.

78. Das Gupta T, Bradfield R. Subungual melanoma: 25-year review of cases. Ann Surg 1965;161:545–52.

79. Papachristou DN, Fortner JG. Melanoma arising under the nail. J Surg Oncol 1982;21:219–22.

80. Heaton K, el-Naggar A, Ensign L, et al. Surgical management and prognostic factors in patients with subungual melanoma. Ann Surg 1994;219: 197–204.

81. Park KG, Blessing K, Kernohan NM. Surgical aspects of subungual malignant melanomas: the Scottish Melanoma Group. Ann Surg 1992;216:692–5.

82. Clarkson JK, McAllister RM, Cliff SH, et al. Subungual melanoma in situ: two independent streaks in one nail bed. Br J Plast Surg 2002;55:165–7.

83. Cochran AM, Buchanan PJ, Bueno RA, et al. Subungual melanoma: a review of current treatment. Plast Reconstr Surg 2014;134:259–73.

Secondary Management of Nonnail Perionychial Deformities
Restoring Aesthetic and Functional Subunits

Nikola Lekic, MD[a], Luis Scheker, MD[b], David Netscher, MD[c,d],*

KEYWORDS

- Fingertip reconstruction • Fingertip deformity • Chronic injuries • Hand flaps

KEY POINTS

- Delayed finger and thumb tip reconstruction should attempt to optimally reconstruct perioncyhial aesthetic and functional units by replacing tissue as closely resembling the original loss as possible.
- Chronic fingertip injuries may be treated with local advancement flaps, staged flaps, and island flaps, whereas a partial toe transfer provides excellent coverage for composite injuries involving multiple subunits or those involving an extensive area.
- Noninnervated flaps, such as cross-finger flaps, heterodigital island flaps, and retrograde homodigital island flaps, tend to regain adequate sensation spontaneously over time with meaningful two-point discrimination.
- To minimize the risk of joint contractures, avoid bringing the fingertip to meet the flap, but rather, advance the flap to the digital tip.

INTRODUCTION: PRINCIPLES AND REQUIREMENTS FOR DELAYED RECONSTRUCTION

There is little published information on secondary reconstruction of chronic fingertip problems. This maybe because patients less frequently present for these problems, either choosing to live with them (sometimes even learning to work around the problem, such as simply excluding that digit from routine use and bypassing it) or because they are not informed about available reconstructive options. Much more is known about the acute treatment of fingertip injuries because the acute injury brings the patient to the emergency room and the acute care hand surgeon.

In the past, for acute injuries, the treatment algorithms were overly simplistic. Choices ranged from secondary healing to cross-finger flap for larger volar angulated pulp wounds and V-Y Atasoy pulp flaps for more dorsally angulated wounds. However, even for acute injuries, there is now a much wider array of potential surgical treatment options (**Fig. 1**).

Possible causes for late digital tip reconstruction may include chronic deformities resulting from (**Fig. 2**):

1. Burn injuries
2. Chemical or radiation injuries, either accidental handling or industrial accidents
3. Residual effects of infections
4. Neglected trauma
5. Tumor resection

One needs to carefully evaluate the specific patient needs and concerns. Even a seemingly trivial

a Department of Orthopaedics, Baylor College of Medicine, 7200 Cambridge Street, Suite 10A, Houston, TX 77030, USA; b Kleinert Institute for Hand and Microsurgery, Department of Plastic Surgery, University of Louisville, 225 Abraham Flexner Way, Suite 700, Louisville, KY 40202, USA; c Baylor College of Medicine; d Weill Cornell Medical College, New York, NY 10065, USA
* Corresponding author. 6624 Fannin Street, Suite 2730, Houston, TX 77030.
E-mail address: Netscher@bcm.edu

Hand Clin 37 (2021) 77–96
https://doi.org/10.1016/j.hcl.2020.09.008
0749-0712/21/© 2020 Elsevier Inc. All rights reserved.

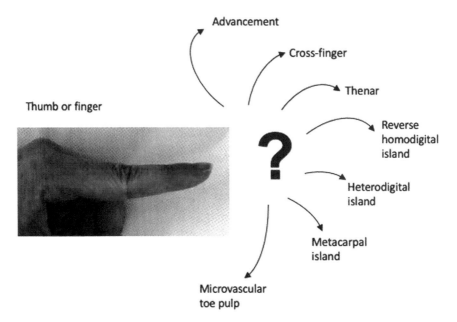

Advancement

Cross-finger

Thenar

Reverse homodigital island

Heterodigital island

Metacarpal island

Microvascular toe pulp

Thumb or finger

?

Fig. 1. Available treatment options for fingertip injuries. The decision in selecting one of these choices depends on the injury, patient's vocational and avocational demands, and optimal function to meet those demands while striving for the best possible aesthetic outcome.

small apical and volar pulp finger deficit may be especially important to a professional musician. However, painful scarring adherent down to underlying bone may be a huge inconvenience even for someone who is less reliant on their hands. A hook nail may be painful and difficult to trim, whereas a nail that is imperfectly adherent at the nail matrix/hyponychial junction may frequently get irritatingly hung up. Likewise, an uncovered nail plate root caused by a retracted and scarred eponychial fold (as occurs in burn injuries) may be a source of discomfort and repeated

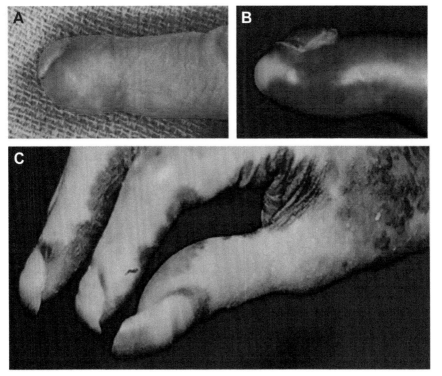

Fig. 2. Examples of chronic fingertip deformities. (*A*) Hook nail. (*B*) Fingertip injury with a nail deformity, painful fingertip, and pulp deficiency. (*C*) Burn patient with retracted eponychium.

infections. Persistent digital neuromas result in pain and dysesthesias. Finally, the distal interphalangeal joint itself needs to be a consideration, especially if fusion is a part of the reconstructive option. In some professions the angle of fusion may be a critical decision.

The functional and aesthetic units of the digital tip are illustrated in **Fig. 3**. The nail and perionychial structures not only have unique aesthetics, but a well-formed nail is also essential for daily functions. Picking up a coin or fastening a small button or clasp become much more difficult tasks without a nail. The paronychium with the smooth transition to the eponychium acts as a cushion on each side of the nail, provides a waterproof and infectious barrier for the nail plate and nail matrix, and provides aesthetic harmony to the fingertip with its smooth subtle tapered contour.

The arrangement of the volar pulp fat pads between fibrous septae that are firmly anchored to bone and the terminal long flexor tendon gives a tactile compressibility and yet a resilience to be able to grip firmly on objects (analogous to a spring mattress). Less sheer is imparted to the fingertip as a result (**Fig. 4**). Volar pulp reconstruction with a fat flap, such as a groin or abdominal flap, has no turgor and just slides as might a jelly and provides poor grip traction (**Fig. 5**).

The epithelium and its deeply anchoring dermis also have several unique characteristics at the digital tip. The dorsal finger has an epidermis that is similar to other parts of the body, but the germinal matrix (lunula and deep surface of the eponychium), cuticle of the eponychium, sterile nail matrix, hyponychium (where the distal nail plate becomes progressively less adherent), and glabrous volar skin all have individual characteristics. Thus, at the critical "watershed" area at the tip of the finger where there is a meeting point of sterile matrix, hyponychium, and glabrous skin, one might better allow secondary healing to enable surface repopulation by cells from each epithelial "zone" much as we have found that a skin graft is a poor method of resurfacing of the sterile nail matrix resulting in failure of nail plate adherence. Likewise, we have found that there is no need to provide lining to the deep surface of a dorsal rotation flap to reconstruct the eponychial fold because the deep surface becomes epithelized by germinal matrix and the reconstructed eponychial fold adheres normally to the nail plate.

When presented with a chronic digital tip deformity, a general principle is to recreate the original defect by excising the deforming scar. Thus, one then has an "acute" injury to reconstruct much as would occur when excising a skin or soft tissue

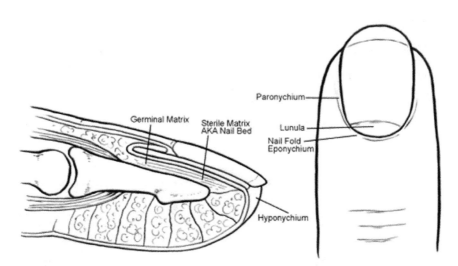

Fig. 3. A side view (*left*) and top-down view (*right*) of functional and aesthetic subunits of the fingertip. The hyponychium at the distal end of the fingertip is the specialized transitional tissue that allows the nail to become increasingly less adherent to the fingertip as the distal sterile matrix of the nail bed merges with the epidermis. The paronychium, coursing along either side of the nail plate not only provides a cushion for fine digital manipulation, but also acts as a barrier against microbial invasion. The eponychium, overlying the proximal end of the nail plate, protects the important germinal matrix and also tapers in transition to the dorsal skin for an aesthetically pleasing finger. In managing perionychial injuries, one should attempt to recreate these subunits so that their original specialized functions and aesthetics may be restored.

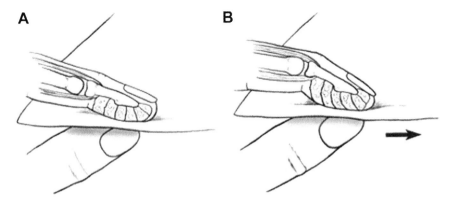

Fig. 4. The fibrous septae originate at the periosteum and paratenon of the long flexor tendons and insert onto the skin. The septae are like springs within a mattress, which compartmentalize the fatty tissue and give the finger a recoil property to allow for fine manipulation of objects. The resting fingertip is seen with its septae (*A*). The fingertip is used to pinch a piece of paper and minimal deformation of the fingertip is observed (*B*). This resistance against displacement is imparted by the fibrous septae, which tether the skin to the deeper structures (bone and tendon).

cancer, or an acute injury for that matter. A thorough release of deforming scar tissue is essential. The reconstructive plan would then depend on:

1. Defect size
2. Specialized reconstructive needs of the wound location
3. Requirements for sensation
4. Need for composite tissue

The goals of treatment of these chronic problems are to obtain a functional, pain-free, sensate, and aesthetically pleasing finger that meets the patient's occupational and recreational demands. Contour the volar pulp, maintain digital length, and avoid nail deformities by providing adequate tip support and respect perionychial subunits. As far as possible, replace like-tissue with like-tissue.

MOST RECENT EVIDENCE FOR OPTIMUM CLINICAL OUTCOME WITH VARIOUS RECONSTRUCTIVE OPTIONS

There is a paucity of meaningful outcome studies. Most of the flap outcome studies are derived from treatment of acute injuries and these have to be extrapolated to reconstruction. Most of those studies evaluated flap reliability and ability to heal a wound and often did not evaluate long-term detailed aesthetic and functional outcome that are specific to the perionychial subunits. However, some studies are more helpful in assessing these outcomes and in noting some reconstructive shortfalls.

The volar pulp V-Y (Atasoy) advancement flap has been used for smaller fingertip injuries. A study of 30 pediatric trauma patients with a

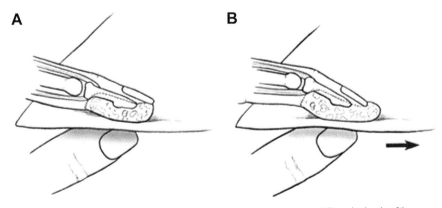

Fig. 5. A fingertip reconstruction with a fat flap, such as a groin or abdominal flap, lacks the fibrous septae of the pulp (*A*). Therefore, the fingertip no longer acts as a spring mattress with adequate recoil, but more like a gel that provides poor grip traction (*B*).

mean follow-up of 4.7 years found no cases of flap necrosis, but other outcomes were less optimistic: 67% had good tactile sensitivity, 50% had hook nail deformity, 73% had hyponychial scarring, and 43% had normal pulp shape.[1] In our opinion, a larger homodigital island flap may produce less wound closure tension and more bulk for larger defects. Also, by providing apical digital coverage but being less concerned with bringing flap skin dorsally, one may allow the subcutaneous exposed flap layers on the dorsal surface to be repopulated by the specialized epithelium of sterile nail matrix, hyponychium, and paronychium.

The long-term outcomes of cross-finger flaps have also been reported with a mean follow-up of 19 years in 22 patients.[2] There were none with painful neuromas and all reported satisfaction with the donor site, and 25% had cold sensitivity. In 36.8% two-point (2PD) sensory testing was worse than the opposite side. Overall, this is a simple reconstruction that seems to enjoy lasting benefits.

Equal success has been reported for antegrade and innervated homodigital island flaps versus homodigital retrograde island flaps with regard to flap survival, cold intolerance, 2PD, time to return to work, interphalangeal joint motion, and DASH (Disabilities of the Arm, Shoulder, and Hand questionnaire) scores.[3] Thus, for small thin flaps to the fingertips, actual flap innervation may be less important. Another study that evaluated patients with volar pulp defects reconstructed by antegrade island flaps with 8-year follow-up found high patient satisfaction, excellent digital active range of motion, grip strength, DASH scores, Semmes Weinstein monofilament testing, and mean 2PD at 5.1 mm.[4]

Partial toe free flap fingertip reconstruction outcomes have been reported in 17 patients with larger wounds.[5] This has the advantage of replacing like with like tissue. No patient reported dysesthesia, resting pain, or cold intolerance. Average 2PD was 10 mm (range, 6–15 mm). Sensate, glabrous tissue reconstruction is possible. Another outcome study involving 246 cases reported good sensory recovery with two having substantially decreased sensation.[6] Although sensory recovery is not always perfect, the most reliable way of resolving painful neuromas is to restore nerve continuity, which is accomplished by an innervated free flap.

Wound healing by secondary intention has often been advocated because of its convenience for acute injuries. It may be suitable for small wounds but is almost certainly unsuitable for managing chronic problems where the deformity has often arisen through scar distortion. However, leaving areas open, provided there is adequate underlying supportive soft tissue, may be advantageous to allow for re-epithelialization of specialized functional epithelium.

AVAILABLE RECONSTRUCTIVE OPTIONS
Skin Grafting

Full- or split-thickness skin grafting is seldom used for secondary reconstruction, except for occasional back grafting to the donor area of a transposition or rotation flap. A hyponychial full-thickness crescentic graft from a toe may be used on occasion for scarred apical hyponychium in the finger or a nail bed graft from a toe for sterile matrix (but generally allowed to re-epithelialize spontaneously).

Local Pedicle Advancement Flaps

These include the volar subcutaneous pedicle V-Y advancement flap (Atasoy) and bilateral (radial and ulnar) V-Y flap as described by Kutler.[7,8] Finally, there is the larger volar Moberg neurovascular flap for thumb tip reconstruction. This is converted into an island for greater advancement by preserving only the neurovascular pedicle. Smaller fingertip injuries are suitable for Atasoy flaps (dorsally angulated) or Kutler flaps (volarly angulated or transverse wounds). The advantage of these flaps over revision amputation is ability to preserve digital length and apical pulp, and minimizes hook nail deformity. Generally, the Moberg flap is suitable for apical thumb pulp wounds less than 1.5 cm.[9]

On the dorsum of the digit, the eponychium may be reconstructed with a rotational flap and there is seldom a need to skin graft the donor site because the proximal aspect of the flap is readily closed with skin redundancy toward the proximal interphalangeal joint.

Staged Flaps

Staged flaps involve bringing the finger toward the donor site and attaching the flap, with subsequent flap division once blood supply ingrowth has occurred in the flap (usually after about 2 weeks). These include the cross-finger flap (originally described by Cronin) and the thenar flap (first described by Gatewood).[10,11] The latter has undergone subsequent modifications, to move the donor site closer to the thumb metacarpophalangeal joint flexion crease to reduce the necessary amount of finger flexion and for ease of donor wound closure. Innervation of the cross-finger flap with the dorsal sensory digital nerve has been described to improve sensation.[12]

The so-called reverse cross-finger flap first described by Pakian and subsequently popularized by Atasoy may be suitable for dorsal finger and perionychial wounds.[13]

Island Flaps

Island flaps are based on a specific axial pattern of blood flow. With a clear understanding of collateral arterial supply (**Fig. 6**), one can plan either antegrade or retrograde arterial flow flaps from the same digit and even heterodigital island flaps from adjacent digits.[14] An added advantage of heterodigital and retrograde homodigital flaps is that the vascular pedicle allows multiple axes of rotation, enabling wound coverage to volar and dorsal aspects of a finger.[15–17] These larger antegrade island flaps allow advancement of up to 1.5 cm and so the original algorithm as to whether or not an injury was volar or dorsal angulating no longer holds absolutely true because these island flaps allow much more versatility.[18–20]

Heterodigital island flaps were described by Littler[21] for sensate thumb coverage from the ring finger. This resulted in several donor site problems but we have described techniques to minimize these problems.[22] For the thumb, a better choice may actually be the heterodigital first dorsal metacarpal artery (Kite) flap as described by Foucher and Braun.[23]

Free Tissue Transfer

A variety of free flaps have been described but most do not provide glabrous skin, nor are they effective at restoring fingertip aesthetics. The notable exception is that the nail unit, perionychial tissues, bone, and sensibility can all be replaced by full toe or partial toe transfers. One must be mindful of not having abnormal shoe wear at the donor site and so the partial great toe transfer would always come from the lateral (inner) side, necessitating, for example, the ipsilateral toe for ulnar sided thumb defects and the contralateral toe for radial sided ones.[24] The medial side of the second toe may sometimes be a better match for finger defects.[5,6,25]

DISCUSSION: MATCHING THE DIGITAL PROBLEM WITH THE OPTIMUM RECONSTRUCTIVE OPTION TO RESTORE AESTHETIC AND FUNCTIONAL SUBUNITS

Hyponychium and Distal Finger Pulp

These wounds may occur in isolation or as part of a much larger digital tip wound. For example, a chronically traumatized finger with hook nail deformity may be corrected by autologous grafting of a toe nail bed to the recipient finger (**Fig. 7**). For central wounds that are too tight to close directly, a unilateral or bilateral Kutler flap brings in tissue from the sides of the finger, providing a nice rounded fingertip with apical padding and hyponychial epithelium. In a female patient, multiple attempts at excising an apical thumb inclusion cyst had previously been undertaken (**Fig. 8**). The fourth excision involved removing an apical wedge of tissue, distal phalanx tip, and sterile matrix. This was nicely contoured with a unilateral Kutler flap. In another case example, a volar oblique fingertip injury was reconstructed using a bilateral Kutler flap (**Fig. 9**). The primary goal is to cover the defect with sensate tissue, maintain length, and recreate the pulp for a functional and aesthetic fingertip. Although this is an example of an acute injury, the same principle may be applied to a chronic fingertip injury.

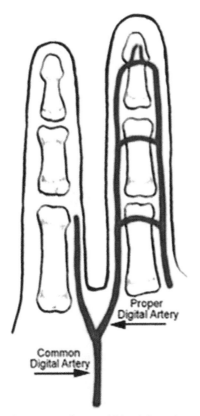

Fig. 6. Illustration of arterial blood flow through the finger. Note the interconnections between the proper digital arteries at the level of the phalangeal necks. Understanding this anatomy is essential when planning for island flaps, especially retrograde flow island flaps.

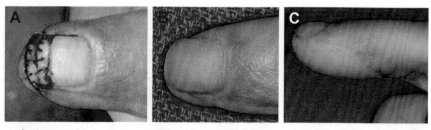

Fig. 7. Image of a hyponychium reconstruction with transfer from a toe donor site (*A*). The patient not only regained the aesthetic appearance of the nail with an adherent nail bed (*B*), but also an optimal functional outcome by being able to maintain his finger length (*C*).

Some of the reasons the volar V-Y Atasoy flap gets a bad reputation for unfavorable aesthetic outcome and even flap necrosis is caused by inadequate flap release and mobilization and closing the wound too tightly. Additionally, it was often a poor reconstructive option when it was more frequently used. Key to successful reconstruction, as with the Kutler flap, is adequate release of the deep fibrous septal attachments to bone. In this case example (**Fig. 10**), the tips of the middle and ring fingers were amputated. The middle finger was treated with a replantation, whereas the ring finger was treated with a V-Y Atasoy flap. Overstretch or accidental division of small nerve branches leads to a dysesthetic fingertip and potential hook nail. If the nail plate is still in place, do not remove it because this gives a firm anchor point for distal sutures.

LARGER VOLAR PULP DEFECTS

Cross-finger flaps and thenar flaps are still useful options. We find the cross-finger flap especially useful, such as after release of Dupuytren contracture, either for the severe initial contracture or for digits that have had multiple prior surgeries. Scarring and extensive neurovascular dissection with previous trauma may prevent axial pattern island flap reconstruction. The thumb can potentially be resurfaced with a cross-finger flap by resting

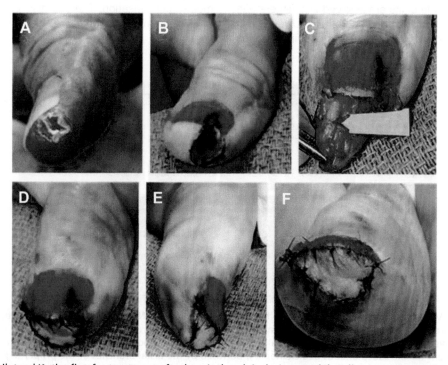

Fig. 8. Unilateral Kutler flap for treatment of a chronic thumb inclusion cyst (*A*). Following a thorough excision of the cyst (*B*), the triangular flap is elevated (*C*) while protecting the neurovascular structures (*blue arrow*). The flap is then transposed to the area of the defect (*D–F*).

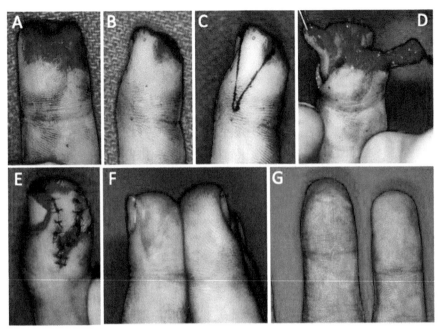

Fig. 9. An example of an acute traumatic fingertip injury (*A, B*) treated with bilateral Kutler flaps. Triangular flaps are raised on either side of the digit (*C*), carefully ensuring that the neurovascular bundles are included (*D*). Following insetting (*E*), and healing, a favorable functional and aesthetic outcome is achieved (*F, G*).

against the index finger and because of the far reach; the thenar flap is useful only for index and middle fingertips. Cross-finger flaps are also useful when multiple digits are involved and fingers can be stacked adjacent to each other. However, it is uncommon for us to use cross-finger flaps

because of the awkwardness of two separate stages, greater risk of finger contracture and stiffness, and long duration before the fingertip has meaningful sensation. There is also the potential risk of harming an otherwise uninjured donor finger.

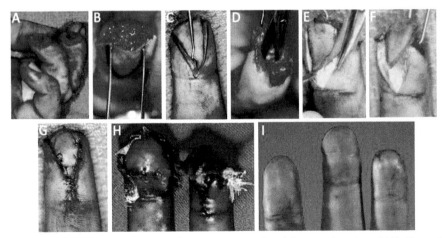

Fig. 10. A V-Y Atasoy flap used to treat a ring fingertip amputation (*A*). Note that the middle fingertip amputation was treated by replantation. The flap is made as wide as the nail structures distally (*B*) and skin incised (*C*). Next, release of the septae off the distal phalanx (*D*) and proximal subdermis (*E*) is required. This allows easy advancement for the subcutaneous pedicle flap (*F*), perfused by the distal branches of the proper digital neurovascular structures. Finally, the proximal donor defect may be closed primarily (*G*) or, if excessive wound tension is of a concern, one may choose to leave the donor defect open to simply allow for secondary healing. One-week (*H*) and long-term (*I*) follow-up demonstrate excellent functional and aesthetic outcomes.

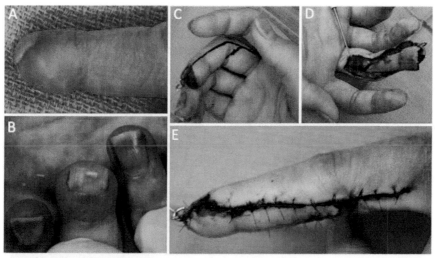

Fig. 11. Hook nail deformity (A, B) treated with an island flap (C–E). Note the retrograde K-wire placed in the distal phalanx (C–E), which functions as a cantilever to elevate the nail bed to decrease hook nail deformity and maximize length while the reconstruction heals.

Our "workhorse" for these larger wounds is the homodigital island advancement flap. The subcutaneous tissue and surface epithelium are more similar to volar pulp than is a cross-finger flap. It is used for coverage of defects up to 1 to 2 cm at the pulp and is advanced by as much as 1.5 cm. Advancement is facilitated by proximal dissection, release of the neurovascular structures, and subsequent medialization of the pedicle on the finger. This flap brings a lot of bulk within the flap island and can provide fingertip support in secondary reconstructions, such as for a hook nail (**Fig. 11**) or chronic fingertip scarring (**Fig. 12**).

Retrograde island flaps are perfused through cross-linking vessels between adjacent ulnar and radial proper digital arteries. One can carry even more soft tissue with these flaps than the advancement island flap, but a disadvantage is that the donor site requires skin grafting. These flaps have multiple degrees of freedom of the axis of rotation and so can reach the volar and dorsal aspects of the fingertip (**Figs. 13** and **14**). Retrograde

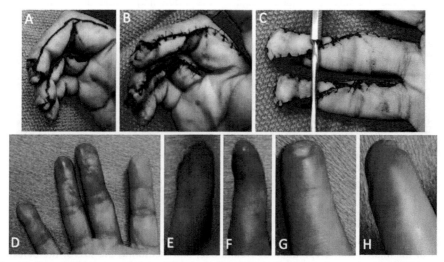

Fig. 12. Chronic fingertip changes of the middle and ring fingers following fingertip necrosis in a patient who had systemic sepsis requiring pressors (A). After debridement of the fingertips and preparation of the wound beds, homodigital island flaps with antegrade blood flow were elevated, advanced, and inset (B, C). The patient demonstrated good functional and aesthetic (D–H) outcomes.

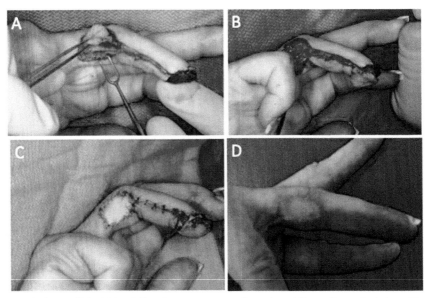

Fig. 13. Retrograde homodigital island flap for treatment of a volar oblique fingertip injury. The flap is first elevated, avoiding damage to the underlying neurovascular structures (*A*). The flap is mobilized by ligating the digital artery proximally and rotating the flap distally around a communicating artery with blood supply provided by the digital artery on the opposite side of the finger, ensuring that the flap is able to reach the injured site (*B*). Following flap insetting, a full-thickness skin graft is applied to the donor site (*C*). Final long-term functional and aesthetic (*D*) outcome.

flaps do not carry a sensory nerve, but as already alluded to, and like the cross-finger flaps, sensory "regrowth" occurs with thin digital flaps.

Finally, for large volar fingertip reconstructions, the heterodigital island flap remains an option, especially when a homodigital flap is not available through scarring or pathology involving the same digit neurovascular structures (**Fig. 15**). Again, we have used this flap for adjacent digit transfer in repeat operations if resurfacing is required for Dupuytren contracture. In the case illustrated (**Fig. 16**), there was an extensive involvement of the middle finger by a vascular malformation. The lesion had recurred three times following prior surgeries. Radical resection required excision of the entire volar pulp to include involved skin. A heterodigital flap from the index finger was used. The dorsal sensory

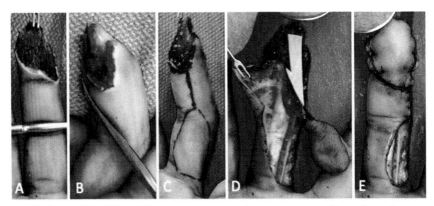

Fig. 14. Retrograde homodigital island flap for treatment of a large volar oblique fingertip injury. Following debridement of the injured site, preparation of wound bed, and measuring the size of the defect (*A, B*), the flap is designed over the proximal phalanx neurovascular bundle (*C*). After ligation of the digital artery proximally, the *blue arrow* (*D*) indicates the communicating artery vascular pedicle around which the flap rotates. Final insetting of the flap to the defect (*E*). The donor site is to be closed with a full-thickness skin graft. This large volar pulp wound would be unsuitable for an advancement island flap.

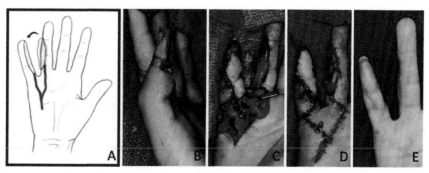

Fig. 15. Illustration of a heterodigital island flap planning (*A*). A case example of a small finger with a large defect of the pulp (*B*) that is treated with a heterodigital island flap (*C*), and placement of a full-thickness skin graft over the donor site (*D*). Long-term follow-up demonstrates a favorable aesthetic outcome (*E*).

nerve branch in the donor skin island was used not only to innervate the reconstructed volar fingertip but also to resolve the painful neuroma and dysesthetic finger. We have modified the Littler method of heterodigital island flap to minimize donor finger morbidity. Do not encroach on the donor finger terminal pulp, leave the proper digital nerve intact, and place the donor site more to the side of the finger.[22]

EPONYCHIUM AND DORSAL SKIN

The eponychium may be retracted in burn scar injuries. Occasionally the eponychium is totally distorted and destroyed by a deforming mucous cyst. A dorsal rotation flap with meticulous insetting distally to precisely restore eponychial anatomy minimizes the risk of scar retraction (**Fig. 17**). More proximally, mobile skin toward the proximal interphalangeal joint allows for donor

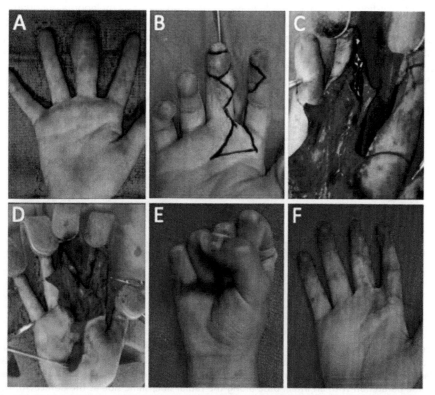

Fig. 16. Heterodigital island flap used to treat a middle finger vascular malformation (*A*). The flap is designed over the adjacent index finger, sparing the donor finger pulp (*B*). Following debridement of the middle finger vascular malformation (*C*), the flap is elevated including the radial digital artery and dorsal sensory nerve branch of the index finger (*D*). Long-term results demonstrate excellent motion and aesthetic outcomes (*E, F*).

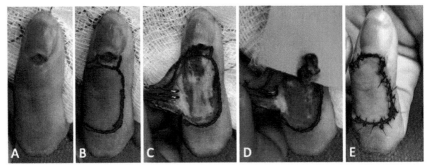

Fig. 17. Rotation flap for reconstruction of the eponychium following excision of a mucous cyst. The mucous cyst is seen at the distal eponychium, partially involving the nail unit (*A*). The three-limbed flap is designed ending just distal to the proximal interphalangeal joint (*B*). The flap is elevated off the extensor tendon paratenon (*C*). Following excision of the mucous cyst (*D*), the flap is rotated and inset distally, recreating the eponychial fold (*E*).

site suture closure, except in the scarred burn patient where skin may be less pliable and require donor skin grafting. A reverse cross-finger flap, as popularized by Atasoy, may be useful for a larger eponychial wound (**Fig. 18**). The recipient area necessitates skin grafting and the adjacent fingers need to be separated at a second stage around 2 weeks later. If nail matrix is resurfaced with a reverse cross-finger flap then simply leave the recipient area open and allow it to spontaneously re-epithelialize and this ultimately leads to an adherent nail.[13,26]

For larger soft tissue wounds over the dorsum of the distal finger, a heterodigital island flap or a retrograde flow homodigital island flap (**Fig. 19**) is transposed to reach these sites.[22] Sometimes with large wounds over the finger dorsum, one may need to accept formal ablation of the nail and then vascularized island tissue transfer. This preserves digital length and important tactile volar surfaces, enabling dorsal soft tissue reconstruction nonetheless even though the nail aesthetics and function may be lost.

In the case of in situ perionychial and subungual cancers, such as melanoma or squamous cell carcinoma, composite excision of the entire nail bed and perionychial tissues down to periosteum leaves a surface that can take a full-thickness skin graft (**Fig. 20**). Again, even though nail function and aesthetics are lost, the appearance is still satisfactory but more important, digital length is preserved.

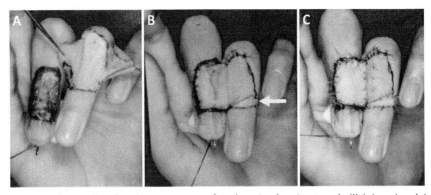

Fig. 18. Reverse cross-finger flap for the treatment of a chronic abrasive treadmill injury involving the eponychium and extensive dorsal finger tissue. Following debridement of the chronic deformity, dissection of a thin skin flap with an intact base along the ulnar side, opposite the defect, the fatty subcutaneous layer is elevated off the paratenon with an intact base along the radial side, same side as the defect (*A*). The fatty subcutaneous layer is turned over the wound, bringing with it a small sliver of skin from the ring finger (*arrow*) for reconstruction of the eponychium (*B*). At completion of the case, a full-thickness skin graft covered the flap on the injured finger and along the small portion of exposed paratenon of the donor finger from where the skin paddle was procured (*C*).

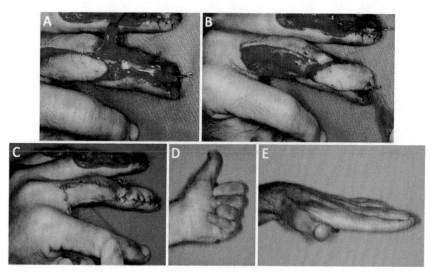

Fig. 19. Wood planer injury to the dorsum of the middle, ring, and small fingers, treated with reverse flow homodigital island flaps to maintain adequate length and to allow volar surfaces to maintain their tactile sensations. After debridement, residual nail bed ablation, and stabilization of the distal phalanx fracture with a K-wire, a radial-sided retrograde flow homodigital island flap is designed and skin incisions made (*A*). The flap is mobilized on its distally based vascular pedicle and turned 180° to cover the dorsal finger defect (*B*). After insetting the flap, a full-thickness skin graft is placed over the donor site (*C*). Long-term follow-up demonstrates a favorable functional and aesthetic outcome (*D, E*).

VERY LARGE PERIONYCHIAL AND COMPOSITE FINGERTIP RECONSTRUCTIONS

Although the medialis pedis and medial plantar artery perforator flaps have been described for providing glabrous donor skin from the foot,[27] the first webspace of the foot and its subtended great toe pulp and second toe pulp flaps are most preferred to provide the closest match, not only for subunits of the perionychium but also for composite tissue and sensory reinnervation. Indeed, chimeric flaps are harvested from lateral great toe pulp and medial second toe, with a common vascular pedicle through the first dorsal

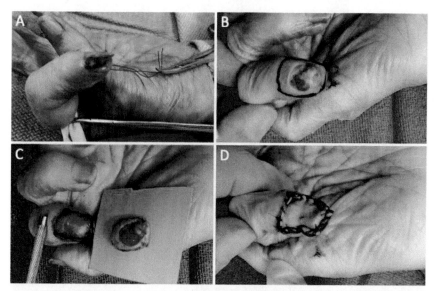

Fig. 20. Squamous cell carcinoma in situ of the perionychium (*A*) treated with composite excision down to periosteum (*B, C*) and full-thickness skin grafting (*D*). Despite the loss of the nail and presumptive loss of aesthetics, the healed appearance is generally satisfactory and, more importantly, the digital length is maintained for optimal function.

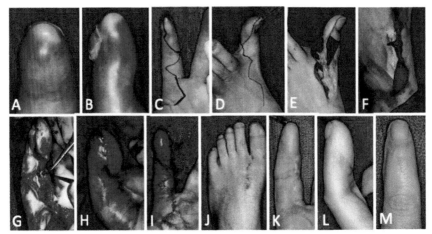

Fig. 21. Partial great toe pulp free tissue transfer for reconstruction of a chronic index fingertip injury. The thin skin flap and its scarring to the underlying bone imposes a painful fingertip with a "woody" character to it (*A, B*), causing the patient much discomfort and avoidance of the finger with object manipulation. A Bruner incision is designed over the volar index finger into the distal palm for access to the neurovascular pedicle (*C*). The lateral great toe donor flap incision is marked, extending proximally onto the dorsal foot for access to the first dorsal metatarsal artery (*D*). The pedicle is isolated (*E*) and the flap is mobilized (*F*). The flap is transferred with vascular anastomosis to the recipient site (*G*) and inset (*H, I*). The donor site healed well with minimal morbidity from scarring (*J*). Long-term follow-up (*K–M*), after a minor revision with a hyponychial free graft from the toe shown in **Fig. 7**, demonstrates a good functional and aesthetic outcome.

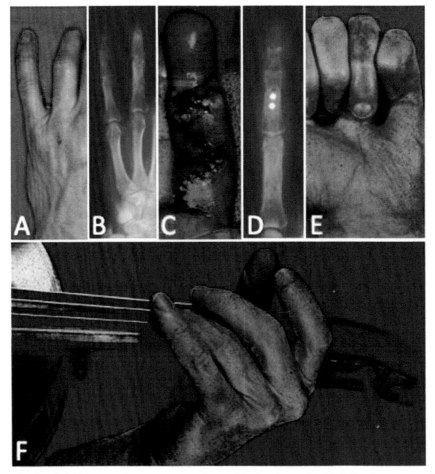

Fig. 22. A professional violinist sustained an amputation to his ring finger (*A, B*). Following a second toe, microvascular transfer to the ring finger (*C, D*), an aesthetic (*E*) and functional (*F*) outcome was achieved.

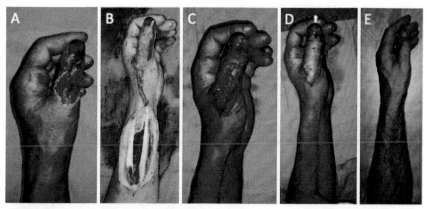

Fig. 23. Extensive dorsal thumb injury involving the eponychium and partial nail unit (*A*). A retrograde flow fascial flap is elevated and mobilized to be able to reach the area of the defect (*B*). The flap is tunneled under a skin bridge and inset onto the recipient site, while the donor site skin is closed primarily (*C*). A full-thickness skin graft is used to cover the fascial flap (*D*). Final long-term follow-up demonstrates an excellent aesthetic outcome (*E*). (*From* Taghinia AH, Carty M, Upton J. Fascial Flaps for Hand Reconstruction. J Hand Surg Am. 2010 Aug;35(8):1351-5; with permission.)

metatarsal artery. An illustrative case of a great toe pulp flap is shown in **Fig. 21**. The patient had a prior avulsion injury to the distal index finger with scarring adherent down to bone and a painful neuroma. The flap gave excellent aesthetic and functional recovery with resolution of the neuroma pain. In another case example, a total ring fingertip loss was replaced by second terminal toe

microvascular transfer (**Fig. 22**). This enabled the professional violinist to return to his musical proficiency.

RECONSTRUCTION OF THUMB DEFECTS

Because the thumb is shorter than the other digits, it is within reach of pedicle regional forearm flaps.

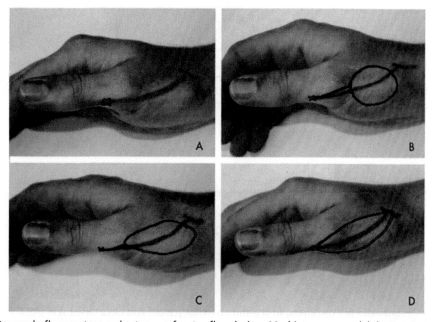

Fig. 24. Retrograde flow metacarpal artery perforator flap design. Markings on a model demonstrate the course of the metacarpal artery perforator with the pivot point marked by the "X"(*A*). Various flaps may be designed, centered over this vessel, which are turned over to cover a distal thumb wound (*B–D*). (*From* Hrabowski M, Kloeters O, Germann, G. Reverse Homodigital Dorsoradial Flap for Thumb Soft Tissue Reconstruction: Surgical Technique. J Hand Surg Am. 2010 Apr;35(4):659-62; with permission.)

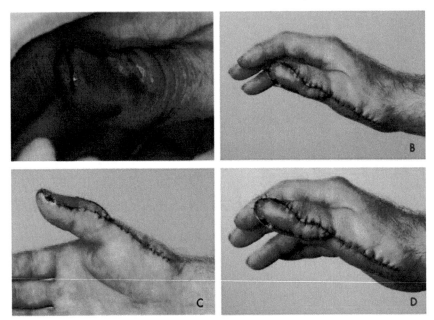

Fig. 25. A case example of an extensive dorsoradial thumb wound (*A*), following a retrograde metacarpal artery perforator flap reconstruction with primary closure of the donor site (*B–D*). (*From* Hrabowski M, Kloeters O, Germann, G. Reverse Homodigital Dorsoradial Flap for Thumb Soft Tissue Reconstruction: Surgical Technique. J Hand Surg Am. 2010 Apr;35(4):659-62; with permission.)

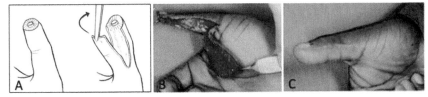

Fig. 26. An illustration of a Moberg flap for thumb coverage (*A*). This patient sustained a radiation injury to his thumb pulp several years prior with a painful scar of the pulp after handling radioactive material with an ungloved hand, for which a Moberg flap was performed (*B*) following debridement of the chronic pulp scar. Final follow-up demonstrates satisfactory functional and aesthetic (*C*) outcomes.

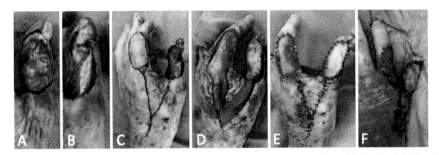

Fig. 27. Invasive squamous cell carcinoma of the thumb perionychium and ulnar-sided skin (*A*). Considering the patient's age and physical demands, the patient desired to avoid amputation of the thumb and elected to proceed with excision of the lesion (*B*), coverage with a first dorsal metacarpal artery flap (*C, D*), full-thickness skin grafting to the donor site (*E*), followed by radiation to help eradicate residual cancerous cells with a presumptive positive margin. Short-term follow-up, which included radiation therapy to the hand, demonstrates a good aesthetic (*F*) and functional outcome.

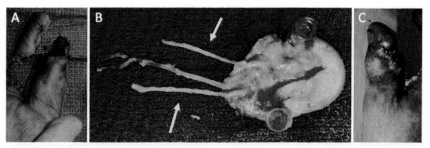

Fig. 28. An example of a partial thumb amputation with extensive pulp involvement (*A*). The amputated tip was prepared for replantation by nerve graft and vein grafting (*arrows*) the arteries on the back table (*B*) for adequate length to be able to perform the replantation with a successful anastomosis (*C*).

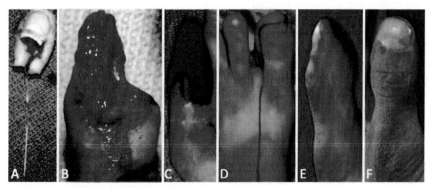

Fig. 29. Thumb tip amputation (*A, B*) with attempted replantation that failed (*C*). The thumb was revised with reconstruction using a partial toe transfer (*D*) with good functional and aesthetic (*E, F*) outcomes.

Table 1
Available surgical options for fingertip reconstructions

	Local Advancement Flaps				Staged Flaps			Island Flaps				Free Flaps
	V-Y Advancement (Atasoy)	Bilateral V-Y Advancement (Kutler)	Moberg	Rotation	Thenar	Cross-Finger	Reverse Cross-Finger	Antegrade Homodigital Artery	Retrograde Homodigital Artery	Heterodigital Artery	First Dorsal Metacarpal Artery	Partial Toe Transfer
Hyponychium & Distal Pulp												
Extensive Pulp & Paronychium												
Eponychium & Dorsal Skin												
Thumb (volar)												
Thumb (dorsal)												
Composite Loss of Multiple Subunits												

This is especially important for larger dorsal degloving injuries to the thumb that may extend all the way out to the nail unit. A radial forearm fascial flap may be ideal as a retrograde flow flap with the recipient area being skin grafted (**Fig. 23**). This actually gives more pleasing recipient aesthetics and avoids an unsightly skin graft at the volar forearm donor site.[28]

For slightly smaller dorsal thumb wounds, but nonetheless too large for cross-finger or heterodigital flaps and where the complexities of a free flap or regional flap might be avoided, metacarpal artery perforator flaps can be retrograde flaps and turned over from the metacarpal area and still allow direct suture wound closure of the donor site (**Fig. 24**). A case example of a radial-sided thumb wound treated with a retrograde metacarpal artery perforator flap is seen in **Fig. 25**.[29]

Reconstructive options for defects at the apex of the thumb and volar pulp depend to some extent on the size. The volar pulp of the thumb is much larger than a finger, and so lends itself well to V-Y Atasoy advancement flaps. A flap not possible on a finger is the Moberg flap whose vascular pedicle includes ulnar and radial digital neurovascular structures. The interphalangeal joint of the thumb is a little more "forgiving" than interphalangeal joints of fingers and so some of the deficiency in flap advancement may also be overcome by a small amount of thumb interphalangeal joint flexion. Distal advancement of up to 2 cm may be possible. Distal reach is increased by making an island of the flap and back-grafting or by V-Y advancement, which avoids a skin graft.[30] In the patient illustrated, he had painful thumb tip scarring from having accidently picked up some radioactive material without protective gloves (**Fig. 26**). After scar excision, the reconstruction was accomplished by Moberg advancement flap.

For larger volar defects, but also for apical and dorsal defects, a heterodigital flap based on the vascularity of the first dorsal metacarpal artery functions well. It is purported to have good sensibility through branches of the superficial radial sensory nerve, but we have found that the sensation is frequently referred back to the dorsum of the index finger. A case example of squamous cell carcinoma involving the thumb perionychium and extensive ulnar-sided skin that was excised and covered with a first dorsal metacarpal artery flap is presented (**Fig. 27**).[23] In an effort to bring sensate skin to the distal thumb pulp, Littler[21] ingeniously proposed bringing a sensate island flap from a less critical tactile area, such as the ulnar aspect of the ring finger. However, we seldom recommend this

option, because of provision of inadequate flap size, donor digit morbidity, and sensation being annoyingly referred back to the donor digit.

For larger volar pulp thumb defects, always try to reattach the avulsed part by replantation if at all possible. This may be technically demanding and require nerve and vein grafting (**Fig. 28**). However, it gives the most assured way of restoring optimum aesthetics and function. Should the amputated part be unusable or if replantation were to fail, then for these large defects a partial toe transfer by far provides the most suitable reconstruction, restoring the aesthetic and functional units (**Fig. 29**).

Clinical care points: complications and their avoidance

Some complication is avoided by following simple surgical "pearls":

1. Flap neurosis: Risk of vascular insufficiency of vascularized pedicle flaps may be minimized by maintaining a substantive fibrofatty "cuff" around the artery, particularly to avoid venous congestion. The pedicle should have adequate length to avoid unnecessary tension. Tourniquet deflation after insetting the flap may allow one to remove certain sutures if believed to be constricting.

2. Decreased fingertip sensation: This may result from iatrogenic nerve injury but may also result from excessive pedicle tension. However, it has also been shown that flaps, which do not carry a nerve, with time assume meaningful 2PD.[31]

3. Joint contractures: Contractures less commonly arise from linear scars crossing joint creases than they do from digital immobilization (as with cross-finger flaps) or inducing digital flexion to enable an island flap to reach its target. Avoid bringing the fingertip to meet the flap but rather reach the flap out to advance to the digital tip by sufficient flap pedicle mobilization.

4. Cold intolerance: This is common and has been reported in 31.8% of cross-finger flaps, 17% of thenar flaps, and 12% of reverse flow island flap reconstructions.[2,32,33] It is uncertain if the cause has a vascular or neural etiology and its presence may be more as a consequence of the original injury rather than the type of reconstruction.

5. Unfavorable aesthetics: With correct reconstructive choice and technical execution, these imperfections should be mild. However, it is not too uncommon to require minor flap debulking and recontouring, or Z-plasty to efface scars.

SUMMARY

Delayed finger and thumb tip reconstruction should try to optimally reconstruct perioncyhial aesthetic and functional units by replacing tissue as closely resembling the original loss as possible. We have tabulated reconstructive options that may be best suited to the digital tip subunit, and size of the defect (**Table 1**). Avoid thinking in terms of a "reconstructive ladder" but rather going directly to the reconstructive choice that seems most suited to the task. Some reconstructive choices may seem more attractive because of their simplicity, but may not necessarily give the best functional and aesthetic result. Free flaps and the newer advancements with vascular island flaps give many more and versatile reconstructive options.

DISCLOSURE

The authors have nothing to disclose.

REFERENCES

1. Haehnel O, Plancq MC, Deroussen F, et al. Long-term outcomes of Atasoy flap in children with distal finger trauma. J Hand Surg Am 2019;44(12):1097. e1-6.
2. Rabarin F, Saint Cast Y, Jeudy J, et al. Cross-finger flap for reconstruction of fingertip amputations: long-term results. Orthop Traumatol Surg Res 2016;102(4 Suppl):S225–8.
3. Gulec A, Ozdemir A, Durgut F, et al. Comparison of innervated digital artery perforator flap versus homodigital reverse flow flap techniques for fingertip reconstruction. J Hand Surg Am 2019;44(9):801. e1-6.
4. Arsalan-Werner A, Brui N, Mehling I, et al. Long-term outcome of fingertip reconstruction with the homodigital neurovascular island flap. Arch Orthop Trauma Surg 2019;139(8):1171–8.
5. Spyropoulou GA, Shih HS, Jeng SF. Free pulp transfer for fingertip reconstruction: the algorithm for complicated Allen fingertip defect. Plast Reconstr Surg Glob Open 2015;3(12):e584.
6. Kim HS, Lee DC, Kim JS, et al. Donor-site morbidity after partial second toe pulp free flap for fingertip reconstruction. Arch Plast Surg 2016;43(1):66–70.
7. Kutler W. A new method for finger tip amputation. J Am Med Assoc 1947;133(1):29.
8. Atasoy E, Ioakimidis E, Kasdan ML, et al. Reconstruction of the amputated finger tip with a triangular volar flap. A new surgical procedure. J Bone Joint Surg Am 1970;52(5):921–6.
9. Moberg E. Aspects of sensation in reconstructive surgery of the upper extremity. The J bone Jt Surg Am volume 1964;46:817–25.
10. Cronin TD. The cross finger flap: a new method of repair. Am Surg 1951;17(5):419–25.
11. Meals RA, Brody GS. Gatewood and the first thenar pedicle. Plast Reconstr Surg 1984;73(2):315–9.
12. Cohen BE, Cronin ED. An innervated cross-finger flap for fingertip reconstruction. Plast Reconstr Surg 1983;72(5):688–97.
13. Atasoy E. Reversed cross-finger subcutaneous flap. J Hand Surg Am 1982;7(5):481–3.
14. Strauch B, de Moura W. Arterial system of the fingers. J Hand Surg Am 1990;15(1):148–54.
15. Lanzetta M, Mastropasqua B, Chollet A, et al. Versatility of the homodigital triangular neurovascular island flap in fingertip reconstruction. J Hand Surg Br 1995;20(6):824–9.
16. Evans DM, Martin DL. Step-advancement island flap for fingertip reconstruction. Br J Plast Surg 1988; 41(2):105–11.
17. Kojima T, Tsuchida Y, Hirase Y, et al. Reverse vascular pedicle digital island flap. Br J Plast Surg 1990;43(3):290–5.
18. Venkataswami R, Subramanian N. Oblique triangular flap: a new method of repair for oblique amputations of the fingertip and thumb. Plast Reconstr Surg 1980;66(2):296–300.
19. Foucher G, Smith D, Pempinello C, et al. Homodigital neurovascular island flaps for digital pulp loss. J Hand Surg Br 1989;14(2):204–8.
20. Foucher G, Khouri RK. Digital reconstruction with island flaps. Clin Plast Surg 1997;24(1):1–32.
21. Littler JW. The neurovascular pedicle method of digital transposition for reconstruction of the thumb. Plast Reconstr Surg (1946) 1953;12(5): 303–19.
22. Pham DT, Netscher DT. Vascularized heterodigital island flap for fingertip and dorsal finger reconstruction. J Hand Surg Am 2015;40(12):2458–64.
23. Foucher G, Braun JB. A new island flap transfer from the dorsum of the index to the thumb. Plast Reconstr Surg 1979;63(3):344–9.
24. Chen J, Bhatt R, Tang JB. Technical points of 5 free vascularized flaps for the hand repairs. Hand Clin 2017;33(3):443–54.
25. Yan H, Ouyang Y, Chi Z, et al. Digital pulp reconstruction with free neurovascular toe flaps. Aesthet Plast Surg 2012;36(5):1186–93.
26. Atasoy E. The reverse cross finger flap. J Hand Surg Am 2016;41(1):122–8.
27. Tsai FC, Cheng MH, Chen HC, et al. Microsurgical medialis pedis flaps for reconstruction of soft-tissue defects in the hand. Ann Plast Surg 2002; 48(1):41–7.
28. Taghinia AH, Carty M, Upton J. Fascial flaps for hand reconstruction. J Hand Surg Am 2010;35(8): 1351–5.
29. Hrabowski M, Kloeters O, Germann G. Reverse homodigital dorsoradial flap for thumb soft tissue

reconstruction: surgical technique. J Hand Surg Am 2010;35(4):659–62.

30. Mutaf M, Temel M, Gunal E, et al. Island volar advancement flap for reconstruction of thumb defects. Ann Plast Surg 2012;68(2):153–7.

31. Lai CS, Lin SD, Chou CK, et al. A versatile method for reconstruction of finger defects: reverse digital artery flap. Br J Plast Surg 1992;45(6):443–53.

32. Regmi S, Gu JX, Zhang NC, et al. A systematic review of outcomes and complications of primary fingertip reconstruction using reverse-flow homodigital island flaps. Aesthet Plast Surg 2016;40(2): 277–83.

33. Rinker B. Fingertip reconstruction with the laterally based thenar flap: indications and long-term functional results. Hand (N Y). 2006;1(1):2–8.

Microsurgical Free Tissue Options for Fingertip Reconstruction

Min Ki Hong, MD, Jin Ha Park, MD, Sung Hoon Koh, MD, PhD,
Dong Chul Lee, MD, Si Young Roh, MD, PhD, Kyung Jin Lee, MD,
Jin Soo Kim, MD, PhD*

KEYWORDS

- Microsurgery • Fingertip • Reconstruction • Free flap • Soft tissue defect • Digit

KEY POINTS

- Reconstructive options for hand injuries, when considering fingertip injuries, the location of damage should be considered.
- The important thing is to use a similar texture, "like with like" tissue.
- One special thing is that the nailbed is located in the dorsum of the fingertip, which has special tissues different from any other part of the finger.

INTRODUCTION

Hand injuries can occur anywhere, anytime in everyday life. In modern society, the use of power tools is indispensable for many jobs, increasing the probability of causing defects or disabilities in the hands.[1] When replantation is not possible, there are various options to reconstruct the hand after injury; however, reconstruction methods are not all the same, and method selection depends on the characteristics, size, and severity of the wound. Therefore, various reconstructive options can be considered for managing each unique patient and injury.

Reconstructive treatment for hand injuries, especially when considering fingertip injuries, can be largely classified into nonmicrosurgical methods and microsurgical methods.[2] Local flaps and skin grafts can be used for relatively minor damage. Local flaps can be selected depending on the damaged area and the size of the defect, including the thenar flap, cross-finger flap, V-Y flap, or Moberg flap.[3,4] However, if in a condition of severe contamination or extensive defect,

reconstruction with these flaps is inadequate. Also, when limitations in motion are expected owing to involvement of the joint, local flap, or skin graft should not be used.

In these cases, microsurgical free tissue transfer is an excellent reconstructive option. Owing to the development of microsurgical technology and equipment, even small vessels in the fingertip can be maneuvered easily compared with the past. When choosing a free flap, the location and size of the defect, a surgeon's experience, microsurgical skill, and preference should be considered. Sensation and appearance of the fingertip are important factors in reconstruction, so whether innervation is possible and appearance after reconstruction should also be considered. With the development of microsurgical skill, many methods for fingertip reconstruction have been introduced. In this article, various surgical methods for treating fingertip defects that have been introduced previously are summarized. The free flaps shown in **Fig. 1** are used for fingertip reconstruction in different locations.

Funding: None.

Department of Plastic and Reconstructive Surgery, Gwangmyeong Sungae General Hospital, 36 Digital-ro, Gwangmyeong 14241, South Korea
* Corresponding author.
E-mail address: hlaze@hanmail.net

Hand Clin 37 (2021) 97–106
https://doi.org/10.1016/j.hcl.2020.09.002
0749-0712/21/© 2020 Elsevier Inc. All rights reserved.

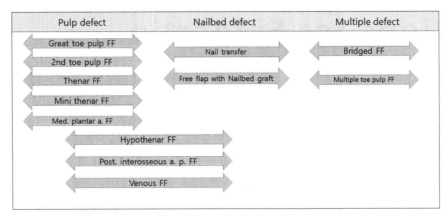

Fig. 1. Use of various free flaps (FF) based on different defect location.

Dorsal and volar sides of fingers have distinctly different properties. This nature is more prominent at the level of the metacarpophalangeal joint, metacarpal bone, wrist, and forearm, but it also shows a clear difference in the fingertip, including the distal phalanx. One special thing is that the nail bed is located in the dorsum of the fingertip, which has special properties different from any other part of the finger. If there is a defect in this area, there is no other method other than to take and graft another nail bed from a different finger or toe, and this becomes impossible when the defect is severe. In addition, in the case of the pulp, it is necessary to make the fingertip in a rounded shape rather than a flat shape, so it is necessary to consider the reconstruction in 3 dimensions.

FREE FLAP OPTIONS
Pulp Defect

Among the fingertip defects, when approaching a pulp defect it is important to consider that this area has a critical role in pinching and grasping. Therefore, to obtain excellent results, sensory recovery must be achieved. Here we review the reconstructive options that can provide recovery of sensation as well as restoration of functional and cosmetic aspects.

Great toe pulp free flap
Toe pulp flap is a very effective flap for reconstructing pulp defects. The greatest advantage of this flap is that it can bring tissue with the same texture as what was lost. The first dorsal metatarsal artery is mainly used as a donor vessel, and because a great toe is used as a donor, a relatively larger flap can be harvested than a second toe pulp flap. Therefore, it can be used to cover large defects in the thumb pulp (**Fig. 2**).[5,6] In

addition, there is an advantage in that the digital nerves of the great toe can be coapted to digital nerve of the finger. Because the scar after toe pulp harvest is located on the foot, the donor site is usually hidden; but, for patients who wear flip flops or sandals often, the scar may be frequently seen, and the cosmetic downside of this donor site becomes more impactful for these patients.

Also, when harvesting larger pulp flaps, donor sites cannot be closed primarily. In this case, a skin graft can be used, or it can be left to heal via secondary intention. However, if left to heal, the condition of donor site will often be poor, and chronic pain or toenail deformity may occur.

Second toe pulp free flap
The second toe pulp flap, like the great toe pulp flap, is useful for reconstructing pulp defects. After the second toe pulp flap was introduced, it became one of the popular surgical options in many hand clinics, including our center. This technique can be a very good option for use with relatively small defects in digits other than the thumb (**Fig. 3**). This tissue has glabrous skin, and the texture is very similar to the finger pulp.[7,8] It can be used not only for reconstruction of defects confined to pulp, but if there are defects that include a little nail bed along with pulp defects, a "like with like" tissue with a pulp and nail bed can be used in toe as an onychocutaneous free flap. Unlike the great toe free flap, most second toe donor sites can be closed primarily, and patient satisfaction with the donor site is high because scars of the donor site occur on the medial side of the toe.

Radial artery superficial palmar branch free flap (Thenar free flap)
The radial artery superficial palmar (RASP) branch free flap (thenar free flap), which uses the

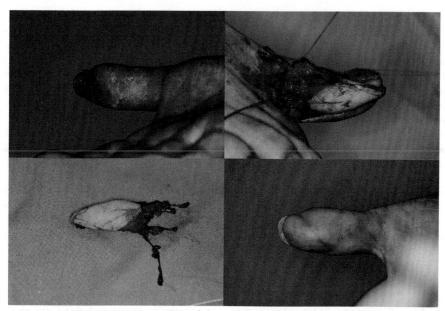

Fig. 2. Great toe pulp free flap. This patient sustained an injury from an electric saw. After debridement of the defect, a great toe pulp free flap was harvested from the medial side of the great toe. The flap inset excellently, and glabrous skin of the toe pulp works similarly to finger pulp as seen in a follow-up photo.

superficial palmar branch of the radial artery as a pedicle, can also be a good reconstruction option to obtain glabrous skin for covering volar defects.[7] It can be used in situations where the defect size is relatively large and difficult to cover with a toe pulp flap. Also, an innervated RASP branch flap can also be used and can provide good sensory recovery at the fingertip.[9]

This RASP free flap has the advantage of not only obtaining tissue with a texture that matches

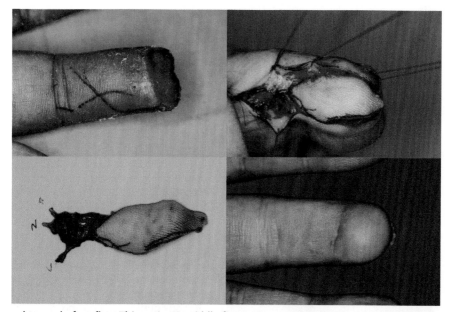

Fig. 3. Second toe pulp free flap. This patient's middle finger tip was amputated with crushing injury. Replantation was performed but subsequently failed. After debridement, a second toe pulp free flap was harvested from the medial side of the second toe. Glabrous skin provides an excellent aesthetic and functional result.

the fingertip, but also harvesting a flap of adequately large dimension that can cover relatively large defects. According to anatomic studies, the superficial palmar branch of the radial artery and the palmar cutaneous branch of the median nerve can always be included into the flap, thereby completing the innervation of the flap. Another advantage of this flap is that the direct skin perforator is in a relatively constant position, so a reliable artery can be almost always obtained. The size of the artery is similar to a digital artery, and it can be anastomosed easily. Also, preparation for surgery is simpler because the entire surgery is performed in a single operative field. The flap can be harvested in the superficial layer from the palmar aponeurosis and can minimize donor morbidity by closing the donor site primarily (**Fig. 4**).

Thenar mini free flap

A thenar mini free flap can be obtained from the metacarpophalangeal flexion crease of the thumb, distal to the classic thenar free flap (**Fig 5**). The radial digital artery of the thumb is used as a pedicle and the flap can be completed using a palmar vein.[10] It is easy to get a relatively small flap and minimizes donor morbidity, so there is almost no donor site complication. Texture and color can be quite similar to the defect site, and this flap can be used with other flaps introduced previously to cover multiple defects.

Hypothenar free flap

The hypothenar free flap is also an ideal choice for coverage of pulp defects (**Fig. 6**). As it was initially described, the flap perforator was found by using a hand-held Doppler device, but the size of the pedicle was not consistent, so some flaps had to be converted to an arterialized venous free flap. Recent technique modifications have identified that a pedicle with sufficient length and diameter can be obtained by using the perforator of the fourth common digital artery with improved reliability. The hypothenar free flap is also appealing because it can be done in a single operative field, and color and texture matching for volar soft tissues is also excellent.[11] However, the diameter of the perforator is often less than 1 mm, so it is necessary to have skilled microsurgical technique for this flap.

Arterialized venous free flap

Arterialized venous free flaps are also an option used by many surgeons to reconstruct fingertips. Usually, this flap is harvested from the forearm using a subcutaneous vein, and anastomosed with the volar digital artery and dorsal vein of the recipient site.[12] However, a unique advantage of this flap concept is that any of the other flaps described can be converted to a venous flap if the pedicle is damaged or circulation is not clear during surgery. The major downside to this flap is that congestion is unpredictable. Additionally,

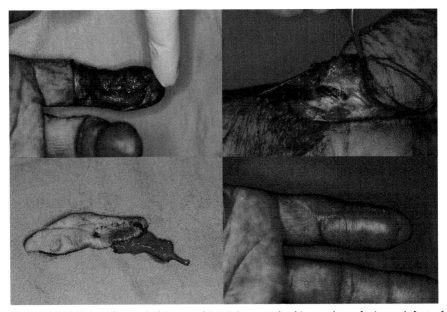

Fig. 4. An innervated RASP free flap. A belting machine injury resulted in a volar soft tissue defect of the index finger with exposure of flexor tendon. It had the right size and location to perform a thenar free flap. From the follow-up photo, you can see that it has a texture similar to native volar skin.

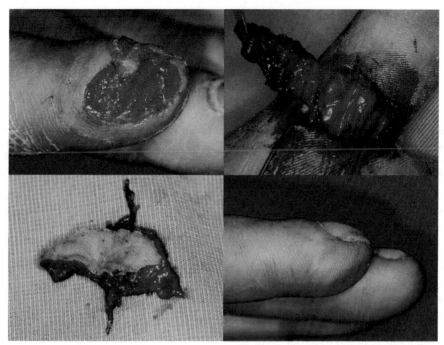

Fig. 5. Thenar mini free flap.

after these flaps heal, instability during pinching or grasping is often noted and is a substantial downside. However, if a good donor site for other free flap options is limited or unavailable, this flap should be considered.

Medial plantar artery perforator free flap

The medial plantar artery perforator free flap (**Fig. 7**) uses the foot as a donor site, similar to the medialis pedis flap. This flap also provides a texture that matches well for covering volar

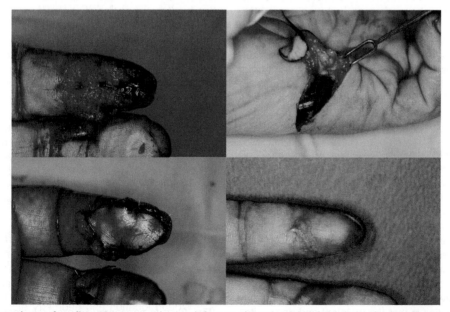

Fig. 6. Hypothenar free flap. This patient had a defect on the volar side of the index finger after injury from a press machine without. Almost all volar soft tissue was absent, so sufficient glabrous skin was needed. Hypothenar free flap was an excellent choice to cover the volar defect.

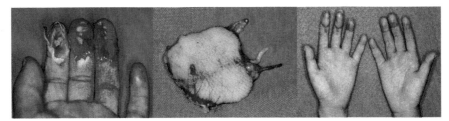

Fig. 7. Medial plantar artery perforator free flap. To cover a volar defect on 3 adjacent fingers, a medial plantar artery perforator free flap was the best choice to provide glabrous skin for 3 fingers. 3 weeks after free flap was performed, survival of the free flap was confirmed. The single free flap was divided and inset to each finger with proper shape and contour for all 3 fingers.

defects.[13] For this flap, the main branch to the foot is not used so as to preserve the major vessels that supply blood to the foot. In the medialis pedis flap, the donor site is often impossible to close primarily, and the location of scar causes pain when wearing shoes. This issue is made better by moving the scar to the plantar surface. Although this change decreased complications associated with the medialis pedis flap, the donor site still is not always able to be closed primarily. Also, the scar is located on the tubercle of the navicular bone, so persistent discomfort can be a problem.

Dorsoulnar perforator free flap
The dorsoulnar perforator free flap uses a dorsoulnar branch off the ulnar artery that can be found 2 to 4 cm proximal to the pisiform. This branch comes from the ulnar artery after passing the flexor carpi ulnaris in the distal forearm. In this flap, a dorsoulnar nerve can almost always can be included, which provides the option for a neurosensory flap. This flap can be performed in a single operative field and has the advantage of being able to elevate a very thin flap with less fatty tissue than other flaps.[14] Also, this flap can be transformed to composite tissue transfer with tendon or nerve. But, transient numbness may occur because of the use of the dorsoulnar nerve.

Posterior interosseous artery perforator free flap
The posterior interosseous artery perforator flap can be designed in various shapes and sizes. It can be used to reconstruct small defects and larger defects and is not only limited to the fingertips.[15–19] This flap is often used for reconstruction of the hand and forearm. Multiple perforators originate from the posterior interosseous artery, so 2 or more flaps can be designed. A wrap-around flap for fingertip defects can also be performed because a relatively large flap can be designed and harvested.

The advantage of this flap in upper extremity reconstruction is that the recipient and donor sites are in a single operative field, which, like many of the other flaps mentioned, allows for the procedure

to be performed with brachial plexus block. Additionally, because the forearm is used as the donor site, the surgery can be performed with a tourniquet applied to the upper arm. The flap is thin and pliable, so it can be made to fit many different shapes and defects and has the advantage that color and texture are similar to the hand or finger.

Free Tissue Reconstruction of Nail Defects

Groin flaps, anterolateral thigh flaps, radial forearm flaps, or dorsalis pedis flaps have traditionally been used to cover dorsal defects. Coverage is reliable, but flap bulkiness is a major challenge. To solve this problem, a flap would need to be thin and be able to be stretched when bending a finger. Flaps to cover dorsal defects that satisfy these conditions are very limited. For many of these defects, using a free fascial flap (eg, anterolateral thigh or lateral arm) and then subsequently putting a skin graft on the incorporated fascial flap is often our option of choice.

However, dorsal defects become far more complicated when the nail bed and/or nail fold are involved. Reconstruction is often done using flaps that do not address partial or complete defects of the nail bed. However, considering the cosmetic aspect, it is good to rebuild the nail bed for dorsal fingertip defects. When there is a partial defect in the nail bed, the best reconstructive option is to use a toe pulp free flap and bring some of the nail bed with it. If there is a complete nail bed defect, a nail bed graft may be performed after a fascial flap; however, free nail transfer may be performed and might be a better option, depending on the defect.

Toe pulp free flap with nail bed transfer
In a situation with a partial defect on the distal or lateral side of the nail bed along with a defect of the fingertip, second toe pulp free flap can be performed with part of the nail bed included in the flap (**Fig. 8**). It is necessary to precisely measure the fingertip nail bed defect, and the free flap should be accurately designed to reconstruct the exact

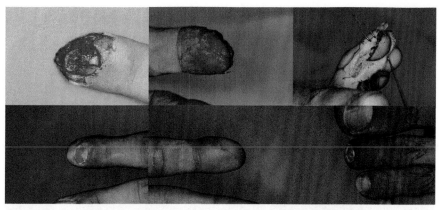

Fig. 8. Second toe pulp free flap with nail bed transfer. This patient had a fingertip injury from a press machine. The defect included about 20% of the distal nail bed. In this case, a second toe pulp free flap including partial nail bed was used for reconstruction of the intact nail bed. The toe nail bed was included in the free flap and precisely matched to the defect of the finger nail bed. During follow-up, the involved toenail and fingernail both grew with satisfactory cosmetic appearance.

defect of the nail bed. The toenail of the donor site tends to grow without any problems after harvest and it does not have notable functional or cosmetic deformity (see **Fig. 8**).

Free nail transfer

When there is complete loss of the dorsal fingertip and nail bed, free nail transfer is a relatively complete method of reconstruction. The size of the second toenail is similar to a fingernail, and it can be transferred to replace a fingernail. In contract to a full the second toe transfer that can leave a cosmetically severe deformity of the foot, free nail transfer is far less extensive and is relatively satisfactory to patients because only the toenail and surrounding soft tissue is transferred (**Fig 9**).

Reconstruction for Multiple Defects

All of the flaps introduced in this article are small to intermediate sized flaps that are limited to specific locations and defects. Alternatively, defects may occur simultaneously in multiple adjacent fingers. In this case, free flaps on each finger can be a burden to surgeons. In addition, in the case of defects over a large area, it is insufficient to provide coverage with only a fascial free flap and skin graft. A sufficient amount of soft tissue is required in wide defects. If there is a wide defect including the interphalangeal joint of the thumb or the distal interphalangeal joint of the fingers, or if there is a defect in the tendon, simply covering it with soft tissue shortens the length of the finger and likely cannot provide satisfactory motion later.

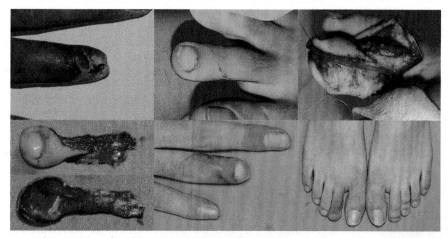

Fig. 9. Free second toenail transfer. This patient had a ring finger without nail growth and with associated deformity of the nail bed. Because the patient wanted full nail growth, a free nail transfer using the second toe was performed. The second toenail was sacrificed to give the nail of the ring finger a complete reconstruction.

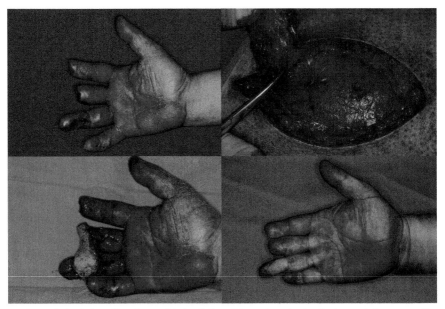

Fig. 10. Anterolateral thigh free flap for multiple digits. This patient had soft tissue defects on adjacent middle and ring fingers. Rather than perform 2 free flaps, it was decided to connect an anterolateral thigh as a bridge. After the flap was incorporated, division was performed 3 weeks after the initial free flap surgery. With this method it was possible to decrease the number of free flaps to one and perform efficient surgery.

Alternatively, there are some flap options that allow for multiple digit reconstruction.

Bridged free flap

If the size of the defect is very large or there is a defect in multiple digits, a larger flap may be needed. In this case, defects can be covered using a sizable free flap such as the anterolateral thigh or lateral arm flap, or moderate sized flaps like the RASP free flap or medial plantar artery perforator free flap. If multiple digits require resurfacing, making a temporary syndactyly with a single free flap is recommended.[20–25] When doing this, the vein can be anastomosed with opposite finger which makes a preferable situation that blood is supplied from one side and drained to the opposite side. Subsequent division is done around 3 to 4 weeks when flap survival becomes clear. It is possible

to then create the ideal shape by trimming and thinning flaps to match the shape of the defect (**Figs. 10** and **11**).

Multiple free flaps for multiple defects

If there are relatively uniform defects on multiple fingers, and the best option for each defect is to use a specific free flap, multiple free flaps can be performed. In particular, when there are 2 or more defects in the volar pulp of each finger, multiple toe pulp free flaps are recommended. Unlike other free flaps, the toe pulp free flap can be harvested from the great toe, second toe, and third toe as donors, and can be used as a donor for up to 6 toe pulp free flaps when using both feet (**Fig 12**). It may be a burden for the surgeon to do multiple free flaps at once, but for surgeons who are familiar with these flaps it can be overall more efficient than

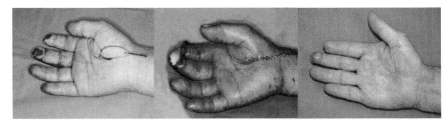

Fig. 11. An innervated RASP free flap for adjacent 2 fingers. This patient had finger pulp and volar soft tissue defects on the index and middle fingers. Because the size of the defect on each finger was relatively small, a large flap was not required. We chose a RASP free flap as the flap with the most appropriate size to cover both defects and provide sensation, and the flap was inset as a bridge across both fingers. Division was done 3 weeks after free flap, and both sides of the flap survived without any complication.

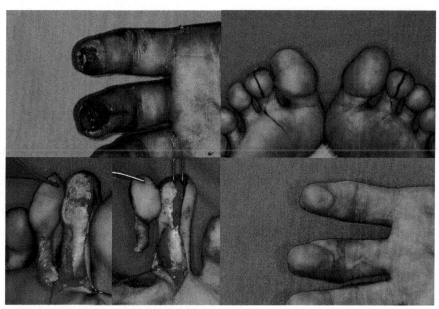

Fig. 12. Multiple second toe pulp free flaps. This patient had fingertip and volar pulp defects with bone exposure on both the small and ring fingers. Both fingers needed glabrous skin for grasping, so second toe pulp free flap was designed to reconstruct a glabrous fingertip on both fingers. Both donor sites were closed primarily, and both fingertips had adequate soft tissue and glabrous skin.

having to return to an operating room to divide a bridged free flap. It also might be less of a challenge for the patient to undergo 1 longer surgery rather than 2 surgeries for a bridged free flap.

SUMMARY

Free flaps for fingertip reconstruction are not limited to 1 or 2 types, but can be selected and used in various ways depending on the defect area or size and the patient's condition. If the defect is not large or the microsurgical experience is insufficient, defects can be covered using local flaps or regional flaps, but more options are available when microsurgical free tissue transfer is possible. This can maintain the length of the finger and restore some sensation. With the development of microsurgery various free flaps have been introduced, but some research results show that there is no distinct difference in quality between various free flaps.[26] However, the author believes there is an efficient flap depending on the location of the defect.

In case of a pulp or volar defect, toe pulp free flap is considered to be the best option for reconstruction. If the flap is harvested with a similar size and location from the toe pulp to match the size and location of the defect, the anatomic similarity can be maintained and reconstruction can provide a good replacement for the lost tissue. Functional and cosmetically good results have been reported in several studies.[27]

Various options are available to cover volar defects. Depending on the size of the defect and surgeon preference, thenar free flaps, hypothenar free flaps, and medial plantar artery perforator free flap can be used to cover volar fingertip defects. In addition to pulp soft tissue, recovery of sensation is an important factor in reconstructing volar defects, Therefore, using a sensate free flap can improve the outcome and increase patient satisfaction. Also, tailoring the flap so it is not too thick or bulky will improve results for grasping or pinching.

Thin and pliable tissue is needed to cover dorsal defects. If the purpose is to cover the defect, any flap mentioned in this article can be used; however, if you consider cosmetic factors as well as the motion of the distal interphalangeal joint and/or reconstruction of the nail complex, the reconstruction options become quite limited. The authors believe that a good option for solving this problem is to perform a fascial free flap followed by skin graft or nail bed graft after incorporation. Fascia only flaps can be harvested by using an anterolateral thigh or lateral arm as a donor. If a skin graft or nail bed graft is performed after survival of the free flap, it can achieve a satisfactory reconstruction both functionally and cosmetically. Alternatively, when reconstructing partial or complete nail complex defects, a free toe pulp with nail bed component (for partial defect) or free nail transfer (for a complete defect) should be considered.

Numerous methods have been used to reconstruct fingertip defects. Depending on the location and size of the defect, there are defects that can be covered with local flaps or regional flaps, but there are cases that better shape and functional results can be obtained by using free flaps. Fingertip reconstruction using a free flap requires highly skillful microsurgical technique, and to reach this, there is a learning curve for surgeons. However, reconstruction using one of the small tailored free flaps discussed in this article can minimize donor site morbidity, facilitate early mobilization, and improve sensory recovery, making these flaps an excellent option even though greater efforts are required.

CLINICS CARE POINTS

- Most importantly, we must have skillful surgical technique, but also confidence to reconstruction. Always pay attention to the arteries and veins that will connect the flap. Anyone can have a successful reconstruction if they operate while paying attention to the basic principles of tissue transfer surgery.

DISCLOSURE

None to declare.

REFERENCES

1. Kim YH, Choi JH, Chung YK, et al. Epidemiologic study of hand and upper extremity injuries by power tools. Arch Plast Surg 2019;46(1):63–8.
2. Bennet N, Choudhary S. Why climb a ladder when you can take the elevator? Plast Reconstr Surg 2000;105:2266.
3. Bickel KD, Dosanjh A. Fingertip reconstruction. J Hand Surg Am 2008;33(8):1417–9.
4. Foucher G, Boulas HJ, Da Silva JB. The use of flaps in the treatment of fingertip injuries. World J Surg 1991;15:458–62.
5. Zheng H, Liu J, Dai X, et al. Free lateral great toe flap for the reconstruction of finger pulp defects. J Reconstr Microsurg 2015;31:277–82.
6. Balan JR. Free toe pulp flap for finger pulp and volar defect reconstruction. Indian J Plast Surg 2016;49(2):178–84.
7. Lee DC, Kim JS, Ki SH, et al. Partial second toe pulp free flap for fingertip reconstruction. Plast Reconstr Surg 2008;121(3):899–907.
8. Lee SH, Cheon SJ, Kim YJ. Clinical application of a free radial artery superficial palmar branch flap for soft-tissue reconstruction of digital injuries. J Hand Surg Eur 2017;42(2):151–6.
9. Yang JW, Kim JS, Lee DC, et al. The radial artery superficial palmar branch flap: a modified free thenar flap with constant innervation. J Reconstr Microsurg 2010;26(8):529–38.
10. Tsai TM, Sabapathy SR, Martin D. Revascularization of a finger with a thenar mini-free flap. J Hand Surg Am 1991;16(4):604–6.
11. Kim KS, Kim ES, Hwang JH, et al. Fingertip reconstruction using the hypothenar perforator free flap. J Plast Reconstr Aesthet Surg 2013;66(9):1263–70.
12. Kong BS, Kim YJ, Suh YS, et al. Finger soft tissue reconstruction using arterialized venous free flaps having 2 parallel veins. J Hand Surg Am 2008; 33(10):1802–6.
13. Huang SH, Wu SH, Lai CH, et al. Free medial plantar artery perforator flap for finger pulp reconstruction: report of a series of 10 cases. Microsurgery 2010; 30(2):118–24.
14. Inada Y, Tamai S, Kawanishi K, et al. Free dorsoulnar perforator flap transfers for the reconstruction of severely injured digits. Plast Reconstr Surg 2004; 114(2):411–20.
15. Ishiko T, Nakaima N, Suzuki S. Free posterior interosseous artery perforator flap for finger reconstruction. J Plast Reconstr Aesthet Surg 2009;62(7):e211–5.
16. Tonkin M, Stern H. The posterior interosseous artery free flap. J Hand Surg Br 1989;14(2):215–7.
17. Carty MJ, Taghinia A, Upton J. Fascial flap reconstruction of the hand: a single surgeon's 30-year experience. Plast Reconstr Surg 2010;125:953–62.
18. Taghinia AH, Carty M, Upton J. Fascial flaps for hand reconstruction. J Hand Surg Am 2010;35: 1351–5.
19. Lee KJ, Kim YW, Kim JS, et al. Nail bed defect reconstruction using a thenar fascial flap and subsequent nail bed grafting. Arch Plast Surg 2019;46(1):57–62.
20. Das De S, Sebastin SJ. Considerations in flap selection for soft tissue defects of the hand. Clin Plast Surg 2019;46(3):393–406.
21. Gosain AK, Matloub HS, Yousif NJ, et al. The composite lateral arm free flap: vascular relationship to triceps tendon and muscle. Ann Plast Surg 1992; 29(6):496–507.
22. Haas F, Rappl T, Koch H, et al. Free osteocutaneous lateral arm flap: anatomy and clinical applications. Microsurgery 2003;23(2):87–95.
23. Gu YD, Zhang GM, Cheng DS, et al. Free toe transfer for thumb and finger reconstruction in 300 cases. Plast Reconstr Surg 1993;91(4):693–700.
24. Henry SL, Wei FC. Thumb reconstruction with toe transfer. J Hand Microsurg 2010;2(2):72–8.
25. Chung KC, Wei FC. An outcome study of thumb reconstruction using microvascular toe transfer. J Hand Surg Am 2000;5(4):651–8.
26. Liu Y, Jiao H, Ji X, et al. A comparative study of four types of free flaps from the ipsilateral extremity for finger reconstruction. PLoS One 2014;9(8): e104014.
27. Gu JX, Pan JB, Liu HJ, et al. Aesthetic and sensory reconstruction of finger pulp defects using free toe flaps. Aesthetic Plast Surg 2014;38(1):156–63.

Pediatric Fingertip Injuries

Scott N. Loewenstein, MD[a], Joshua M. Adkinson, MD[b],*

KEYWORDS

- Fingers • Pediatric • Soft tissue injuries • Crush injuries • Amputation • Nails • Bone fractures
- Open fractures

KEY POINTS

- Pediatric fingertip injuries are common and represent a major source of trauma in children.
- Nail bed injuries with concomitant distal phalanx fractures are common.
- Although a variety of options are available for soft tissue reconstruction of the fingertip, the intrinsic healing potential in children often allows for an initially conservative approach.
- The presence of a physis results in unique fracture patterns (eg, Seymour fracture), and these require a thoughtful approach to treatment.
- Replantation distal to the distal interphalangeal joint in children is technically difficult, and acceptable long-term outcomes can be obtained with composite grafting in young children.

BACKGROUND

Fingertip injuries in children most commonly result from a crush mechanism,[1–6] and door jambs frequently are implicated.[1,7] Although children of all ages may sustain these injuries, there is a peak at approximately 2 years old.[1,4,7] At this age, children have developed sufficient gross and fine motor skills to explore their environment, but rational decision making and consequence awareness lag behind, which puts their fingers at risk. Furthermore, a common presentation involves a parent or sibling closing the door without realizing that the child's finger is in the door jamb.

The longer digits are more susceptible to injury because they protrude furthest from the hand: the middle and ring fingers are the most commonly injured digits, and the thumb and small finger are the least commonly injured digits in children.[1,8] A single digit frequently is injured, although multiple digits are at risk, especially in cases of a sliding window falling onto the hand.[1] Other causes of nontraumatic fingertip injuries, including burn, frostbite, and hair tourniquet syndrome, are not expanded on in this review.

EVALUATION

The evaluation of pediatric fingertip injuries begins with a complete history and physical examination. Often, these patients present acutely to an emergency department (ED), and the initial provider follows advanced trauma life support protocol to assess for other injuries. Most pediatric fingertip injuries, however, occur in the absence of other trauma. Midazolam and intranasal fentanyl can facilitate examining the child that is anxious or in pain. Reassurance helps alleviate guilt in a parent or caregiver who may have caused the injury and builds a rapport that can be leveraged to examine and treat the child. Building a relationship with the patient and caregiver helps facilitate the physical examination.

Dried blood causes the bandage applied at home or ED to be adherent to the patient (ie, "blood cast") and difficult to remove for examination. Soaking the dressing in warm, soapy water

[a] Division of Plastic Surgery, Integrated Plastic Surgery Residency Program, Indiana University School of Medicine, 545 Barnhill Drive, Emerson Hall, Suite 232, Indianapolis, IN 46202, USA; [b] Division of Plastic Surgery, Sidney and Lois S. Eskenazi Hospital, Indiana University School of Medicine, 545 Barnhill Drive, Emerson Hall, Suite 232, Indianapolis, IN 46202, USA
* Corresponding author.
E-mail address: jadkinso@iu.edu

Hand Clin 37 (2021) 107–116
https://doi.org/10.1016/j.hcl.2020.09.009
0749-0712/21/© 2020 Elsevier Inc. All rights reserved.

can make it less painful during removal. If the child does not trust the provider, asking the parent or the child to remove the bandage may help accomplish the task. As an adjunct, 3% hydrogen peroxide applied with a cotton-tipped applicator removes blood and facilitates visualizing the damage.

Once the wound is visible, the provider can perform a careful appraisal of the injury. The alignment of the distal phalanx is assessed to ensure there is no deviation in the radioulnar or dorsovolar planes. Hematoma under the nail plate should be evaluated for, which may suggest nail bed laceration. Capillary refill in the distal finger pulp is assessed as are the statuses of the perionychia and nail plate. Proximal nail plate subluxation can be associated with a displaced germinal matrix and nail bed; these coexisting conditions may be overlooked by an inexperienced provider.

In the young patient, motor and tendon examination is performed by asking the child to grab an object, observing them during activity, squeezing on the flexor aspect of the forearm, and passively flexing and extending their wrist to observe cascade during tenodesis maneuvers. Parents and caregivers can assist with examination if the child is reluctant to comply. Sensation can be assessed by having the child close their eyes, turn their head away, and report when they feel the provider touching them. Frequently, decreased sensation is present with isolated fingertip injuries, but in the authors' experience most blunt injuries with sensory changes can be monitored and have long-term restoration of protective normal or near-normal sensation.

Half of pediatric fingertip injuries have an associated fracture[1]; therefore, nearly all should undergo a radiograph. Fractures involving the physis can be subtle, so extreme care should be taken while assessing the bone segments proximal and distal to the physis on radiograph. Sometimes, the extent of soft tissue damage cannot be determined in the ED, so operative exploration under sedation must be performed prior to definitive repair.

ANESTHESIA

Once the provider determines that a repair is indicated, the appropriate anesthesia, treatment environment, and timing must be chosen. The child's ability to keep the finger motionless during the procedure is a key determinant of the anesthesia technique employed. The repair may be performed with a digital block and conscious sedation. Performing surgery in the ED may be more convenient for the patient, because parents can be present

and the patient does not need to transfer to the operating room. Conversely, performing the procedure in the operating room is more convenient for the surgeon because personnel are able to assist with the procedure and the anesthesia team can administer monitored anesthesia care or general anesthesia.

A digital block can be performed through a volar or dorsal approach. The volar approach may be less desirable in children because passing the needle through thick glabrous skin frequently elicits more pain. Using a 27-gauge or 30-gauge needle and injecting slowly minimize pain. Distracting patients by talking to them and rubbing skin at a different site also can help decrease the perceived intensity of pain. Two adjuncts for pain relief in children are applying vapocoolants during injection, and a topical eutectic 1:1 mixture of topical lidocaine and prilocaine cream covered by an occlusive dressing for 20 minutes prior to injection.

The authors almost exclusively use local anesthetic without epinephrine, even though studies have shown digital blocks with a low dose of epinephrine (1:200,000) are safe, even in neonates.[9] Although epinephrine facilitates hemostasis through vasoconstriction, the digit frequently remains pale white at the end of the procedure, which is disconcerting and requires monitoring for return of normal perfusion. Because there have been reported cases of digital necrosis requiring amputation in adults who receive digital blocks with epinephrine,[10] phentolamine[11] must be available to address prolonged digital ischemia. Furthermore, application of an elastic drain as a finger tourniquet provides adequate hemostasis for the procedure and can be removed to immediately restore perfusion.

The use of digital block as the primary mode of anesthesia has the greatest utility in older patients (>6 years of age). Younger patients rarely are candidates for treatment under a digital block alone because of shorter attention spans and difficulty remaining motionless during the procedure. For patients between 6 years and 12 years old, approximately 50% tolerate the procedure with local anesthesia only. Most children older than 12 years of age tolerate the procedure with local anesthesia only.

The authors have a low threshold to recommend conscious sedation, monitored anesthesia care, or general anesthesia if there is any concern that the child will not tolerate the procedure under local anesthesia only. The authors occasionally have experienced paradoxic agitation with certain agents used for conscious sedation, such as ketamine, and this must be considered when considering conscious sedation. General anesthesia clearly is the most effective modality of anesthesia, but for many acute fingertip injuries it may be impractical to employ.

PULP MANAGEMENT

Management of pediatric fingertip soft tissue injuries depends on whether the nail apparatus is involved. For injuries involving nonperionychial structures, surgical specialists seldom are consulted because simple closure with absorbable sutures is sufficient. The authors cannot overemphasize the importance of using absorbable sutures in children. It prevents the traumatic experience of awake suture removal or the unnecessary anesthetic risk of suture removal under anesthesia. At times, there is skin loss, and primary closure of the skin is not possible. In the absence of frank bone exposure, healing by secondary intention provides acceptable aesthetic and functional results. Most wounds managed conservatively close within a few weeks.

The authors' preferred dressing uses antibiotic ointment (bacitracin, 500 U/g, with polymyxin polymyxin B, 10,000 U/g) to the incision line to decrease infection risk,[11] followed by bismuth-impregnated petroleum gauze, 4 × 4 inch gauze, and a gauze wrap. The wrap continues into the palm and then the wrist, which helps to prevent it from falling off. The authors loosely wrap a compressive, self-adherent elastic wrap to secure the dressing further. Young children have a tendency to place their fingers in their mouth and a bulky dressing decreases the risk of wound contamination with oral bacterial flora.

If the distal phalanx is frankly exposed, coverage with healthy tissue is recommended to prevent osteomyelitis. Similarly, exposed tendon has minimal capacity to heal by secondary intention and requires coverage with vascularized tissue. Normally, the adjacent advancement flaps are elevated to cover the exposed area and the remainder allowed to heal by secondary intention. The distal phalanx also can be trimmed judiciously to allow it to settle under proximal soft tissue padding. In a minority of cases, a more complicated reconstruction is necessary to ensure the bone is covered with durable soft tissue.

For transverse or volar oblique pediatric fingertip injuries, flaps may be advanced in a V-to-Y fashion using a similar technique employed in adults.[12] Using this flap in children provides epicritical tactile sensitivity in 67% but results in a hook nail deformity in 73% and normal pulp shape in only 43% of children who receive it.[13] Avoiding over-advancing sterile matrix helps prevent hook nail

deformity. Erroneously elevating this flap from its vascular supply is a risk for complications. In practice, it is difficult to advance these flaps adequately to cover fingertip wounds. As such, the authors rarely utilize this reconstructive option in children.

The authors prefer reconstructing large transverse or volar oblique finger pulp defects with thenar or hypothenar flaps. Children are less susceptible to immobilization-related stiffness, which can be a concern when using this technique in adults. This is performed in the operating room under general anesthesia and tourniquet control as follows (**Fig. 1**):

1. The injured digit is flexed toward the thenar eminence or thenar crease to ensure appropriate flap design and reach. To account the hemispheric nature of the flap inset, the authors add approximately 50% more length to the flap than the recipient site requires.
2. The skin is incised and a proximally based flap of skin, subcutaneous fat, and thenar fascia is elevated and sutured to the recipient site.
3. The flap can be divided and inset as early as 12 days[14] due to a favorable healing potential in children.

In a study of 16 children receiving a thenar flap for finger reconstruction, the total active range of motion was 248° and static 2-point discrimination was 7 mm.[14] The authors' experience is consistent with previous studies indicating that satisfactory postoperative range of motion and protective sensation are achievable.

The authors' second choice for transverse or volar pulp defects requiring reconstruction is cross-finger flaps. Compared with adults treated in this manner, complications are rare in children. One study of cross-finger flaps found that no children had clinically significant postoperative numbness (vs 21% of adults) or stiffness (vs 28% of adults), and fewer had hyperesthesia (6% of children vs 38% of adults) and cold intolerance (8% of children vs 66% adults).[15] Static postoperative 2-point discrimination was a favorable, 7 mm to 8 mm in 88%.[15] The most frequent complication is hyperpigmentation of the donor site (82%). When choosing this reconstructive option, the potential for growth restriction from scarring on the donor digit should be considered, especially in younger children with considerable longitudinal digital growth remaining.

When restoration of sensation is paramount, such as for critical contact surfaces of the thumb and index finger, a variety of sensory flaps are available. Homodigital island flaps are performed similarly in children as in adults[16] and have

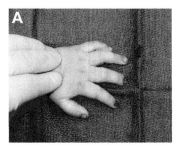
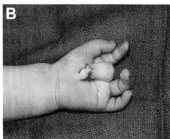

Fig. 1. Thenar flap to reconstruct a fingertip amputation. (*A*) A transverse tip amputation of the middle finger with protruding, exposed distal phalanx requires soft tissue coverage over the bone. (*B*) A thenar flap is elevated and inset to cover the exposed distal phalanx and the flap is divided 2 weeks later.

demonstrated restoration of sensibility, even in toddlers.[17] For the thumb, the Moberg neurovascular advancement flap and first dorsal metacarpal artery flap are performed in a manner similar to adults. For most children, however, sensory flaps are unnecessary. The developing central and peripheral nervous systems have substantial neuroplasticity, and noninnervated flaps generally develop protective sensation.

PERIONYCHIA AND NAIL BED MANAGEMENT

Pediatric fingertip injuries commonly involve the nail bed. Because the nail plate may obscure evaluation of the underlying nail bed, suspicion for injury should be high. Findings correlated with nail bed lacerations are subungual hematoma, injury proximal to the eponychial fold, subluxation of the proximal nail plate, oozing of blood from underneath the nail plate, eponychial fold laceration, and nail plate avulsion (including split nail).[18] Half of nail bed injuries have an underlying tuft fracture,[19] so it is important to obtain an radiograph of the finger if nail bed laceration is suspected. Management of the nail bed and perionychia is controversial and guided by limited evidence, so recommendations vary widely.

Subungual hematomas are common after a crush injury to the fingertip, and the provider must determine the utility of nail plate removal and repair of a possible nail bed laceration. Typical risk factors for a clinically significant nail bed laceration that may guide nail plate removal in adults, such as increasing size of hematoma or distal phalanx fracture,[20] have not been universally observed in children. Most children treated with observation or trephination for hematoma evacuation without nail bed repair generally do not develop clinically significant nail plate deformity.[19,21,22] This nonoperative approach avoids the risks of surgery, decreases the cost of treatment by 4-fold,[19] and confers excellent cosmetic results in most cases.[22] Even if there is an underlying laceration, an intact nail plate serves as a splint for adequate soft tissue healing in most

cases. In cases of trephination performed, the technique is as follows:

1. A heated paper clip, needle, or pen-tip cautery is applied to the nail plate until a drainage hole is created.
2. The finger is irrigated or soaked in water until the underlying hematoma is evacuated.
3. A bandage is placed to absorb any further drainage and to keep the nail clean.

Nail plate removal for exploration and suture repair of an underlying nail bed laceration may be necessary for larger isolated nail bed lacerations and lacerations that involve the adjacent perionychium. The authors prefer 6-0 fast-absorbing suture on a taper needle to repair the nail bed in children (**Fig. 2**). A taper needle causes less trauma to the fragile nail bed than a cutting or reverse cutting needle, and the fast-absorbing gut suture is less inflammatory than other alternative suture options. Suture repair has a high rate of satisfaction (8.9/10) and a low complication rate (7%).[7]

If the nail bed is trephinated or the nail plate is removed during the management of the fingertip injuries, traditional wisdom recommends postoperative antibiotics to prevent osteomyelitis.[19] A 2016 meta-analysis, however, failed to find any infection-preventing benefit in patients of all ages, and there were no cases of osteomyelitis.[23]

Whether or not to replace the nail plate after nail bed trauma or repair also is a matter of some debate. Proponents state that it helps to splint the nail bed repair, splint any associated distal phalanx fracture, and prevent eponychial scarring. Furthermore, it results in less pain with the first dressing change.[24] Conversely, it may increase infection by preventing drainage, delay wound healing, and result in more follow-up visits.[25,26] Currently, a multicenter randomized controlled trial is ongoing to assess the value of nail plate replacement,[26] and this may provide valuable data to drive treatment of this common problem. If the nail plate is removed and replaced as a splint,

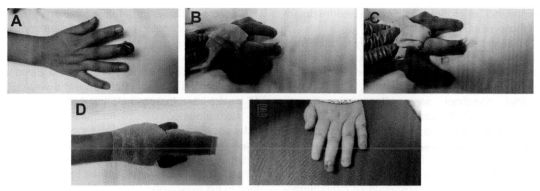

Fig. 2. Nail bed laceration. (*A*) Crush injury in a child demonstrating subluxation of the nail plate and laceration to the nail bed. (*B*) The nail bed is repaired with 5-0 absorbable suture. An Esmarch bandage is used as a finger tourniquet. (*C*) The nail plate is replaced to protect the repair. (*D*) An external splint is secured in place with a self-adherent, elastic wrap. (*E*) Early postoperative follow-up shows typical healing.

patient and caregivers must be counseled that it is expected for the nail plate to fall off before the new nail replaces it.

When replacing the nail plate with suture, the authors perform 2-point or 3-point fixation to secure the nail plate: 1 horizontal mattress suture starting in the nail plate and exiting the apex of the proximal nail fold pulls the nail plate anatomically under the eponychial fold, and 1 or 2 simple sutures distally through the nail plate and skin to secure it in place. The authors frequently use a nonadherent gauze instead of the nail plate, especially when the nail plate is traumatized substantially. This option is faster, avoids passing cicatrix-generating sutures through the apex of the eponychial fold, and enables dressing replacement to decrease bioburden.

Using cyanoacrylate glue for nail bed repair is an appealing alternative to suture repair in the pediatric population. It is faster than placing sutures and potentially obviates a local anesthetic injection or conscious sedation. In 1 prospective randomized controlled study of 40 patients, nail bed repair with cyanoacrylate glue was statistically and clinically significantly faster than suture repair (9.5 minutes vs 27.8 minutes, respectively; *P*<.003).[27] In another prospective series of 30 children, excellent and good cosmetic results were obtained in 100% of patients (25 patients and 6 patients, respectively).[5] A recent systematic review failed to identify differences in outcomes between cyanoacrylate glue and suture repair among patients of all ages, and the investigators conclude that "using a medical adhesive is as effective as suturing nail bed injuries in children."[28] Although these outcomes data are encouraging, the authors do not feel that it justifies universal application of cyanoacrylate glue in all pediatric fingertip injuries. It may trap bacteria in the wound and prevent

drainage. Secondly, cyanoacrylate glues are cytotoxic to fibroblasts during curing, which is of concern in cases of poor skin apposition. As such, the authors feel that the only role for glue in pediatric fingertip injuries is in the setting of clean nail bed trauma without an associated skin injury.

For pediatric fingertip injuries complicated by full-thickness nail bed loss, split-thickness nail bed grafts have been effectively employed on the day of injury in children.[6] Donor sites include noninjured parts of the nail bed in the same finger or the uninjured great toe.[6] In 1 study, all pediatric patients treated this way were very satisfied or satisfied, and only 2 had a subsequent nail deformity. Types of secondary nail plate deformities in children are similar to adults.[6,29] Because of the favorable healing potential in children, the authors prefer to allow secondary intention healing in the setting of nail bed loss, and implement split sterile matrix grafting only for nail nonadherence in the unsatisfied or symptomatic patient.

MANAGEMENT OF AN ASSOCIATED FRACTURE

The distal phalanx is the most commonly fractured bone of the hand in children less than 8 years.[30] The most common type of distal phalanx fracture involves the tuft. The management of distal phalangeal fractures differs from that of adults due to the presence of the physis; once the physis is closed, fractures may be treated in a manner similar to adults. Approximately one-third of distal phalanx fractures in children have an associated complication, such as joint stiffness, osteomyelitis, acute infection, nail deformity, physeal arrest, persistent mallet deformity, and swan neck deformity.[31] The high complication rate underscores the importance of proper identification and treatment of these injuries.

Fixation techniques are limited by fracture fragment size and growth disturbance; percutaneous pinning is the most commonly employed technique. For distal phalanx fractures, a single longitudinal Kirschner wire often is sufficient; however, crossing and transverse orientations also may be employed, if necessary. Some investigators describe using an 18-gauge hypodermic needle advanced into the soft, cartilaginous bone of young children, but the authors' preference is Kirschner wires.[32] Transosseous or circumferential suture fixation also may be effective for distal phalanx fractures in children. Many surgeons replace the nail plate to splint the fracture fragments, in addition to or instead of splinting, citing advantages identified in an adult biomechanical study,[33] but this not always is unnecessary.

Providers can fashion custom external splints from thermoplastic polyurethane, plaster, and fiberglass. Due to lower blood pressures, children are more susceptible to ischemia from compressive splints and dressings, so it is paramount that enough pressure is applied to the finger to secure the splint but not so tight that it exceeds tissue perfusion pressure. Self-adherent elastic wraps are effective for maintaining splint or dressing position but have a narrow therapeutic index. When applied too tightly, they can have devastating ischemic complications, which may require amputation.[34]

Mallet Finger

In children, a majority of mallet fingers seeking clinical attention have an associated fracture (80%).[35] Treatment of these injuries is especially challenging in children because of their low capacity to adhere to the strict immobilization regimen required for uncomplicated healing. In a study of pediatric mallet fingers, treatment non-compliance was associated with a higher incidence of extensor lag (67% versus 11% of compliant patients; $p<0.05$) and other complications (50% versus 8% of compliant patients, $p<0.05$).[35]

In some children, operative repair of a bony mallet deformity may be preferred. Various pinning techniques are described for pediatric mallet fingers.[36] The authors' preference is a single longitudinal Kirschner wire with or without an extension block pin. Outcomes are related to time to treatment, with 12% of patients having extensor lag and 9% having complications when treated within 28 days, compared with 25% and 19%, respectively, when treated after 28 days. Interfragmentary pinning also has been shown to be effective[36] but can be technically difficult in children.

Closed soft tissue mallet finger management in children is complicated by poor treatment compliance. In these cases, Kirschner wire fixation may be preferred to ensure adequate healing of tendon to bone. The Kirschner wire is cut and allowed to sink below the skin for later removal 8 weeks to 12 weeks later. In open soft tissue mallet injuries, a dermatotenodesis technique[37,38] (terminal extensor tendon and skin are reapproximated en masse in a single layer of suture) can be employed. Often, the authors combine this with Kirschner wire immobilization with the distal interphalangeal joint in full extension.

Seymour Fracture

A Seymour fracture is a displaced distal phalanx fracture involving the physis with an associated nail bed injury. The injury may present similarly to a mallet finger and can be misdiagnosed as a simple fracture. These injuries occur most commonly from finger impaction against another child or ball during play.[39] Reduction is prevented by germinal matrix entrapped between fracture fragments; therefore, injuries usually are treated with open reduction and extraction of the nail bed. Early recognition and treatment within 24 hours significantly decreases the risk for infection and improves outcome.[18,39,40] Treatment involves incision and extraction of the nail bed, fracture reduction with or without percutaneous stabilization,[41] and antibiotics.

Although in some settings successful management can be performed in the ED,[41] the authors prefer operating room management for access to anesthesia, fixation equipment, and fluoroscopy. The procedure is performed as follows (**Fig. 3**):

1. The nail plate is removed and the eponychial fold is reflected proximally via radial incisions.
2. The germinal matrix is extracted from fracture site by hyperflexing the distal fracture fragment and carefully elevating the fragment with a freer elevator. Extreme care must be taken to preserve any intact nail bed that is entrapped in the fracture site.
3. A Kirshner wire is passed anterograde through the center of the hyperflexed distal fracture fragment, the fracture is reduced, and the Kirshner wire is passed retrograde through the proximal epiphysis and into the middle phalanx (or proximal phalanx of the thumb).
4. The nail bed is repaired, the wound is dressed, and a splint is applied.

Complications from treating Seymour fractures include nail dystrophy, physeal disturbance, unplanned operating room procedures, and

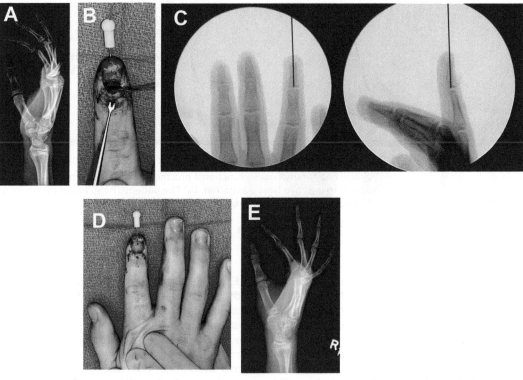

Fig. 3. Seymour fracture of the index finger in a 14-year-old boy. (*A*) Seymour fracture radiograph. (*B*) The eponychial fold is incised and reflected proximally, the nail matrix is extracted with a freer elevator, and a Kirshner wire fixates the reduction. (*C*) Intraoperative fluoroscopy confirms adequate reduction and fixation. (*D*)The nail plate is used to stent the proximal nailfold and splint the fracture. (*E*) Radiographs at 1 postoperative month demonstrate signs of healing.

medication side effects. Antibiotics are recommended because these are considered open fractures. In 1 series, a median 7-day course of cephalexin prevented infection in 94% of patients.[41]

Seymour fractures frequently are missed at initial presentation; this delay increases the risk for infection. In a study of Seymour fractures with a delayed diagnosis, antibiotics were protective against nonunion (33.3% vs 5.1%, respectively; odds ratio 0.11; $P = .008$), even when controlling for operative intervention.[39] Clindamycin may be more effective than oral cephalexin for delayed Seymour fracture (0/18 failures vs 4/16 failures, respectively; $P = .039$).[39] Recent evidence shows that when presenting with radiographic evidence of osteomyelitis, most can be treated effectively with 4 weeks to 6 weeks of antibiotics alone.[39,40] When operative incision and drainage is performed, methicillin-sensitive *Staphylococcus aureus* is the most commonly identified microbe intraoperatively.[40]

MANAGEMENT OF AMPUTATIONS

Door jamb entrapment is by far the most common cause of pediatric fingertip amputations distal to the distal interphalangeal joint (or interphalangeal joint of the thumb).[15,42] Initial management should follow the standard principles of amputation, including wrapping the amputated part in a moistened dressing and placing in a bag in an ice water slurry prior to arriving to the hospital. Replantation distal to the distal interphalangeal joint is technically challenging in children due to small vessel caliber. Composite grafting of amputated fingertips, however, has a higher rate of success in children compared with adults.

The survival of a composite graft is related to several factors. Although longer ischemia time generally is believed to have a negative impact on survival, the exact duration of time at which irreversible damage occurs is unclear. In 1 study, all composite grafts replaced in less than 5 hours from amputation survived whereas none of those replaced after 5 hours of ischemia time survived.[43] Another study found no difference in graft survival when the procedure was performed within 6 hours of the injury compared with those performed between 6 hours and 24 hours. The same study, however, reported that no grafts performed after

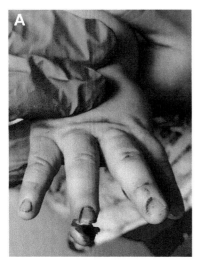 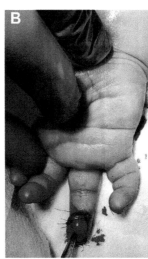

Fig. 4. Subtotal amputation of a fingertip. (*A*) Child at presentation of subtotal fingertip amputation. (*B*) Fingertip repaired demonstrating mild venous congestion. No further intervention was pursued and healing was uneventful.

24 hours survived.[44] Given the lack of high-quality data to drive clinical practice, the authors attempt to perform composite grafting as early as possible but accept that timing may not necessarily correlate with graft survival.

Patient age is an important variable possibly affecting composite graft survival. Butler and colleagues[45] found patients less than 4 years old had a composite graft (distal to distal interphalangeal joint) survival of 14% compared with 3% if greater than 4 years of age ($P = .02$). This finding was corroborated by Greig and colleagues.[26] Conversely, Eberlin and colleagues[42] did not find age to be related to graft survival. Age also may be considered a surrogate for the size and metabolic demand of the amputated segment, where younger patients have smaller grafts and thus a shorter distance for nutrients to travel. Given these data, it may be concluded that composite grafting is more likely to be successful in younger patients with smaller amputated segments. It also is worth noting that crush injuries are more likely to survive than avulsion injuries.[44]

Generally speaking, when a part is not replantable, the authors nonetheless will reattach the segment as a composite graft even if there is a high likelihood of failure, as follows (**Fig. 4**):

1. Perform a thorough irrigation and conservative debridement of the wound and amputated part.
2. Remove subcutaneous fat from the distal fragment in order to decrease the distance for nutrients to diffuse to the fingertip.
3. Suture the amputated segment to the donor site with simple, interrupted, 4-0 or 5-0 absorbable sutures.
4. Dress the wound and instruct the patient to follow-up every 1 week to 2 weeks until healed.

Expectation management is essential, because most composite grafts appear dusky at the first postoperative visit and complete graft take at this visit is the exception rather than the rule.[2,44] Nevertheless, many fingers have near normal form over time because re-epithelialization can occur even under nonviable grafts. On average, pediatric patients rate finger appearance at 3.5/5 and rate satisfaction with appearance as 4/5 after composite grafting.[44] Toe-to-thumb composite-free tissue transfer has been described for pulp reconstruction, but the authors have found that local reconstructive options are equally effective with lower morbidity.[46]

CLINICS CARE POINTS

- Plain radiographs should be obtained in most patients with nailbed injuries since half of patients have an underlying fracture.
- Most children with pulp injuries can be managed with local wound care unless there is bone or tendon exposure.
- Many children have difficulty adhering to the strict immobilization regimen required for prevention of mallet finger associated extensor lag. As such, thorough counseling and/or operative management should be strongly considered.
- Early recognition and treatment of a Seymour fracture, where the germinal matrix becomes entrapped in the fracture, decreases the risk for infection and improves outcomes.
- Expectation management for composite grafting of amputated finger tips is essential since most grafts appear non-viable at their first postoperative appointment, but heal satisfactorily in young children.

DISCLOSURE

The authors have nothing to disclose.

REFERENCES

1. Satku M, Puhaindran ME, Chong AK. Characteristics of fingertip injuries in children in Singapore. Hand Surg 2015;20(3):410–4.
2. Murphy AD, Keating CP, Penington A, et al. Paediatric fingertip composite grafts: do they all go black? J Plast Reconstr Aesthet Surg 2017;70(2):173–7.
3. Rai A, Jha MK, Makhija LK, et al. An algorithmic approach to posttraumatic nail deformities based on anatomical classification. J Plast Reconstr Aesthet Surg 2014;67(4):540–7.
4. Macgregor DM, Hiscox JA. Fingertip trauma in children from doors. Scott Med J 1999;44(4):114–5.
5. Langlois J, Thevenin-Lemoine C, Rogier A, et al. The use of 2-octylcyanoacrylate (Dermabond(®)) for the treatment of nail bed injuries in children: results of a prospective series of 30 patients. J Child Orthop 2010;4(1):61–5.
6. Rohard I, Subotic U, Weber DM. Primary reconstruction of fingernail injuries in children with split-thickness nail bed grafts. Eur J Pediatr Surg 2012; 22(4):283–8.
7. Pearce S, Colville RJ. Nailbed repair and patient satisfaction in children. Ann R Coll Surg Engl 2010; 92(6):483–5.
8. Yorlets RR, Busa K, Eberlin KR, et al. Fingertip injuries in children: epidemiology, financial burden, and implications for prevention. Hand (N Y) 2017; 12(4):342–7.
9. Mantilla-Rivas E, Tan P, Zajac J, et al. Is epinephrine safe for infant digit excision? a retrospective review of 402 polydactyly excisions in patients younger than 6 months. Plast Reconstr Surg 2019;144(1): 149–54.
10. Zhang JX, Gray J, Lalonde DH, et al. Digital necrosis after lidocaine and epinephrine injection in the flexor tendon sheath without phentolamine rescue. J Hand Surg Am 2017;42(2):e119–23.
11. Heal CF, Banks JL, Lepper PD, et al. Topical antibiotics for preventing surgical site infection in wounds healing by primary intention. Cochrane database Syst Rev 2016;11:Cd011426.
12. Atasoy E, Ioakimidis E, Kasdan ML, et al. Reconstruction of the amputated finger tip with a triangular volar flap. A new surgical procedure. J Bone Joint Surg Am 1970;52(5):921–6.
13. Haehnel O, Plancq MC, Deroussen F, et al. Long-term outcomes of atasoy flap in children with distal finger trauma. J Hand Surg Am 2019;44(12):1097. e1–6.
14. Barr JS, Chu MW, Thanik V, et al. Pediatric thenar flaps: a modified design, case series and review of the literature. J Pediatr Surg 2014;49(9): 1433–8.
15. Thomson HG, Sorokolit WT. The cross-finger flap in children: a follow-up study. Plast Reconstr Surg 1967;39(5):482–7.
16. Wang B, Chen L, Lu L, et al. The homodigital neurovascular antegrade island flap for fingertip reconstruction in children. Acta orthopaedica Belgica 2011;77(5):598–602.
17. Varitimidis SE, Dailiana ZH, Zibis AH, et al. Restoration of function and sensitivity utilizing a homodigital neurovascular island flap after amputation injuries of the fingertip. J Hand Surg Br 2005;30(4):338–42.
18. Gibreel W, Charafeddine A, Carlsen BT, et al. Salter-Harris fractures of the distal phalanx: treatment algorithm and surgical outcomes. Plast Reconstr Surg 2018;142(3):720–9.
19. Roser SE, Gellman H. Comparison of nail bed repair versus nail trephination for subungual hematomas in children. J Hand Surg 1999;24(6):1166–70.
20. Simon RR, Wolgin M. Subungual hematoma: association with occult laceration requiring repair. Am J Emerg Med 1987;5(4):302–4.
21. Seaberg DC, Angelos WJ, Paris PM. Treatment of subungual hematomas with nail trephination: a prospective study. Am J Emerg Med 1991;9(3):209–10.
22. Meek S, White M. Subungual haematomas: is simple trephining enough? J Accid Emerg Med 1998;15(4): 269–71.
23. Metcalfe D, Aquilina AL, Hedley HM. Prophylactic antibiotics in open distal phalanx fractures: systematic review and meta-analysis. J Hand Surg Eur vol 2016;41(4):423–30.
24. Dove AF, Sloan JP, Moulder TJ, et al. Dressings of the nailbed following nail avulsion. J Hand Surg Br 1988;13(4):408–10.
25. Miranda BH, Vokshi I, Milroy CJ. Pediatric nailbed repair study: nail replacement increases morbidity. Plast Reconstr Surg 2012;129(2):394e–6e.
26. Greig A, Gardiner MD, Sierakowski A, et al. Randomized feasibility trial of replacing or discarding the nail plate after nail-bed repair in children. Br J Surg 2017;104(12):1634–9.
27. Strauss EJ, Weil WM, Jordan C, et al. A prospective, randomized, controlled trial of 2-octylcyanoacrylate versus suture repair for nail bed injuries. J Hand Surg Am 2008;33(2):250–3.
28. Edwards S, Parkinson L. Is fixing pediatric nail bed injuries with medical adhesives as effective as suturing?: a review of the literature. Pediatr Emerg Care 2019;35(1):75–7.
29. Ashbell TS, Kleinert HE, Putcha SM, et al. The deformed finger nail, a frequent result of failure to repair nail bed injuries. J Trauma 1967;7(2):177–90.
30. Rajesh A, Basu AK, Vaidhyanath R, et al. Hand fractures: a study of their site and type in childhood. Clin Radiol 2001;56(8):667–9.

31. Lankachandra M, Wells CR, Cheng CJ, et al. Complications of distal phalanx fractures in children. J Hand Surg Am 2017;42(7):574.e1–6.

32. Rha E, Lee M, Lee J, et al. Treatment of mallet fracture using a percutaneous fixation technique with an 18-gauge needle. Acta Orthop Belg 2015;81(2):296–302.

33. Wang W, Yu J, Fan CY, et al. Stability of the distal phalanx fracture - a biomechanical study on the importance of the nail and the influence of fixation by crossing Kirschner wires. Clin Biomech (Bristol, Avon) 2016;37:137–40.

34. Makarewich CA, Lang P, Hutchinson DT. Digital ischemia after application of self-adherent elastic wrap dressing: a case series. Pediatrics 2018;141(1):e20163067.

35. Lin JS, Samora JB. Outcomes of splinting in pediatric mallet finger. J Hand Surg Am 2018;43(11):1041.e1–19.

36. Reddy M, Ho CA. Comparison of percutaneous reduction and pin fixation in acute and chronic pediatric mallet fractures. J Pediatr Orthop 2019;39(3):146–52.

37. Ferrari GP, Fama G, Maran R. Dermatotenodesis in the treatment of "mallet finger". Arch Putti Chir Organi Mov 1991;39(2):315–9.

38. Kardestuncer T, Bae DS, Waters PM. The results of tenodermodesis for severe chronic mallet finger deformity in children. J Pediatr Orthop 2008;28(1):81–5.

39. Samade R, Lin JS, Popp JE, et al. Delayed presentation of seymour fractures: a single institution experience and management recommendations. Hand (N Y) 2019. https://doi.org/10.1177/1558944719878846. 1558944719878846.

40. Reyes BA, Ho CA. The high risk of infection with delayed treatment of open Seymour fractures: Salter-Harris I/II or Juxta-epiphyseal fractures of the distal phalanx with associated nailbed laceration. J Pediatr Orthop 2017;37(4):247–53.

41. Lin JS, Popp JE, Balch Samora J. Treatment of acute Seymour fractures. J Pediatr Orthop 2019;39(1):e23–7.

42. Eberlin KR, Busa K, Bae DS, et al. Composite grafting for pediatric fingertip injuries. Hand (N Y) 2015;10(1):28–33.

43. Moiemen NS, Elliot D. Composite graft replacement of digital tips. 2. A study in children. J Hand Surg Br 1997;22(3):346–52.

44. Borrelli MR, Dupre S, Mediratta S, et al. Composite grafts for pediatric fingertip amputations: a retrospective case series of 100 patients. Plast Reconstr Surg Glob Open 2018;6(6):e1843.

45. Butler DP, Murugesan L, Ruston J, et al. The outcomes of digital tip amputation replacement as a composite graft in a paediatric population. J Hand Surg Eur vol 2016;41(2):164–70.

46. Jones NF, Clune JE. Thumb amputations in children: classification and reconstruction by microsurgical toe transfers. J Hand Surg Am 2019;44(6):519.e1–10.

Fingertip Injuries in Athletes, Musicians, and Other Special Cases

Bryan Bourland, DO[a,b], Eric Astacio, MD[a,c], Abdo Bachoura, MD[d],
John D. Lubahn, MD[a,*]

KEYWORDS

• Athlete • Musician • Fingertip • Jersey finger • Mallet finger

KEY POINTS

• Management of fingertip injuries in athletes is optimized by consideration of the sport, the playing position, timing within the season, level of competition, and the patient's goals.
• Mallet and jersey fingers are common injuries in athletes and may be treated in several different ways, based on the nature of the injury and the timing of presentation, as well as the athlete's demands.
• Management of fingertip injuries in musicians is optimized by consideration of how the musician handles his/her instrument and the specific requirements of the injured digit in the context of musical performance.
• The decision on how to best obtain fingertip coverage depends on the size, shape, and location of the defect, the requirements for sensibility, the musician's demands, the surgeon's comfort level, and the available resources.

ATHLETES

Fingertip injuries in athletes may arise secondary to a myriad of causes on the field and may occur in virtually any sport. Management of fingertip injuries in athletes presents a unique scenario for hand surgeons, because treatment necessitates consideration of the sport, the playing position, the timing within the season, the level of competition, and the patient's goals.[1] Two of the most common fingertip injuries in athletes are mallet and jersey fingers.

MALLET FINGER

Mallet finger occurs secondary to an eccentrically applied flexion force on a hyperextended distal phalanx. Radiographs are recommended to determine whether the injury is a soft tissue (avulsion of the terminal tendon) or a bony mallet (avulsion of the terminal tendon with its bony insertion), as bony mallets generally heal quicker than soft tissue mallets. Closed soft tissue injuries or those that involve a small dorsal bone fragment of the distal phalanx can be treated nonoperatively with distal interphalangeal joint (DIPJ) extension splinting or casting. The region immobilized spans the fingertip and DIPJ and allows for proximal interphalangeal joint (PIPJ) motion. Cylinder casting is the most common and best tolerated treatment of mallet fingers in the senior author's practice. A polyurethane material is used, and patients are instructed to wear the cast 24/7 for 6 weeks. For competition and practice, the cast should be

[a] UPMC Hamot, Erie, PA, USA; [b] Texas Tech University Health Sciences Center, Lubbock, TX, USA; [c] Hospital Metropolitano, San Juan, PR, USA; [d] University of Central Florida/HCA Healthcare, Ocala, FL, USA
* Corresponding author. Hand, Microsurgery and Reconstructive Orthopaedics, 300 State Street, Suite 205, Erie, PA 16507.
E-mail address: jdlubahn@jdlubahn.com

Hand Clin 37 (2021) 117–123
https://doi.org/10.1016/j.hcl.2020.09.012
0749-0712/21/© 2020 Elsevier Inc. All rights reserved.

held in place with tape and changed frequently. Volar or dorsal splints may also be used but require the patient to maintain the finger in full extension if the splint needs to be changed. Care should be taken to avoid direct pressure on the dorsal skin or hyperextension of the DIPJ to avoid skin ischemia. Good outcomes require 6 to 8 weeks of immobilization in bony mallet injuries and 12 weeks in tendon only mallet fingers. In most cases, the athlete continues to wear the splint when participating in his/her sport.

Bony mallet injuries with involvement of greater than one-third of the articular surface may result in loss of joint congruency and volar subluxation of the DIPJ. Closed reduction and extension of the DIPJ should be attempted, along with DIPJ extension splinting or casting. Radiographs should be performed after reduction and immobilization to guide further treatment. If persistent subluxation is visible or substantial joint incongruity, operative management may be considered. Closed reduction and percutaneous extension block pinning is currently a popular treatment[2] or in rare cases, open reduction and internal fixation. Open treatment comes with the caveat of a higher complication rate.[3] Most patients prefer nonoperative treatment, as there is less time away from the sport. Percutaneous Kirschner-wire (K-wire) fixation of the DIPJ in extension has been advocated by some investigators but casting or splinting is still required to protect the K-wire from bending or breaking. When this technique is used, the authors recommend placing the K-wire obliquely across the joint so it can be removed in either direction if it bends or breaks.

Outcomes are generally good with nonoperative treatment of mallet injuries, although athletes should be counseled about the possibility of residual extension lag of 5 to 10° and with bony mallet, a dorsal prominence over the proximal part of the distal phalanx. The risks of neglected mallet finger should be discussed with the athlete, and these risks include the development of a persistent flexion deformity of the DIPJ, swan neck deformity of the finger, and DIPJ osteoarthritis.

Seymour Fracture

In skeletally immature patients, an open fracture of the distal phalanx through the epiphysis can appear similar to a mallet finger. This injury is commonly referred to as a "Seymour fracture"[4] and is a Salter-Harris type I or II fracture. The injury is sustained from an axial load, such as awkwardly catching a basketball. Patients often state that they "jammed" their finger when the ball strikes them on the tip of an extended finger. The nail

plate may seem to have a fracture line through it, but blood may conceal the extent of injury (**Fig. 1**A, B). A high index of suspicion is required to make this diagnosis because on examination the findings may be subtle and unimpressive, unlike crush injuries of the fingertip, which are obvious. A delayed or missed injury that goes untreated may lead to nail deformity, infection, and osteomyelitis.[5]

The diagnosis is made by a detailed physical examination of the injured digit. A true lateral radiograph of the involved finger, rather than the whole hand, will avoid overlapping digits and reveal the Salter-Harris fracture (**Fig. 1**C). This is visualized as a step-off and dorsal displacement of the distal phalanx relative to the epiphysis. Treatment is usually operative and necessitates nail plate removal, irrigation, and gentle debridement of the fracture, removal of the interposed nail matrix from the fracture site, open reduction, commonly fixation, and nail bed repair (**Fig. 1**D, E).

Jersey Finger

The flexor digitorum profundus (FDP) attaches to the volar metaphysis and occupies 20% of the area of the distal phalanx.[6] Disruption of this insertion most commonly occurs when a sudden hyperextension force is applied to an actively flexed DIPJ leading to avulsion of the FDP. This commonly occurs while grasping the jersey of a player who quickly pulls away. These injuries are described as zone 1 flexor tendon injuries and may be purely tendon avulsion or associated with bony fractures of the distal phalanx. This injury leads to loss of active flexion of the DIPJ, a hyperextended DIPJ, and inability to make a full fist secondary to the affected digit (**Fig. 2**A, B).

The most common classification system used for jersey finger injuries is the Leddy and Packer classification, which is useful for diagnostic and treatment purposes.[7] Type I injuries are characterized by FDP tendon avulsion from its insertion on the distal phalanx. If both the long and short vinculum are ruptured as well, the profundus tendon may retract into the palm leaving the tendon with a relatively poor blood supply. These injuries should be treated promptly in 7 to 10 days to avoid tendon contraction and preserve viability. In type II, the FDP tendon retracts to the level of the PIPJ. In these, the long vinculum is still preserved, and the FDP has some nutrition. These do not warrant the same urgency for repair as type I. In type III, there is a large bony avulsion fracture from the FDP insertion. The tendon and fracture fragment are usually found at the distal margin of the A4

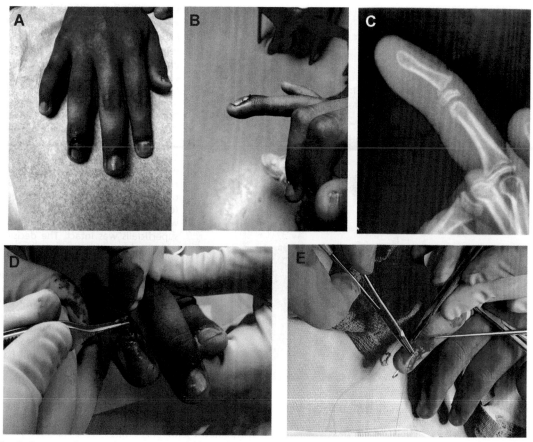

Fig. 1. Seymour fracture in an 11-year-old boy. The open fracture may be easily missed due to the benign appearance of the fingertip (*A, B*). The fracture is best visualized on the lateral view. The fracture line seems to involve the epiphysis and metaphysis, consistent with a Salter-Harris type II fracture (*C*). The open fracture through the physis and the laceration in the nail bed are best visualized by removal of the nail plate and elevation of the proximal nail fold. (*D*). In this case, following irrigation and gentle debridement, the fracture was reduced and pinned, and the nail bed repaired with 5-0 chromic suture (*E*).

pully or the Chiasm of Camper. In type IV, there is a double avulsion injury where there is a distal phalanx fracture as in a type III along with a tendinous avulsion off of that bony fragment. To determine the type of jersey finger, routine radiographs are recommended. If no fracture is visible, these can be supplemented with ultrasound or MRI to confirm the diagnosis and aid in accurate preoperative localization of the tendon.

Several different surgical techniques are available to treat acute avulsion injuries of the FDP tendon. The techniques most commonly used by hand surgeons include either the pull-out suture technique or tendon repair with suture anchor.[8] Type III injuries require internal fixation of the avulsed fragment. Type IV injuries require internal fixation of the avulsed fragment along with tendon incorporation into the avulsed fragment. Common treatment complications include

adhesion formation, stiffness, joint contractures, and quadrigia if an FDP tendon with a common muscle belly (long, ring, small finger) is advanced greater than 1 cm.

Some athletes may present with chronic injuries once their playing season has ended (greater than 4–6 weeks after the initial injury). In these instances, treatment is based on the patient's symptoms and demands. In type II and III injuries, delayed primary repair can be attempted. If the athlete is concerned about range of motion of the DIPJ and loss of dexterity, staged FDP tendon reconstruction is an option. If the athlete wishes to return to play as quickly as possible and is not concerned about the loss of dexterity, nonoperative treatment may be suggested. FDP excision is recommended when the injury is chronic and the patient is experiencing painful adhesions and mechanical irritation (**Fig. 2**C). DIPJ fusion is

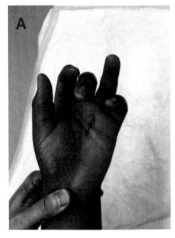
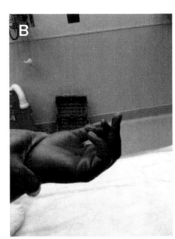
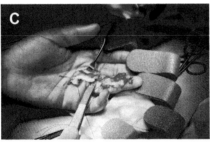

Fig. 2. A 15-year-old healthy boy with a jersey finger, sustained an injury to his left ring finger 45 days before presentation while playing football. Physical examination of the digit revealed tenderness at the base of the finger and A2 pulley, no palpable lump, no active FDP function; passive DIP motion -10° to 60°, PIP active motion 0° to 45°, passive PIP 0° to 95°, 6 cm to the distal palmar crease (A, B). Intraoperatively, the incision was extended to A1 pulley where the FDP was found contracted and could only be advanced to the PIPJ level (C). Intrathecal synovial adhesions were released. The flexor digitorum superficialis was intact. The decision was made to excise the FDP and allow the patient to resume immediate return to activities with a sublimis finger. With an untreated profundus avulsion, hypertrophic synovitis within the flexor sheath can interfere with superficialis gliding and produce a PIPJ flexion contracture. Seven weeks after surgery, the patient had no pain and no functional limitations. His active range of motion was 0° to 95° at the PIP. DIP hyperextension of 10° remained and his active digital closure was within 1 cm of the distal palmar crease.

recommended as a reliable option to treat symptomatic DIPJ hyperextension.

Athletes can expect to return to play in approximately 3 to 6 months, depending on the treatment selected, and once they have functional active range of motion, minimal or no pain, and a reasonable grip strength.

MUSICIANS

According to the United States Bureau of Labor Statistics, approximately 175,600 musicians were employed in 2019.[9] The overwhelming number of hand injuries in musicians are overuse injuries and are thought to comprise 75% to 85% of injuries in this patient population.[10–12]

Traumatic fingertip injuries in musicians make up the minority of injuries but require special considerations. In general, the treating surgeon should attempt to maintain fingertip length, sensibility, and mobility.[13,14] Although revision amputations are often simpler procedures, the shortening of the digit can alter a professional musician's career substantially. Therefore, revision amputations to obtain soft tissue coverage or primary nail bed ablations may not be the optimal initial treatment

option. When dealing with musicians, the treating hand surgeon should consider the use of various local, regional, or free tissue for coverage.

The literature on fingertip injuries in musicians and their capacity to return to musical performance is scarce.[14] In general, it is thought that this patient population benefits from restoration of anatomy to enable the restoration of function. Prior to initiation of treatment, the surgeon should aim to understand how the musician handles his or her instrument and what the functions of the involved digit are, with respect to musical performance. For example, the radial border of the fingertip, which is generally considered to be a noncritical sensory area, may be critical to a drum player using a traditional left underhand grip (**Fig. 3**). Pianists on the other hand, require less in the way of interphalangeal motion but need full motion and accuracy from metocarpophalangeal joint control.[15]

The presence of a nail plate is not only important for cosmetic reasons but serves to improve pulp sensibility and fine prehension.[14] Nail bed injuries, which are often associated with distal phalangeal fractures, should be treated in a manner that will restore the nail apparatus. This

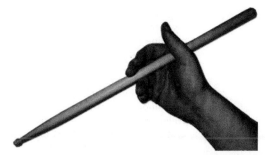

Fig. 3. The ulnar border of the long and the radial border of the ring fingertips, which are generally considered to be noncritical sensory areas, may be critical to a drum player using a traditional left underhand grip.

may require careful nail plate removal and repair of the nail matrix in the operating room under controlled settings, as opposed to an emergency room repair.

Fingertip sensation may be restored in several different methods, varying in complexity (**Fig. 4**). These techniques include simple dressing changes, dermal matrix,[16] nonmicrosurgical neurosensory flaps,[17] and free toe pulp reconstruction.[18] Although the specific techniques are beyond the scope of this article, the decision on how to best obtain coverage depends on the

size, shape, and location of the defect, the requirements for sensibility, the patient's demands, the surgeon's comfort level, and available resources. **Fig. 5** illustrates a partial fingertip amputation in a pianist in a local chamber orchestra. He was treated with a cross-finger flap and had return of functional sensation.

Distal fingertip replantation should be attempted in these patients, especially if the resources and expertise are available and the zone of injury is narrow. Although these replantations are technically difficult, if they succeed they provide a near normal appearance.[14] Often, the FDP remains attached to the metaphysis and does not need to be repaired, and sensory recovery is satisfactory.

Hand therapy for edema control and early motion is desirable in order to minimize posttraumatic adhesions and contractures. Musicians are generally very motivated patients and are compliant with postoperative rehabilitation.[13]

OTHER SPECIAL CASES

Individuals whose occupations depend on fine manual tasks, and who are unable to comply with the use of splints, may benefit from surgical treatment. For example, surgeons, dentists, or cooks, whose livelihood depends on manual tasks, are considered special cases. Mallet fingers, which are generally treated nonoperatively for 8 to

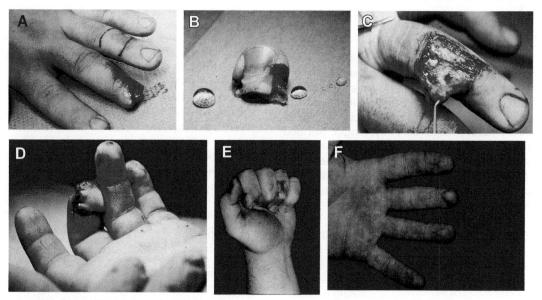

Fig. 4. An injury to a 32-year-old pianist who sustained an index finger distal amputation on a table saw (*A, B*). The sensate volar pulp was lost and in order to maintain the tip of the finger with reasonably sensate skin, a cross-finger flap was selected (*C, D*). The flap was left in place for 3 weeks, then divided, and active range of motion begun. Remarkably good sensation returned, and by 6 months he had returned to playing the piano in his church (*E, F*).

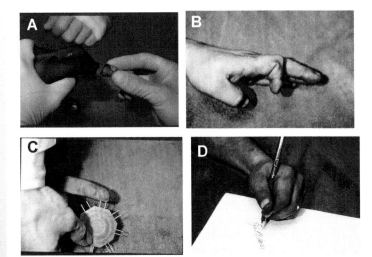

Fig. 5. A 34-year-old man in otherwise good health who amputated his left dominant index finger in a machine press (*A*). Although replantation of single digit and an index finger are both relative contraindications to replantation, a young otherwise healthy individual who wants the finger replanted and who is willing to incur potential increase in cost and is committed to at least a 6-week period of rehabilitation and time off work may be a good candidate for rehabilitation and may regain meaningful 2-point discrimination and function (*B–D*).

12 weeks with an orthosis, could be treated with a buried K-wire in order to enable the professional to resume their line of work and have more reliable healing. As noted for athletes, the K-wire needs to be placed obliquely, so that if it breaks in the joint it can be retrieved from either direction. Surgeons may also be treated with a sterilized dorsal alumafoam splint, which is applied with Steri strips after scrubbing. Although this may sound tedious, it avoids the risk of a buried K-wire holding the DIPJ in extension, as a buried K-wire across the DIPJ is subject to bending, breaking, or infection.

SUMMARY

In many instances, these "special" cases are treated using the same approaches and algorithms as any other patient. However, it is important to consider adjusting the treatment plan to address various potential issues including unique sensory requirements, dexterity, length, nail bed and plate, and ability to tolerate treatment (eg, splinting vs pinning a mallet deformity) when managing fingertip and nail bed injuries in athletes, musicians, and other patients with similar unique needs.

DISCLOSURE

The authors have nothing to disclose.

REFERENCES

1. Bachoura A, Ferikes AJ, Lubahn JD. A review of mallet finger and jersey finger injuries in the athlete. Curr Rev Musculoskelet Med 2017;10(1):1–9.
2. Hofmeister EP, Mazurek MT, Shin AY, et al. Extension block pinning for large mallet fractures. J Hand Surg Am 2003;28(3):453–9.
3. Lubahn JD. Mallet finger fractures: a comparison of open and closed technique. J Hand Surg Am 1989; 14(2 Pt 2):394–6.
4. Seymour N. Juxta-epiphysial fracture of the terminal phalanx of the finger. J Bone Joint Surg Br 1966; 48(2):347–9.
5. Reyes BA, Ho CA. The high risk of infection with delayed treatment of open Seymour fractures: Salter-Harris I/II or juxta-epiphyseal fractures of the distal phalanx with associated nailbed laceration. J Pediatr Orthop 2017;37(4):247–53.
6. Chepla KJ, Goitz RJ, Fowler JR. Anatomy of the flexor digitorum profundus insertion. J Hand Surg Am 2015;40(2):240–4.
7. Leddy JP, Packer JW. Avulsion of the profundus tendon insertion in athletes. J Hand Surg Am 1977;2(1):66–9.
8. Chu JY, Chen T, Awad HA, et al. Comparison of an all-inside suture technique with traditional pull-out suture and suture anchor repair techniques for flexor digitorum profundus attachment to bone. J Hand Surg Am 2013;38(6):1084–90.
9. Bureau of Labor Statistics, U.S. Department of Labor, Occupational Outlook Handbook, Musicians and Singers. Available at: https://www.bls.gov/ooh/entertainment-and-sports/musicians-and-singers.htm. Accessed September 6, 2020.
10. Slade JF 3rd, Mahoney JD, Dailinger JE, et al. Wrist and hand injuries in musicians: Management and prevention. J Musculoskelet Med 1999;16(9):542. Gale Academic OneFile, Accessed September 6, 2020.
11. Sheibani-Rad S, Wolfe S, Jupiter J. Hand disorders in musicians: the orthopaedic surgeon's role. Bone Joint J 2013;95B(2):146–50.

12. Cayea D, Manchester R. Instrument-specific rates of upper-extremity injuries in music students. Med Probl Perform Art 1998;13(1):19–25.

13. Winspur I. Special operative considerations in musicians. Hand Clin 2003;19(2):247–58.

14. Dumontier C. Distal replantation, nail bed, and nail problems in musicians. Hand Clin 2003;19(2):259–72.

15. Amadio PC, Russotti GM. Evaluation and treatment of hand and wrist disorders in musicians. Hand Clin 1990;6(3):405–16.

16. Jacoby SM, Bachoura A, Chen NC, et al. One-stage Integra coverage for fingertip injuries. Hand (N Y) 2013;8(3):291–5.

17. Slutsky D. Neurosensory pedicled flaps to the hand. Atlas Hand Clin 2005;10:141–70.

18. Spyropoulou GA, Shih HS, Jeng SF. Free pulp transfer for fingertip reconstruction-the algorithm for complicated Allen fingertip defect. Plast Reconstr Surg Glob Open 2016;3(12): e584.

Understanding and Measuring Long-Term Outcomes of Fingertip and Nail Bed Injuries and Treatments

Kenneth R. Means Jr, MD*, Rebecca J. Saunders, PT, CHT

KEYWORDS

- Outcome measures • Fingertip • Nail bed • Injury • Injuries • Trauma

KEY POINTS

- There are many outcome measures to choose from when caring for or studying fingertip and nail bed trauma and treatments.
- This article outlines general outcome measures principles as well as guidelines on choosing, implementing, and interpreting specific tools for these injuries.
- It also presents recent results from the literature for many of these measures, which can help learners, educators, and researchers by providing a clinical knowledge base and aiding study design.

This article provides frameworks for identifying and using different outcome measures for fingertip and nail bed injuries and treatments. It considers fingertip injuries as those that occur at or distal to the distal interphalangeal (DIP) joint. Much of what it presents is extrapolated from publications on general hand trauma because of the paucity of such information solely focusing on fingertip and nail bed injuries. It presents advantages and disadvantages for each evaluation tool as applicable, which is helpful for providers, educators, and investigators who manage, teach about, and study these injuries. Present publications provide useful information toward this goal, but knowledge gaps remain. Most studies present a small retrospective series, and true long-term, and comparative, results are rarely reported.[1] Also, classifications and assessments are often incompletely defined, limiting comparison across past as well as future efforts. Thus, there is a lack of definitive evidence and consensus for most outcome measures and treatments for these

patients. This article focuses on the last 5 years of available information, recognizing that substantial and influential contributions predate this period.

A complete review of outcome measures and their use in research is beyond the scope of this article. **Table 1** lists pertinent terms and definitions that are helpful as a reference in broadly understanding psychometric, or clinimetric, characteristics of outcome measures. Throughout the article, a simple analogy for measuring a finger joint's range of motion (ROM) is used as an example for interpreting outcome measures and their characteristics.

Before presenting the various outcome measures available, it is important for educators and researchers to recognize and select classification schemes for fingertip and nail bed injuries. The authors think an ideal classification should be useful in clinical and research settings; be easy to conceptualize but comprehensive, including applicability to amputation and nonamputation injuries;

The Curtis National Hand Center @ MedStar Union Memorial Hospital, Baltimore, MD, USA
* Corresponding author. The Curtis National Hand Center @ MedStar Union Memorial Hospital, 3333 North Calvert Street, JPB#200, Baltimore, MD 21218.
E-mail address: kenneth.means@medstar.net

Hand Clin 37 (2021) 125–153
https://doi.org/10.1016/j.hcl.2020.09.011
0749-0712/21/© 2020 Elsevier Inc. All rights reserved.

Table 1
Psychometric (clinimetric) terms and definitions for characteristics of outcome measures

Outcome Characteristic Psychometric (Clinimetric) Term	Definition
Validity	Degree to which an outcomes tool measures what it is intended to measure
Content validity	Degree to which an outcomes tool comprehensively and relevantly applies to intended patients and their clinical states
Construct validity	Degree to which results of an outcomes tool apply to the patient's clinical state, or a related hypothesis; indicated in part by correlation with other tools measuring the same clinical state/hypothesis (convergent validity) and lack of correlation with other tools measuring different clinical states/hypotheses (divergent validity)
Face validity	Degree to which the individual parts of an outcomes tool seem to apply to the patient's clinical state
Criterion validity	Degree to which an outcomes tool relates to an established gold standard criterion; often applied when comparing a shortened version of an outcomes tool with its original version
Responsiveness	Degree to which an outcomes tool is able to detect meaningful changes (ie, improving or worsening) in a patient's clinical state and the degree to which the outcomes tool is able to distinguish between patients who have meaningfully changed and those who have not
Reproducibility	Degree to which results of an outcomes tool are replicable; determined by several attributes listed below
Reliability	Degree to which results of an outcomes tool, despite its measurement error, are able to consistently establish a patient's clinical state and distinguish between patients in different clinical states
Test-retest reliability	Degree to which results of an outcomes tool remain consistent and applicable when repeatedly administered to patients who remain in the same clinical state over a specified time
Intrarater and inter-rater reliability	Degree to which an outcomes tool measures what it is intended to measure across the same (intrarater) or different (inter-rater) examiners for the same patient during the same visit, or for the same patient who remains in the same clinical state over time
Internal consistency	Degree to which individual parts of an outcomes tool relate to each other and in turn measure the same clinical state
Measurement error (aka agreement)	Degree to which an outcomes tool generates different results, because of its inherent variability, during repeated use for the same clinical state; reported as an absolute value in the same units as the outcomes tool result and often expressed as the SEM; eg, the SEM for finger joint ROM with a device may be $\pm 4°$, during which time the patient's finger ROM has not changed, such as with using the device for repeated measurements within an hour of each measurement with no intervening treatment

(continued on next page)

Table 1
(continued)

Outcome Characteristic Psychometric (Clinimetric) Term	Definition
MDC (aka SDC or true change)	The smallest possible change in result for an outcomes tool not caused by random chance or measurement error; dependent on number of individual parts included in the outcomes tool and range of potential results for each part and calculated from the associated SEM; always larger than the SEM for the outcomes tool
MIC (aka MCID or MID)	The smallest change in an outcomes tool result for a patient that is thought to indicate a meaningful change in the clinical state, representing a clinically meaningful improvement or worsening and an opportunity for altering or continuing current management
Measurement error rating for an outcomes tool	The difference between MIC and MDC (MIC minus MDC) for an outcomes tool that indicates its appropriateness for a particular use; (+) values indicate appropriate to use for that clinical situation; (−) values indicate inappropriate to use, or should be used with caution, for that clinical situation; eg, if a 5° ROM change is considered to be relevant for patient care or a particular study (MIC) and a measuring device is only able to reliably detect 10° of ROM change (MDC), then 5–10 = −5 and that device is not ideal for that patient population or study because any changes in ROM between 5° and 10° measured by the device could indicate relevant clinical changes or changes caused by measurement error or random chance

Abbreviations: aka, also known as; MDC, minimal detectable change; MIC, minimal important change; MID, minimal important difference; ROM, range of motion; SDC, smallest detectable change; SEM, standard error of measurement.
Data from Refs.[2–8]

combine indicators of damaged anatomic structures, including skin, nail elements, tendons, and skeletal structures, as well as the trauma mechanism, with relative weighting values for each of these factors; have a scoring system that correlates with outcomes that are performance and patient based; guide treatment; and have adequate confirmation of validity and reliability via formal evaluation. To date, we are unaware of such a classification system. **Table 2**, presents the most relevant commonly used systems, although there are others available that investigators may favor.[9,10] Of note, nearly all of these classifications have been modified or repurposed to varying degrees when used by other researchers, as seen in the table references (**Box 1**). All of them also have limited, if any, formal evaluation of their usage. The authors recommend the Allen classification as likely the most generalizable for fingertip and nail bed injuries, whether amputated or not; the Zook if focusing on nail bed injuries alone;

and the Hirase for amputation/replantation given its delineation of arterial zones of injury and repair.

It is tempting but unrealistic to simply state what the ideal outcomes measure is for all fingertip and nail bed injuries. Even a cursory literature review reveals a seemingly unending number of assessments from which to choose. On our review through the past 5 years alone we encountered more than 35 potential tools at the clinician's and researcher's disposal, each with its proponents and detractors. The challenge is to be appropriately selective to not exhaust patients, providers, or readers. Rather than merely assigning a single evaluation method for all patients, thoughtful clinicians and investigators consider several key questions or factors. These factors include the age of their population; the anatomic structures that are injured, treated, and how; whether it is a work-related injury; whether patients are able to return to work, to the same or different occupation, and how important that is from their, their patients',

Table 2
Fingertip and nail bed injury classification schemes

Classification System Name	Classification Basis	Classification Values	Advantages	Disadvantages	References
Allen (Fig. 1)	Anatomic injury levels based on structures involved and whether trauma was clean or crush	Zone I: pulp only Zone II: pulp and nail bed distal to lunula/germinal matrix and not bone Zone III: pulp, nail bed distal to lunula/germinal matrix, and distal phalanx Zone IV: pulp, nail bed at or proximal to lunula/germinal matrix, and distal phalanx	• Widely used in research • Includes some injury mechanisms • Somewhat guides treatment • Simple and practical • Somewhat prognostic for nail bed deformities • Likely best face validity for uses other than amputations	• Incompletely described in original publications • Anatomic and injury gaps in described zones • No accounting for flexor/extensor tendon status	11,12
Foucher	Amputation anatomic level	Zone I: from at or just distal to the FDS insertion on the middle phalanx to the DIP joint Zone II: between the DIP joint and the nail fold Zone III: distal to the nail fold	Partially includes tendon status	Zone sequencing is in reverse of most other systems	13
HISS (aka Campbell HISS)	Anatomic structures injured	Values assigned by injured structures per digit, including skin, skeleton, tendon, and nerves; total sum of all digits multiplied by different constants for each digit; ranges from 0 to 826 with higher scores indicating worse severity:	• Strong negative correlation with Tamai functional score (−.77) • Some correlation with DASH • Mostly objective	• Awkward scoring range and qualitative grading assignments with likely ceiling effect • Constants assigned to each digit generated empirically without formal validation	14–16

		0–20 = minor 21–50 = moderate 51–100 = severe >100 = major			
Hirase	Amputation anatomic level based on arterial structures at each level	Zone I: distal to termination of all digital arterial branches Zone IIa: between level where central artery branches off the distal digital arch and zone 1 Zone IIb: at the level of the distal digital arch (around the level of the nail fold) Zone III: between the DIP joint and zone IIb (ie, proximal to the distal digital arch, at the level of both proper digital arteries)	• More detailed for fingertip levels • Informs surgical care options based on level of arterial repair possible	• Solely anatomic • Unknown until surgical dissection completed • Inconsistent use of different categories across studies • Some studies use mix of vascular, soft tissue, and skeletal levels to distinguish zones • Poor face validity for usage other than amputation/replantation	11,17
Ishikawa: Modified-Ishikawa subdivides zone 1 into a (distal to all nail elements) and b (from midnail to zone 1a) and combines zones 3 and 4 into a single zone 3 (**Fig. 2**)	Amputation anatomic level: 4 zones from the fingertip to the DIP joint	Zone 1: from midnail distal Zone 2: from proximal edge of nail fold to zone 1 Zone 3: from midpoint between DIP joint and zone 2 to zone 2 Zone 4: from DIP joint to zone 3	Subcategorizes fingertip amputations and nail bed involvement • Might account for flexor vs extensor involvement, although not created, described, or studied as such • Widely used in research	• Solely anatomic • Created only for amputations • Inconsistent use of different categories across studies • Possible overlap between zones for the same or different evaluators (intrarater and inter-rater reliability issues)	18–22

(continued on next page)

Table 2
(continued)

Classification System Name	Classification Basis	Classification Values	Advantages	Disadvantages	References
Tamai[a]	Amputation anatomic level; 5 zones described for entire length of fingers and thumb	Zone I: amputation distal to the nail fold Zone II: amputations between the nail fold and DIP joint All other zones are proximal to DIP joint	• Widely used clinically and in research • Simple	• Anatomic injury levels not as detailed as others for fingertips • Created only for amputations	23
Yamano	Amputation mechanism and injury severity	• Clean cut • Blunt cut (aka moderate crush) • Severe crush or avulsion (some studies separate these mechanisms into 2 categories)	• Simple • Mechanism of injury prognostic of replantation survival	• Incompletely described in original publications • Only described for partial or complete amputations • Subjective differentiations between categories • No scoring system • Inconsistent use of different categories across studies	11,24,25
Zook Nail Bed Injury Categorization (see Box 1)	Includes categories of anatomic injury level, injury mechanism, and use of nail plate substitute with subsections in each category	See **Box 1**	• Relatively comprehensive for nail bed injuries • Widely used in research	• Complex for regular clinical use • Overlap between injury categories • Incompletely described in publications • No scoring system	26

Abbreviations: DASH, Disabilities of the Arm, Shoulder and Hand; FDS, flexor digitorum superficialis; HISS, Hand Injury Severity Score.
[a] The same classification was described in publications before Tamai's; however, since Tamai's publication, it has usually been attributed as such.

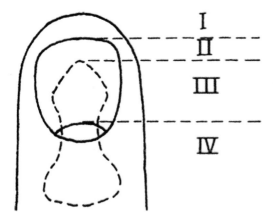

Fig. 1. Allen fingertip injuries classification zones. (*From* Allen MJ. Conservative management of finger tip injuries in adults. The Hand 1980;12(3):257-65; with permission.)

or society's standpoint; whether they are concerned with impairment, disability, or both; and whether satisfaction with the care process, treatment, or outcomes is important and how it will be assessed.

To gain a comprehensive evaluation of fingertip injuries, it is appealing to combine patient-reported outcome measures (PROMs) with measured outcomes, some of which are termed performance-based outcome measures (PBOMs). PROMs can be affected by psychosocial factors, often more so than by injury severity factors.[27] Although frequently thought to be more objective than PROMs, PBOMs can also be influenced by patient effort or other psychosocial elements and may correlate poorly with PROMs.[2,28,29] However, there are few truly objective tools available, such as determining residual digit or nail length or finger pulp thickness.[30] The authors suggest PBOMs and PROMs be considered for what they can each bring to the clinical or research setting; one should not replace the other.

Box 1
From Zook Categorization of Injuries, with some reordering and clarification

Categories

Nail bed only involved

Nail bed and fingertip involved

Distal phalanx fracture present

Cause of injury (list mechanism)

Type of injury

    Laceration

    Stellate laceration

    Severe crush

    Avulsion

Site of injury

    Involvement of distal one-third of nail bed (sterile matrix)

    Involvement of middle one-third of nail bed (sterile matrix)

    Involvement of proximal one-third of nail bed (sterile matrix)

    Involvement of palmar nail fold (germinal matrix)

    Involvement of dorsal nail fold (eponychium)

Material used to temporarily replace nail plate

    Original nail plate

    Silicone sheet

    Adaptic (or other) gauze

    Other*

    None*

Asterisks and ( ) indicate that it was not part of the original description.
Adapted from Zook E.G., Guy R.J., Russell, R.C. A study of nail bed injuries: Causes, treatment, and prognosis. J Hand Surg Am. 1984 9:247-52; with permission.

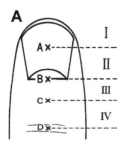

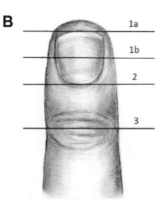

Fig. 2. (*A*) Ishikawa (size adjusted for comparison). (*B*) Modified-Ishikawa fingertip amputation classifications. ([*A*] *Adapted from* Suzuki Y, Ishikawa K, Isshiki N, et al. Fingertip replantation with an efferent A-V anastomosis for venous drainage: clinical reports. Br J Plast Surg. 1993 Apr;46(3):187-91, with permission; and [*B*] *From* Moiemen NS, Elliot D. Composite graft replacement of digital tips. 2. A study in children. J Hand Surg Br. 1997 Jun;22(3):346-52; with permission.)

Table 3
Objective, pseudo-objective, and performance-based outcome measures

Measured Outcome/PBOM	Outcome Range and Meaning	Relevant or Representative Values in Fingertip/Nail Bed Trauma Across Studies	Advantages	Disadvantages	References
AROM and/or PROM	MCPs 0°–80° PIPs 0°–110° DIPs 0°–80° Total 0°–270° Higher scores indicate better motion; often reported as % of contralateral	Mean DIP AROM after fingertip revision amputation ~65° Single fingertip Tamai zone 1 amputations: replant mean TAM ~70%, SD 13, range 42–96; homodigital flap with or without bone/nail bed composite mean ~80%, SD 14, range 45–100 (SSD) Allen III/IV fingertip amputation homodigital flap mean TAM 260°, SD 23° (97%)	• Simple • Track over time • Patient valued	• Time consuming • Tedious • Error-prone • Not easily compiled • Inconsistent correlation with impairment and disability	5,8,31–34
Digit strength via key pinch	Measured in absolute kilograms or pounds; often reported as mean of 3 measurements; often reported as % of contralateral	Single fingertip Tamai zone 1 amputations: replant mean 60%, SD 25, range 17–100; homodigital flap with or without bone/nail bed composite mean ~80%, SD 12, range 60–100 (SSD)	• Simple • Track over time • Patient valued • Good test-retest reliability	Recordings not easily compiled	32,35
Digit strength via lateral tip pinch	Measured in absolute kilograms or pounds; often reported as mean of 3 measurements; often reported as % of contralateral	NA	• Simple • Track over time • Patient valued • Good test-retest reliability	Recordings not easily compiled	35

Hand strength via grip (Jamar Hand Dynamometer most commonly used): some use same setting for all patients (2 or 3 most common), others use whichever setting patients think allows them to generate most power	Measured in absolute kilograms or pounds; often reported as mean of 3 measurements; often reported as % of contralateral	Allen III/IV fingertip amputation homodigital flap, mean 33 kg, SD 13 (91%)	Simple, tracking over time, patient valued, good test-retest reliability	Recordings not easily compiled	33,35
Digit sensation via S2PD	2 mm to >15 mm; higher numbers indicate worse sensory nerve density of slowly adapting fibers; often compared with contralateral uninjured digits	Mean 7 mm for fingertip replantation; mean 5.6 mm for fingertip revision amputation Foucher zone 2/3 amputations: replant mean 4.5 mm (range 2–7 mm); reverse homodigital flap with composite bone/nail bed graft mean ~6 mm (range 2–9 mm) For cross-finger flap ~50% equal to contralateral, ~30% 2 mm worse than contralateral, ~10% 4 mm worse than contralateral Allen III/IV fingertip amputation homodigital flap, mean 5 mm, SD 1.7, range 2–8	• Simple • Track over time	• Poor inter-rater and intrarater reliability and responsiveness • Questionable validity	13,30,31,33,36–39

(continued on next page)

Table 3
(continued)

Measured Outcome/ PBOM	Outcome Range and Meaning	Relevant or Representative Values in Fingertip/Nail Bed Trauma Across Studies	Advantages	Disadvantages	References
Digit sensation via M2PD	2 mm to >15 mm; higher numbers indicate worse sensory nerve density of quickly adapting fibers; often compared with contralateral uninjured digits; results typically smaller than for S2PD	Foucher zone 2/3 amputations replanted mean ~4 mm; for those treated with reverse homodigital flap with composite bone/nail bed graft mean ~5 mm	Returns earlier after nerve injury/repair compared with S2PD	• More difficult to perform and for patients to report • Not as widely used	13,40
Digit Sensation via SWMs	Grade 0: cannot detect any sized filaments Grade 1: can detect 6.65 filament = deep pressure sensation Grade 2: can detect 4.56 filament = absent protective sensation Grade 3: can detect 4.31 filament = diminished protective sensation Grade 4: can detect 3.61 filament = diminished light touch sensation Grade 5: can detect 2.83 filament = normal touch and pressure sensation	For cross-finger flaps ~60% equal to contralateral/grade 5, ~40% 1 grade worse than contralateral/ grade 4 Single fingertip Tamai zone 1 amputations: replant mean 4.0, SD 0.7, range 2.4–5.1, homodigital flap with or without bone/nail bed composite mean 3.4, SD 0.4, range 2.4– 4.0 (SSD) Allen III/IV fingertip amputation homodigital flap median 2.83 (~60% 2.83, ~30% 3.61, ~10% 4.31); MIC 0.7	• Track over time • Quantitative and qualitative scales via Touch-Test Sensory Evaluator instructions • Shown to correlate with hand dexterity • More responsive than S2PD	• Tedious recording not easily compiled over time • Lack of validity for grading scale and qualitative descriptions • Use of mean for summary reporting inappropriately implies continuous measures, whereas in practical use SWM testing has discrete ordinal values so reporting proportions/percentages and medians is more appropriate	30,32–34,36,37,39,41

Measure	Scale/Description		Findings	Advantages	Limitations	Ref
Sensation via MRCC scale	S0: absent sensation S1: deep pain sensation (S1+: superficial pain sensation) S2: superficial pain and some touch sensation (S2+ = S2 level + hyperesthesia) S3: intact touch sensation without hyperesthesia, S3+ = S3 level + some recovery of S2PD (715 mm) and M2PD (4–7 mm) S4: normal sensation (S2PD 2–6 mm and M2PD 2–3 mm) ( ) = common modifications	NA		• Widely used for decades • Track recovery over time	• Incomplete gradations within and between categories often lead to modifications in practice or research • Limited usage in fingertip/nail bed injury reports	40,42–44
Residual digit length vs contralateral	NA		Longer digit length correlates with greater pinch power (r = 0.68, SS) and patient satisfaction	• Simple • Objective • Patient valued	• Unknown disability significance • No correlation with Purdue Pegboard Test	37
Residual visible nail length vs contralateral	NA		Longer visible nail correlates with greater patient satisfaction r = 0.65 (SS) 55% length of normal nail cutoff for patient satisfaction benefits Allen III/IV fingertip amputation homodigital flap mean 1.8 mm shorter, SD 0.6, range 1–3	• Simple • Objective • Patient valued	• Unknown functional significance • No correlation with Purdue Pegboard Test	33,37

(continued on next page)

Table 3
(continued)

Measured Outcome/ PBOM	Outcome Range and Meaning	Relevant or Representative Values in Fingertip/Nail Bed Trauma Across Studies	Advantages	Disadvantages	References
Presence of nail deformity	Multiple descriptive terms (hook, in-grown, split, grooved, rough, uneven, pitted, horn, synechia, narrowing, widening, thinning, thickening, liftoff, and so forth)	24% for fingertip replantation Allen III/IV fingertip amputation treated with homodigital flap and nail preservation: 64% hook nail	Simple descriptive use	• Difficult to categorize and subcategorize • Substantial overlap or coexistence of deformities	37,38
Zook Fingernail Appearance Classification (see **Table 4**)	Identifies number of major and minor variations for injured fingernail compared with normal contralateral fingernail in 5 categories: nail shape, adherence, surface, splitting, and eponychium status; sum of variations determines qualitative grade for each injured fingernail (see **Table 4**)	Nail bed composite graft from amputated part or donor toe 36% excellent, 23% very good, 18% good, 9% fair, 14% poor; inter-rater reliability 0.36 (95% CI 0.09–0.68)	• Relatively comprehensive • Widely used in research	• Evaluator bias • Low inter-rater reliability • Different interpretations of scoring • Incomplete qualitative grading scale may minimize or mislead on impact for patient • Complex and time consuming for regular clinical use	26,45,46
Lim Hook Nail Classification (**Fig. 3**)	Finger divided into 4 zones viewed from lateral side; whichever zone the fingernail ends in is degree of hook nail; range 0 (normal) to 4 (worst possible)	Allen III/IV fingertip amputation homodigital flap 36% grade 0, 27% grade 1, 32% grade 2, 5% grade 3	Very specific	Very specific	33,47

Measure	Description	Example results	Advantages	Limitations	References
Vancouver Scar Scale	Total score based on 4 elements: vascularity, pigmentation, pliability, and height; higher scores indicate worse scar appearance	Allen III/IV fingertip amputation homodigital flap mean 0.6, range 0–3	Photo-based option	• Rater bias • Poor face validity for fingertip injuries	33
Volar Pulp Ratio	Ratio of normal volar pulp to injured or reconstructed volar pulp on lateral view radiographs (however, the authors suggest reporting this instead as a ratio or percentage of injured pulp relative to normal pulp for interpretability)	14% of fingertip replantations with some amount of pulp atrophy; for cross-finger flaps mean ratio of 1.03 (range 0.85–1.25)	• Objective • Patient valued for aesthetics	Unknown functional significance	30,38
Fingertip survival after replantation	Complete Partial (%) None	Overall 76% complete survival Yamano type 1 = 100% complete Yamano type 2 = 75% complete Yamano type 3 = 70% complete Foucher zone 2/3 86% survival Tamai zone 1 90%–100% survival	Patient, surgeon, and society valued	• Evaluator bias • Conflicting reports of functional correlation	13,25,32
Local flap survival	Complete Partial (%) None	98% for reverse homodigital island flaps	• Affects future care • Partial determinant of treatment success	Rater bias in determining percentage	48

(continued on next page)

Table 3
(continued)

Measured Outcome/ PBOM	Outcome Range and Meaning	Relevant or Representative Values in Fingertip/Nail Bed Trauma Across Studies	Advantages	Disadvantages	References
Fracture union or nonunion, and if nonunion symptomatic or not	Radiographic evidence of bone healing a certain length of time since injury or treatment (some indicate as a nonunion if no healing at >3 mo and others if none at >6 mo)	NA	Impact on patient symptoms, recovery time, and medical costs	Rater bias especially based on time from injury and diagnosis of nonunion	—
Purdue Pegboard Dexterity Test	Number of pegs, or peg pairs for both hands, inserted in 30 s ; a single testing session is typically done with dominant hand for 30 s, then nondominant for 30 s, then both for 30 s; averages of 2–3 testing sessions recommended for increased reliability; assembly score also used = number of pin-washer-collar assemblies completed in 60 s	Single fingertip Tamai zone 1 amputations: replant mean 18, SD 6, range 7–28; homodigital flap with or without bone/nail bed composite mean 22, SD 8, range 7–45	• Widely used clinically and in research for decades • Good assessment of finger dexterity • Good test-retest reliability (ICC 0.66 to >0.80) • Normative values available for age/gender/hand-dominance/vision differences	Can be affected by neuromuscular and psychosocial factors, patient vision, and practice effect	8,32,34,35,37,49,50

	Description	Interpretation	Strengths	Limitations	References
Jebsen-Taylor Hand Function Test	Combined time for 7 tasks: stacking checkers; simulated page turning and eating; lifting small, large/light, and large/heavy objects; and handwriting Lower times indicate better dexterity with the tasks	Cutoff time maximizing sensitivity and specificity for injured hands ~37 s and for uninjured hands ~33 s (excluding handwriting portion)	• Therapist familiarity • Commonly used in research and practice • Good/excellent reliability and validity • SS correlations with strength, amputation level, AMA impairment rating, DASH, qDASH, MHQ, and bMHQ —ICC 0.77–0.97	• Handwriting portion often excluded because of hand dominance dependence • Effects of age and sex undetermined • Lack of validity and responsiveness for effect of surgery • Unknown MIC	1,8,29,51
Tamai Hand Function	0–100 points with higher scores indicating better function 0–39 poor 40–59 fair 60–79 good 80–100 excellent ROM 20 pts ADLs 20 pts Sensation 20 pts Satisfaction 20 pts Symptoms 10 pts Appearance 10 pts	Median score 67–78 for those able to RTW vs 39 for those unable to RTW (SSD)	• Combines PBOMs and PROMs • Historically popular	• Evaluator bias • Lack of clinimetric characterization	15,23
Sollerman Hand Function Test	20 tasks simulating ADLs; each scored from 0 (unable to complete) to 4 (completed appropriately within 20 s)	NA	• Some association with ROM, VAS pain, and disability • Strong association with VAS function	• Not as widely used or studied • Possible examiner bias • Lengthy	8,52

(continued on next page)

Table 3
(continued)

Measured Outcome/ PBOM	Outcome Range and Meaning	Relevant or Representative Values in Fingertip/Nail Bed Trauma Across Studies	Advantages	Disadvantages	References
AMA Guides to the Evaluation of Permanent Impairment (important to note which edition when using)	% of normal digit, hand, upper extremity, whole person	$r = 0.38$ correlation with DASH (SS) $r = -0.24$ correlation with MHQ (SS)	• Used to determine permanent partial impairment for worker's compensation patients • Contains some truly objective elements • Correlates well with Jebsen-Taylor Hand Function Test	• Simplistic • Not evidence based • Contains no patient-rated measures other than pain reporting • Rater and patient biases • Limited testing of validity • Weak to moderate correlation with disability assessments	1,53
Time off work	Reported as days, weeks, months, or years from the time of injury/treatment to RTW, either to prior or different job and to prior or reduced work hours	Single fingertip Tamai zone 1 amputations: replant 4 mo ± 4; revision amputation 1 mo ± 1 (SSD) Foucher zone 2/3 amputations: replant 81 d (range 78–93) Allen III/IV fingertip amputation homodigital flap mean 6.1 wk, SD 3.3, range 1–12 Reverse homodigital with composite bone/ nail bed graft 82 d (range 80–95 d) Mean 7 wk for fingertip revision amputation	Patient and society valued	• Strongly influenced by psychosocial factors that may or may not be related to the anatomic injury • Currently lacks differential weighting for returning to same vs different job and same vs different work hours	27,31,33,48

				35
Functional Capacity Evaluation	Formal evaluation of a patient's work-specific capabilities and limitations	NA	• Follows standardized protocols tailored to patient's specific work environment • Performed by skilled/trained assessors • Can partially account for patient effort • Can develop recommendations for work accommodations or other interventions	• Typically only available for patients covered under worker's compensation insurance • Lengthy and expensive • No scoring system per se, which limits its use as a research tool

Abbreviations: ADLs, activities of daily living; AMA, American Medical Association; AROM, active digit ROM; bMHQ, Brief Michigan Hand Questionnaire; CI, confidence interval; ICC, intra-class correlation coefficient (measure of test-retest reliability); MCP, metacarpophalangeal; M2PD, moving 2-point discrimination; MRCC, Medical Research Council classification; PIP, proximal interphalangeal; pts, points; qDASH, Quick Disabilities of the Arm, Shoulder, and Hand; RTW, return to work; S2PD, static 2-point discrimination; SS, statistically significant; SSD, statistically significantly different; SWM, Semmes-Weinstein monofilaments; TAM, total active motion; VAS, visual analog scale.

Table 4
From Zook Categorization of Fingernail Result Compared to Contralateral, with some reordering and clarification

Classification Categories and Ratings	Check Boxes	
	Major Variation	Minor Variation
Nail Shape		
Identical to opposite		
Shorter		
Narrower		
Longitudinal curve		
Transverse curve		
Nail Adherence		
Complete		
≥2/3 but not complete		
≥1/3 but <2/3		
<1/3		
Nail Surface		
Identical to opposite		
Slightly rough		
Very rough		
Longitudinal ribs		
Transverse grooves		
Nail Split		
Absent		
Present		
Eponychium		
Identical to opposite		
Notched		
Synechia		
Total Number of Checked Boxes	Major	Minor

For research purposes, an assessor independent of the patient's care should perform and record PBOMs. Few PBOMs have well-established clinimetric properties for hand trauma in general, and even less so for fingertip and nail bed injuries. PROMs have more widely reported psychometric values for hand, fingertip, and nail bed trauma, although definite knowledge gaps remain. Another advantage of PROMs is they are administered with minimal or no direct human contact, minimizing potential bias and influence. The Core Outcomes Measures in Effectiveness Trials (COMET) report notes that the most site-specific and disease-specific tools should be used when possible. However, no single PROM is likely to satisfy all situations or users for research or clinical applications.[3] Most measures were initially developed for other conditions, such as carpal tunnel syndrome or arthritis, and subsequently validated to varying degrees for hand trauma.

For approaches pertinent to fingertip and nail bed injuries, **Table 3** list the properties and advantages/disadvantages of commonly used

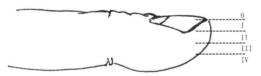

Fig. 3. Lim hook nail classification. The finger is divided into 4 zones when viewed from the lateral side; whichever zone the tip of the fingernail ends in is the reported degree of hook nail. (*From* Arsalan-Werner A, Brui N, Mehling I, et al. Long-term outcome of fingertip reconstruction with the homodigital neurovascular island flap. Arch Orthop Trauma Surg. 2019 Aug;139(8):1171-1178, with permission.)

measured outcomes and PBOMs. Relevant recent examples of each measure being used in studies on fingertip and nail bed trauma are also provided (**Table 4**). **Table 5** does the same for PROMs.

For many of the objective outcome measures, pseudo-objective outcome measures, or PBOMs in **Table 3**, it is ideal to have a certified hand therapist (CHT) perform and record them, especially when doing so for research purposes. CHTs are well educated on standardizing these measures to minimize bias and variability between assessments for different patients or at different times, decreasing measurement error. Furthermore, CHTs perform these tests as part of their daily clinical practice and are thus able to complete them accurately and efficiently. CHTs can also train other research personnel on how to appropriately perform these evaluations. This article presents reasons for choosing, and recommended methods for carrying out, some of these assessments. It covers covers the use of static 2-point discrimination (S2PD), moving (dynamic) 2-point discrimination (M2PD), and Semmes-Weinstein monofilaments (SWMs) because the authors use them routinely in practice and for research purposes. For these sensory tests, the patient's hand/digit should rest on a towel or similar support so movement during testing is minimized and avoids inadvertent detection caused by movement rather than sensation. Patients are also asked to close their eyes during sensory examinations. S2PD assessment in the digital nerve distributions is the most commonly used sensory measure. This assessment correlates with the density of slowly adapting nerve fibers. For compressive neuropathies, S2PD is often the last measure to become abnormal and therefore is not sensitive to early disease. However, for traumatic injuries such as this article is concerned with, S2PD is a baseline indicator of sensory loss that is easy to track during recovery. Commercial tools are available, or a paperclip can be bent to use the 2 free ends at varying distances measured with a ruler.[75]

For fingertip injuries, each digital nerve should be tested individually. It is helpful to first test an uninjured digit so patients become familiar with the tool and understand the instructions. The examiner alternates randomly between a single point and both points touching the skin longitudinally in a single, radial or ulnar, digital nerve distribution. The examiner applies just enough pressure with the points to barely indent and blanch the skin, and then the points are quickly taken away from the skin. When applying 2 points, the examiner must take care to apply the same amount of pressure with each point. The patient is asked to reply after each touch whether they detect 1 or 2 points.

The examiner starts with a 5-mm spread, identifying normal sensation. If the patient is unable to detect the difference between 1 point and 2 points at this spread, the examiner gradually tests larger and larger spreads when applying 2 points. The examiner continues to quickly alternate randomly between applying a single point and 2 points in successively larger 2-point spreads until the patient is able to distinguish between the application of 1 versus 2 points, or it becomes clear that the patient is unable to even distinguish when there is a greater than 15-mm spread between the 2 points. Whatever was the smallest 2-point spread the patient was able to distinguish from a single point is recorded as the S2PD. If a patient is unable to distinguish a greater than 15 mm spread between the 2 points, the authors advocate recording this as 16 mm rather than "not available" or similar so as to not lose meaningful patient data.[76]

M2PD assesses the density of quickly adapting sensory nerve fibers and returns sooner during peripheral nerve recovery compared with S2PD. During the examination, the evaluator alternately and randomly moves 1 or 2 points along the skin in the digital nerve distribution. The points are applied with just enough pressure to blanch the skin. The smallest 2-point spread the patient is able to distinguish from a single point is recorded as the M2PD. Again, results greater than 15 mm are recorded as 16 mm.

SWMs measure so-called threshold sensation, an indication of the smallest amount of stimulation required to generate a sensory response. This measure is an indicator of clinically relevant light touch sensation. Compared with S2PD, SWMs are more sensitive in detecting early sensory disturbances and more responsive in signaling sensory recovery. They also correlate better with manual dexterity, including for fingertip injuries. The examiner starts with the smallest monofilament in the set and applies it to the skin in one of the patient's digital nerve distributions. The examiner applies just enough force to bend the monofilament. The patient replies whenever the monofilament is detected. If the patient is unable to detect the initial monofilament, successively larger (thicker) monofilaments are used until determining the smallest one the patient is able to detect, which is recorded as the result. Again, if patients are unable to detect even the largest monofilament, then a value at or higher than the largest monofilament is recorded to indicate no meaningful sensation rather than excluding the patient's results.[77]

For measuring digital joint ROM after a fingertip or nail bed injury, the authors recommend using the smallest manual goniometer available. Some evaluators place the goniometer along an envisioned midaxis of the measured digit; however, the authors recommend placing it along the dorsum of the digit. Although edema and deformity may influence this method, we still find it more consistent between measurements and examiners. The metacarpophalangeal (MCP) and proximal interphalangeal (PIP) joint ROMs are easily measured with handheld goniometry; however, the DIP joints are much more difficult to measure reliably with composite fist flexion. Instead, if possible, the patient should actively extend the MCP joints as much as is achievable while then maximally flexing the PIP and DIP joints. This intrinsic-minus position allows the use of a handheld goniometer on the DIP joints. Alternatively, the authors have used photogoniometry to measure DIP joint motion, although there are limits to its applicability and agreement with manual goniometry, especially for nonborder digits.[77] For this approach, a lateral side-view picture is taken of the digit in maximum extension and maximum flexion. Digital angle measurements of each joint are then taken and recorded. Where we find this approach more appealing is in following patients longitudinally to demonstrate to them, and document, how they progress regarding motion and appearance. This approach is especially helpful if the images are logged in the electronic medical record or a radiology system, both of which we use in practice.

Strength measurements following fingertip and nail bed injuries and treatments are helpful adjuncts to clinical practice and research. Patients appreciate seeing their progress during strengthening efforts. This progress can help them regain confidence and self-efficacy following their injuries. Strength assessments can also help patients get a sense of whether they are ready to return to certain activities. For example, patients may think they are capable of returning to heavy-duty work or even aggressive athletic or recreational activities; however, a pinch or grip strength less than 10% of their uninvolved side helps signify they could benefit from further rehabilitation to safely return to such high-intensity behaviors. The authors currently use non–scientifically established but clinically useful strength estimates to help guide patients, therapists, trainers, employers, and other providers following such injuries. For example, for activities of daily living, a good goal is to have at least 50% strength compared with the contralateral and with adequate comfort during assessments. For high-level athletic and heavy-duty work, greater than 75% strength is recommended, depending on

the nature of their endeavor. These estimates also offer good targets to strive toward, again helping with confidence and self-efficacy. For work scenarios, a formal functional capacity evaluation may be needed to obtain as thorough a determination of a patient's capabilities and limitations as possible.

For evaluations in clinical practice and research work, the authors commonly measure hand grip, tip pinch, and key pinch strength. Using a consistent approach, as with the other methods discussed earlier, is key to minimizing measurement variance. Examiners should routinely have patients tested with their extremities in the same positions as best as possible. This approach entails having patients' upper arms at their sides, elbows flexed 90°, and wrists in neutral rotation. From this position, grip strength is assessed with a dynamometer. There are several grip-size positions available on dynamometers. Some investigators choose to always use the same grip-size setting when carrying out a research project. However, the authors think it is more clinically applicable, and thus useful for research purposes also, to have patients use the setting on which they think they can generate maximum grip strength. The formal protocol for independent medical examinations of worker's compensation or other medicolegal patients, permanent impairment ratings, functional capacity evaluations, or work hardening programs is to have the patient rapidly alternate from the injured to the uninjured side for a total of 3 measurements per side. If there is minimal variation for each side's individual readings (eg, <5%), this is thought to indicate good, consistent effort on the patient's part and thus a reasonable estimate of grip strength on each side. In this case, the average of the 3 readings on each side is recorded as the result. If there are large variations for 1 or both sides' individual readings, this can indicate poor, inconsistent effort or pain that limits the accuracy of the strength estimate. In this case, the range of the readings is recorded, and a note is made of the inconsistent readings. Tip pinch and key pinch strength are measured and recorded in a similar fashion using a pinchmeter. The authors measure tip pinch between the thumb and each injured finger, whenever clinically appropriate and safe to do so. For routine clinical purposes not involving worker's compensation or other medicolegal evaluations, the rapid alternating approach is typically deferred and single maximum effort recordings are used.

One general approach for deciding which outcome measures to use is to consider face validity for the injuries or treatments that are being managed or studied. This approach is especially

Table 5
Patient-rated outcome measures

PROM	Outcome Range and Meaning	Relevant or Representative Values in Hand Trauma	Relevant or Representative Values in Fingertip/ Nail Bed Trauma Across Studies	MIC (aka MCID)	Advantages	Disadvantages	References
DASH	0–100 Higher scores indicate more disability	Initial 61 ± 20, final 19 ± 10 ES 0.67–1.66 SRM 0.84–1.40; $r = 0.38$ correlation with AMA impairment rating (SS)	Single fingertip Tamai zone 1 amputations: replant mean 8, SD 5, range 2.2–17.5, homodigital flap with or without bone/nail bed composite mean 7, SD 8, range 0–31.8 Allen III/IV fingertip amputation homodigital flap mean 16 r>0.60 correlation with MHQ	Unknown for fingertip/ nail bed injuries; for hand trauma and general hand/upper extremity conditions MIC 5–19; SEM ~ 5	• Widely studied and used • Represents the upper extremity as a whole • Good reliability, validity, and responsiveness: MICs>MDCs for most constructs • Moderate to good correlation with grip strength and pain	• Global upper extremity rather than hand specific • Lengthy • Lacks responsiveness for hand trauma • Ceiling effect • Weak to moderate correlation with impairment ratings	3,4,8,32,33,54-57
qDASH	0–100 Higher scores indicate more disability	Median score 15 for those able to RTW; 49 for those unable to RTW (SSD)	Fingertip injuries mean initial score 35, SD 18, range 0–93; mean at 1 mo 17, SD 17, range 0–75 (SSD) Tamai zone 1: revision amputations mean 7 ± 5; replantations 2 ± 3 (SSD) ICC = 0.94; Cronbach α = 0.90; r = 0.61 correlation between qDASH and days off work	Unknown for fingertip/ nail bed injuries; for hand trauma and general hand MIC 8– 26; MDC at 90% CI ~13–28 (note this is not ideal given some of the reported MDC range values are higher than the reported MIC range values)	• 19 fewer questions than DASH with acceptable criterion validity • Good correlation with Jebsen-Taylor Test	• Likely lacks responsiveness for hand-specific trauma • Unscorable if more than 1 question not answered	3,15,27,35,48,58
MHQ	0–100 Higher scores	Initial 66 ± 13, final 87 ± 33 ES 0.84–1.89	r>0.60 correlation with DASH	Unknown for fingertip/ nail bed injuries; for hand trauma and	• Widely studied and used	Lengthy	3,4,37,54-59

(continued on next page)

Table 5
(continued)

PROM	Outcome Range and Meaning	Relevant or Representative Values in Hand Trauma	Relevant or Representative Values in Fingertip/Nail Bed Trauma Across Studies	MIC (aka MCID)	Advantages	Disadvantages	References
	indicate better outcomes	SRM 1.05–1.84; r = –0.24 correlation with AMA impairment rating (SS)		general hand/wrist disorders MIC 8–15	• Good reliability, validity, and responsiveness • More responsive than DASH or DHI • Hand/wrist specific • MICs>MDCs		
bMHQ	0–100 Higher scores indicate better outcomes	NA	NA	Unknown for fingertip/nail bed injuries; most use MHQ values given high criterion validity	• 62 fewer questions than full MHQ and as responsive • Excellent criterion validity with MHQ (r = 0.99) • Good correlation with Jebsen-Taylor Test	No bilateral/hand dominance inclusion as in full MHQ	60
DHI	0–90 Higher scores indicate worse activity limitations	Initial 52 ± 21, final 6 ± 15 ES 1.68 SRM 1.48	NA	NA	• Shorter than some other full-version PROMs (18 questions) • Some use in hand trauma	• Developed for rheumatoid arthritis • Atypical scoring range • Not as widely used/studied	55
VAS for pain	0–10 (aka Numeric Rating Scale) or 0–100 Higher scores indicate worse pain	—	Fingertip injuries mean initial 2.8, SD 2.3, range 0–8; mean at 1 mo 1.2, SD 1.2, range 0–6 (SSD) Allen III/IV fingertip amputation homodigital flap mean 1.2	Not clearly defined for hand trauma; for general use MIC typically 1–2 for 0–10 scale and 10–20 for 0–100 scale	• Simple • Commonly used • Track over time, option for nonlanguage bias • Patient valued • Strong correlations between the 0–10 and 0–100 scales • Pain intensity correlates with depression and disability	• Floor and ceiling effect • Oversimplified approach to patient pain and how different patients are affected differently • Changes in patient pain level are likely nonlinear and thus not completely characterized by a linear construct	27,33,61–63

PSEQ	0–60 Higher scores indicate better self-efficacy 10 questions answered on 0–6 point Likert scales	For general hand practice patients, including those with trauma diagnoses mean score 48, SD 12, range 9–60	Fingertip injuries mean initial 50, SD 11, range 13–60; mean at 1 mo 55, SD 8.7, range 17–60 (SSD)	NA	• High test-retest reliability (r = 0.79) and internal consistency (Cronbach α = 0.92) • Correlation with qDASH, pain, depression (PHQ), and length of time off work • May be best predictor of patient-rated disability • Good criterion validity for shorter 2-question PSEQ-2 version with 0–12 score range	Ceiling effect	27,64
Cold Intolerance Symptom Severity	4–100 Higher scores worse 6 questions re: feeling cold and impact; each question has own scale; >30 total score indicates cold intolerance	For local flaps mean 28, range 4–66 For digital nerve injuries mean 35, range 3–91 For hand fractures mean 23 For general upper extremity trauma median 44, IQR 25–55, range 10–95	NA	Normative values for healthy asymptomatic volunteers suggests scores >30–50 are clinically relevant; MIC NA	• Good reliability and validity • Correlation with DASH	• Lengthy • Very specific • Complex scoring	65–72
Patient-rated VAS for appearance	0–10 or 0–100 Higher scores indicate better appearance	NA	Visible nail lengthening via eponychial flap mean 7.5 ± 1.5; revision amputation 5.9 ± 1.5 (SSD)	NA	• Simple • Commonly used • Track over time • Patient valued • Correlation with patient satisfaction	Lack of formal psychometric evaluation	37

(continued on next page)

Table 5
(continued)

PROM	Outcome Range and Meaning	Relevant or Representative Values in Hand Trauma	Relevant or Representative Values in Fingertip/ Nail Bed Trauma Across Studies	MIC (aka MCID)	Advantages	Disadvantages	References
Patient-rated VAS for satisfaction with outcome	0–10 Higher scores indicate greater satisfaction with treatment or outcome	NA	Homodigital flap fingertip reconstruction mean 8.7, SD 1.4	NA	• Simple • Commonly used • Patient valued • Correlation with aesthetic outcome	• Incomplete assessment of patient satisfaction • Lack of formal psychometric evaluation	33,67,73
PHQ-9	0–27 Higher scores indicate greater depression 9 questions: 5 = mild depression; 10 = moderate depression; 15 = moderately severe depression; 20 = severe depression; score of 10 or higher estimates as a major depression diagnosis	For general hand practice patients, including those with trauma diagnoses, mean score per question = 0.39 ± 0.49	Fingertip injuries mean initial 2.8, SD 3.9, range 0–17; at 1 mo mean 1.6, SD 3.6, range 0–20 (SSD)	NA	• Correlation with qDASH, pain, PSEQ, and length of time off work • High test-retest reliability and internal consistency • Cronbach α = 0.89 • Good criterion validity for shorter 2-question PHQ-2 version with 0–6 score range	• Floor effect • Patient and provider reluctance or lack of resources to use as an outcome tool and act on its results	27,74

Abbreviations: DHI, Duruöz Hand Index; ES, effect size; IQR, interquartile range; MHQ, Michigan Hand Questionnaire; PHQ, Patient Health Questionnaire; PSEQ, Pain Self-Efficacy Questionnaire; SD, standard deviation; SRM, standardized response mean.

Adapted from Zook EG, Guy RJ, Russell RC. A study of nail bed injuries: Causes, treatment, and prognosis. J Hand Surg Am 1984;9:247-52; *Data from* Koh SH, You Y, Kim YW, et al. Long-term outcomes of nail bed reconstruction. Arch Plast Surg 2019;46(6):580–588.

useful for fingertip and nail bed trauma where complete psychometric testing of assessment tools is lacking. Face validity indicates that the clinician has appraised the outcomes construct to determine what, if any, components are pertinent to the patients. Clinicians or researchers can use this approach for any potential outcomes measure. Of course, face validity helps clinicians assess an outcomes measure's applicability to their patients or studies, but it does not ensure that the outcomes measure is inclusive of everything the assessor wishes to gauge. However, time spent considering and discussing what critical elements the chosen outcome measures will and will not capture is time well spent for clinicians and investigators. This article presents a fingertip and nail bed injuries face validity review of 4 of the most commonly used and studied PROMs in hand surgery: the Disabilities of the Arm, Shoulder and Hand (DASH), Quick DASH (qDASH), Michigan Hand Questionnaire (MHQ), and Brief MHQ (bMHQ). The DASH and MHQ have been in use for more than 20 years. The qDASH and the bMHQ have had criterion validity testing in that they have been validated against a gold standard; in this case their parent forms the DASH and MHQ, respectively.

The DASH questionnaire has 30 questions, each with a 5-point rating scale.[78,79] There is a conversion calculation so the final score ranges from 0 to 100, with higher numbers indicating worse disability. The authors consider 28 of the DASH questions applicable to patients with fingertip and nail bed injuries, provided the trauma is isolated to the fingertip with no shoulder or other upper extremity issues. Understanding an outcome measure's minimal important change (MIC) is critical to implementing it appropriately, and this holds true for the DASH. For all outcome measures, the MIC can vary across patient groups, comorbidities, conditions or injuries, treatment types, and clinical timelines.[75,80] Also, the method used to calculate an MIC affects its point estimate, thus MICs for outcome measures should be given as ranges to reflect the imprecision of the point estimates generated.[81,82] Given the lack of DASH MIC evaluation for patients with fingertip and nail bed injuries in isolation, the authors recommend using the general minimal clinically important difference range of greater than 5 to 15 commonly quoted across multiple conditions and treatments, and considering the standard error of measurement of ~5.[8,83] There are also 2 separate optional work and sport components that accompany the DASH with 4 additional questions each, all of which have face validity for patients with fingertip and nail bed trauma.

The qDASH has 11 questions, each with the same 5-point scale as the DASH, and all 11 questions have face validity for patients with fingertip and nail bed damage. There is a calculation conversion for the qDASH so the scoring range is also 0 to 100. The MIC for the qDASH among different patients and conditions is between 8 and 26 points.[8,80] A significant concern in using the qDASH is poor responsiveness. The lower responsiveness for qDASH is attributed to low correlations with global estimates of change evaluations.[84]

In contrast with the DASH, the MHQ considers the hand and wrist in isolation from the rest of the upper extremity, allows for assessment of bilateral hands, and includes patient-rated aesthetic and satisfaction elements. In 1 comparison between MHQ, DASH, and qDASH, the MHQ had good performance across the most psychometric categories, although none of the tools entirely fulfilled all aspects.[3] The full MHQ has the same 37 questions for patients' right and left sides for a total of 74 questions. Each question is answered on a 5-point scale and the final scoring range is 0 to 100, with higher numbers indicating better outcomes. For face validity, the authors consider 35 of 37 questions relevant to patients with fingertip and nail bed injuries. The MIC for the MHQ across different patients and diagnoses, including trauma, is between 8 and 15. To lessen responder burden, the bMHQ evaluates each side in isolation and has 12 total questions. It has near-perfect criterion validity compared with the MHQ for unilateral conditions or constructs.[61] We consider 11 of those questions germane to fingertip and nail bed trauma.

When implementing any outcome measures, clinicians should consider the timing of administering them relative to the patient's clinical course. At a minimum, the authors recommend doing so at the patient's first presentation and monthly until discharge. If midterm outcomes are important, such as for assessing nail growth and aesthetics, then additional evaluations 4 and 12 months after initial presentation are also required, at a minimum. Long-term outcomes that may change over an extended period of time are more important for research purposes when assessing cold intolerance, psychological and functional adaptations, and disability, and should be done at yearly intervals until reaching a plateau for the outcome measure. The authors consider plateau points reached once 2 consecutive measurements over a predetermined time interval decrease to within the minimal detectable change (MDC) range for that outcome. For example, following a fingertip injury, unless patients normalize and are ready for discharge sooner, we measure their ROM at first presentation and then monthly for 4 total months. At that time, patients have commonly reached tissue equilibrium, provided their clinical examinations are consistent with having met that milestone. It is some variable time beyond that point that a true plateau for ROM is achieved. The MDC for measuring a finger joint's ROM with a handheld goniometer is commonly, although not definitively,[5,85] held to be greater than 5° to 10°, with measurement error and random chance accounting for any changes less than that. So, once the patient has reached tissue equilibrium at least 4 months after presentation, any 2 consecutive ROM measurements over 1-month intervals that are within 5° to 10° of each other is considered the ROM plateau and the final result.

It is also important to be aware that anatomic injury and objective measures may not, and often do not, correlate with patient disability or how patients rate their outcomes. Again, combining patient-rated and anatomic functional measures may be the best approach.[2] A patient's psychological status also, not surprisingly, significantly affects the patient's outcome measures and quality of life.[56] Some investigators state that a patient's psychological status, especially having a depressive mood, has a larger impact on the patient's subsequent disability, pain, and time off work than does the anatomic nature of the patient's fingertip injuries.[27] Investigators also report minimal correlation between patient-rated disability and evaluator-rated impairment following hand injuries, indicating that individual patient factors other than extent of injury are important to consider.[54] Cognitive behavior therapy, medications, empathetic care, and ensuring and engendering adequate support systems are all helpful for these patients. It is ideal to have a behavioral health or behavioral pain specialist present or readily available by referral for patients with trauma. Doing so can positively affect patient care and outcomes, and decrease health care costs overall.[86]

This article provides approaches and references that the authors have found helpful for clinical practice and research activities. By doing so, it outlines a knowledge base for those who care for and study patients with fingertip and nail bed injuries and also indicates where evidence gaps remain.

DISCLOSURE

The authors have no commercial or financial conflicts of interest or funding sources related to the material presented in this article.

REFERENCES

1. Giladi AM, McGlinn EP, Shauver MJ, et al. Measuring outcomes and determining long-term disability after revision amputation for treatment of traumatic finger and thumb amputation injuries. Plast Reconstr Surg 2014;134(5):746e–55e.
2. Giladi AM, Ranganathan K, Chung KC. Measuring Functional and Patient-Reported Outcomes After Treatment of Mutilating Hand Injuries: A Global Health Approach. Hand Clin 2016;32(4):465–75.
3. Wormald JCR, Geoghegan L, Sierakowski K, et al. Site-specific Patient-reported Outcome Measures for Hand Conditions: Systematic Review of Development and Psychometric Properties. Plast Reconstr Surg Glob Open 2019;7(5):e2256.
4. Dacombe PJ, Amirfeyz R, Davis T. Patient-Reported Outcome Measures for Hand and Wrist Trauma: Is There Sufficient Evidence of Reliability, Validity, and Responsiveness? Hand (N Y) 2016;11(1):11–21.
5. van Kooij YE, Fink A, Nijhuis-van der Sanden MW, et al. The reliability and measurement error of protractor-based goniometry of the fingers: A systematic review. J Hand Ther 2017;30(4):457–67.
6. Terwee CB, Bot SD, de Boer MR, et al. Quality criteria were proposed for measurement properties of health status questionnaires. J Clin Epidemiol 2007;60(1):34–42.
7. Prinsen CAC, Mokkink LB, Bouter LM, et al. COSMIN guideline for systematic reviews of patient-reported outcome measures. Qual Life Res 2018;27(5):1147–57.
8. van de Ven-Stevens LA, Munneke M, Terwee CB, et al. Clinimetric properties of instruments to assess activities in patients with hand injury: a systematic review of the literature. Arch Phys Med Rehabil 2009;90(1):151–69.
9. Lemmon JA, Janis JE, Rohrich RJ. Soft-tissue injuries of the fingertip: methods of evaluation and treatment. An algorithmic approach. Plast Reconstr Surg 2008;122(3):105e–17e.
10. Evans D, Bernardis C. A new classification for fingertip injuries. J Hand Surg Br 2000;25:58–60.
11. Venkatramani H, Sabapathy SR. Fingertip replantation: Technical considerations and outcome analysis of 24 consecutive fingertip replantations. Indian J Plast Surg 2011;44(2):237–45.
12. Allen MJ. Conservative management of finger tip injuries in adults. Hand 1980;12(3):257–65.
13. Sir E, Aksoy A, Kasapoğlu Aksoy M. Comparisons between long-term outcomes of the use of reposition flaps and replantations in fingertip amputations. Ulus Travma Acil Cerrahi Derg 2018;24(5):462–7.
14. Mink van der Molen AB, Ettema AM, Hovius SE. Outcome of hand trauma: The hand injury severity scoring system (HISS) and subsequent impairment and disability. J Hand Surg Br 2003;28:295–9.

15. Matsuzaki H, Narisawa H, Miwa H, et al. Predicting functional recovery and return to work after mutilating hand injuries: usefulness of Campbell's Hand Injury Severity Score. J Hand Surg Am 2009;34(5):880–5.

16. Campbell D, Kay S. The hand injury severity scoring system. J Hand Surg 1996;21B:295–8.

17. Hirase Y. Salvage of fingertip amputated at nail level: new surgical principles and treatments. Ann Plast Surg 1997;38(2):151–7.

18. Suzuki Y, Ishikawa K, Isshiki N, et al. Fingertip replantation with an efferent A-V anastomosis for venous drainage: clinical reports. Br J Plast Surg 1993;46(3):187–91.

19. Ishikawa K, Kawakatsu M, Arata J, et al. Classification of the amputation level for the distal part of the finger: 10 years study. J Jpn Soc Surg Hand 2001; 18:870–4.

20. Moiemen NS, Elliot D. Composite graft replacement of digital tips. 2. A study in children. J Hand Surg Br 1997;22(3):346–52.

21. Butler DP, Murugesan L, Ruston J, et al. The outcomes of digital tip amputation replacement as a composite graft in a paediatric population. J Hand Surg Eur Vol 2016;41(2):164–70.

22. Borrelli MR, Landin ML, Agha R, et al. Composite grafts for fingertip amputations: A systematic review protocol. Int J Surg Protoc 2019;16:1–4.

23. Tamai S. Twenty years' experience of limb replantation–review of 293 upper extremity replants. J Hand Surg Am 1982;7(6):549–56.

24. Yamano Y. Replantation of fingertips. J Hand Surg Br 1993;18(2):157–62.

25. Dadaci M, Ince B, Altuntas Z, et al. Assessment of survival rates compared according to the Tamai and Yamano classifications in fingertip replantations. Indian J Orthop 2016;50(4):384–9.

26. Zook EG, Guy RJ, Russell RC. A study of nail bed injuries: causes, treatment and prognosis. J Hand Surg Am 1984;9:247–52.

27. Bot AGJ, Bossen JKJ, Mudgal CS, et al. Determinants of disability after fingertip injuries. Psychosomatics 2014;55(4):372–80.

28. Wittink H, Rogers W, Sukiennik A, et al. Physical functioning: self-report and performance measures are related but distinct. Spine 2003;28(20):2407–13.

29. Sears ED, Chung KC. Validity and responsiveness of the Jebsen–Taylor hand function test. J Hand Surg Am 2010;35(1):30–7.

30. Rabarin F, Saint Cast Y, Jeudy J, et al. Cross-finger flap for reconstruction of fingertip amputations: Long-term results. Orthop Traumatol Surg Res 2016;102(4 Suppl):S225–8.

31. Wang K, Sears ED, Shauver MJ, et al. A systematic review of outcomes of revision amputation treatment for fingertip amputations. Hand 2013;8:139–45.

32. Nakanishi A, Omokawa S, Kawamura K, et al. Tamai Zone 1 Fingertip Amputation: Reconstruction Using a Digital Artery Flap Compared With Microsurgical Replantation. J Hand Surg Am 2019;44(8):655–61.

33. Arsalan-Werner A, Brui N, Mehling I, et al. Long-term outcome of fingertip reconstruction with the homodigital neurovascular island flap. Arch Orthop Trauma Surg 2019;139(8):1171–8.

34. Nakanishi A, Kawamura K, Omokawa S, et al. Predictors of Hand Dexterity after Single-Digit Replantation. J Reconstr Microsurg 2019;35(3):194–7.

35. Hollak N, Soer R, van der Woude LH, et al. Towards a comprehensive Functional Capacity Evaluation for hand function. Appl Ergon 2014;45(3):686–92.

36. Chen QZ, Sun YC, Chen J, et al. Comparative study of functional and aesthetically outcomes of reverse digital artery and reverse dorsal homodigital island flaps for fingertip repair. J Hand Surg Eur Vol 2015;40(9):935–43.

37. Chen HY, Hsu CC, Lin YT, et al. Functional and aesthetic outcomes of the fingertips after nail lengthening using the eponychial flap. J Plast Reconstr Aesthet Surg 2015;68(10):1438–46.

38. Sebastin SJ, Chung KC. A systematic review of the outcomes of replantation of distal digital amputation. Plast Reconstr Surg 2011;128:723–37.

39. Fonseca MCR, Elui VMC, Lalone E, et al. Functional, motor, and sensory assessment instruments upon nerve repair in adult hands: systematic review of psychometric properties. Syst Rev 2018;7(1):175.

40. Dellon AL. The moving two-point discrimination test: clinical evaluation of the quickly adapting fiber/receptor system. J Hand Surg 1978;3:474–81.

41. Boudard J, Loisel F, El Rifaï S, et al. Fingertip amputations treated with occlusive dressings. Hand Surg Rehabil 2019;38(4):257–61.

42. Wang Y, Sunitha M, Chung KC. How to measure outcomes of peripheral nerve surgery. Hand Clin 2013; 29(3):349-361.

43. Novak C, Kelly L, Mackinnon S. Sensory recovery after median nerve grafting. J Hand Surg 1992;17A: 59–68.

44. Rosén B, Lundborg G. A model instrument for the documentation of outcome after nerve repair. J Hand Surg Am 2000;25(3):535–43.

45. Greig A, Gardiner MD, Sierakowski A, et al, NINJA Pilot Collaborative. Randomized feasibility trial of replacing or discarding the nail plate after nail-bed repair in children. Br J Surg 2017;104(12):1634–9.

46. Koh SH, You Y, Kim YW, et al. Long-term outcomes of nail bed reconstruction. Arch Plast Surg 2019; 46(6):580–8.

47. Lim GJ, Yam AK, Lee JY, et al. The spiral flap for fingertip resurfacing: short-term and long-term results. J Hand Surg Am 2008;33(3):340–7.

48. Regmi S, Gu J, Zhang N, et al. A Systematic Review of Outcomes and Complications of Primary Fingertip Reconstruction Using Reverse-Flow Homodigital Island Flaps. Aesthetic Plast Surg 2016;40:277–83.

49. Wittich W, Nadon C. The Purdue Pegboard test: normative data for older adults with low vision. Disabil Rehabil Assist Technol 2017;12(3):272–9.

50. Buddenberg LA, Davis C. Test-retest reliability of the Purdue pegboard test. Am J Occup Ther 2000;54:555–8.

51. Sığırtmaç İC, Öksüz Ç. Investigation of reliability, validity, and cutoff value of the Jebsen-Taylor Hand Function Test. J Hand Ther 2020. [Epub ahead of print].

52. Schoneveld K, Wittink H, Takken T. Clinimetric evaluation of measurement tools used in hand therapy to assess activity and participation. J Hand Ther 2009;22(3):221–35.

53. Farzad M, Asgari A, Dashab F, et al. Does Disability Correlate With Impairment After Hand Injury? Clin Orthop Relat Res 2015;473(11):3470–6.

54. Dogu B, Usen A, Kuran B, et al. Comparison of responsiveness of Michigan Hand Outcomes Questionnaire, Disabilities of the Arm, Shoulder and Hand Questionnaire, and Duruöz Hand Index in patients with traumatic hand injury. J Back Musculoskelet Rehabil 2019;32(1):111–7.

55. Horng YS, Lin MC, Feng CT, et al. Responsiveness of the Michigan Hand Outcomes Questionnaire and the Disabilities of the Arm, Shoulder, and Hand questionnaire in patients with hand injury. J Hand Surg Am 2010;35(3):430–6.

56. Yoon AP, Kaur S, Chou CH, et al, FRANCHISE Group. Reliability and Validity of Upper Extremity Patient-Reported Outcome Measures in Assessing Traumatic Finger Amputation Management. Plast Reconstr Surg 2020;145(1):94e–105e.

57. Maia MV, de Moraes VY, Dos Santos JB, et al. Minimal important difference after hand surgery: a prospective assessment for DASH, MHQ, and SF-12. SICOT J 2016;2:32.

58. Franchignoni F, Vercelli S, Giordano A, et al. Minimal clinically important difference of the disabilities of the arm, shoulder and hand outcome measure (DASH) and its shortened version (QuickDASH). J Orthop Sports Phys Ther 2014;44(1):30–9.

59. London DA, Stepan JG, Calfee RP. Determining the Michigan Hand Outcomes Questionnaire minimal clinically important difference by means of three methods. Plast Reconstr Surg 2014;133(3):616–25.

60. Waljee JF, Kim HM, Burns PB, et al. Development of a brief, 12-item version of the Michigan Hand Questionnaire. Plast Reconstr Surg 2011;128(1):208–20.

61. Myles PS, Myles DB, Galagher W, et al. Measuring acute postoperative pain using the visual analog scale: the minimal clinically important difference and patient acceptable symptom state. Br J Anaesth 2017;118(3):424–9.

62. Tashjian RZ, Deloach J, Porucznik CA, et al. Minimal clinically important differences (MCID) and patient acceptable symptomatic state (PASS) for visual analog scales (VAS) measuring pain in patients treated for rotator cuff disease. J Shoulder Elbow Surg 2009;18(6):927–32.

63. Badalamente M, Coffelt L, Elfar J, et al. American Society for Surgery of the Hand Clinical Trials and Outcomes Committee. Measurement scales in clinical research of the upper extremity, part 1: general principles, measures of general health, pain, and patient satisfaction. J Hand Surg Am 2013;38(2):401–6.

64. Briet JP, Bot AG, Hageman MG, et al. The pain self-efficacy questionnaire: validation of an abbreviated two-item questionnaire. Psychosomatics 2014;55(6):578–85.

65. Sun YC, Chen QZ, Chen J, et al. Prevalence, characteristics and natural history of cold intolerance after the reverse digital artery flap. J Hand Surg Eur Vol 2016;41(2):171–6.

66. Li M, Huang M, Yang Y, et al. Preliminary Study on Functional and Aesthetic Reconstruction by Using a Small Artery-only Free Medial Flap of the Second Toe for Fingertip Injuries. Clinics (Sao Paulo) 2019;74:e1226.

67. Nijhuis TH, Smits ES, Jaquet JB, et al. Prevalence and severity of cold intolerance in patients after hand fracture. J Hand Surg Eur Vol 2010;35(4):306–11.

68. Töre NG, Gömüşsoy M, Oskay D. Validity and reliability of the Turkish version of the Cold Intolerance Symptom Severity Questionnaire. Turk J Med Sci 2019;49(4):1221–7.

69. Carlsson IK, Rosén B, Dahlin LB. Self-reported cold sensitivity in normal subjects and in patients with traumatic hand injuries or hand-arm vibration syndrome. BMC Musculoskelet Disord 2010;11:89.

70. Ruijs AC, Jaquet JB, Daanen HA, et al. Cold intolerance of the hand measured by the CISS questionnaire in a normative study population. J Hand Surg Br 2006;31(5):533–6.

71. Carlsson IK, Nilsson JA, Dahlin LB. Cut-off value for self-reported abnormal cold sensitivity and predictors for abnormality and severity in hand injuries. J Hand Surg Eur Vol 2010;35(5):409–16.

72. Kim AR, Kim DY, Kim JS, et al. Application of cold intolerance symptom severity questionnaire among vibration-exposed workers as a screening tool for the early detection of hand-arm vibration syndrome: a cross-sectional study. Ann Occup Environ Med 2019;31:6.

73. Graham B. Defining and Measuring Patient Satisfaction. J Hand Surg Am 2016;41(9):929–31.

74. Bot AG, Becker SJ, van Dijk CN, et al. Abbreviated psychologic questionnaires are valid in patients with hand conditions. Clin Orthop Relat Res 2013;471(12):4037–44.

75. Finnell JT, Knopp R, Johnson P, et al. A calibrated paper clip is a reliable measure of two-point discrimination. Acad Emerg Med 2004;11(6):710–4.

76. Means KR Jr, Rinker BD, Higgins JP, et al. A Multicenter, Prospective, Randomized, Pilot Study of Outcomes for Digital Nerve Repair in the Hand Using Hollow Conduit Compared With Processed Allograft Nerve. Hand (N Y) 2016;11(2):144–51. https://doi.org/10.1177/1558944715627233.

77. Meals CG, Saunders RJ, Desale S, et al. Viability of Hand and Wrist Photogoniometry. Hand (N Y). 2018;13(3): 301–4. https://doi.org/10.1177/1558944717702471.

78. Hudak PL, Amadio PC, Bombardier C. Development of an upper extremity outcome measure: the DASH (disabilities of the arm, shoulder and hand) [corrected]. The Upper Extremity Collaborative Group (UECG). Am J Ind Med 1996;29:602–8.

79. Available at: http://www.dash.iwh.on.ca/

80. Ozer K, Malay S, Toker S, et al. Minimal clinically important difference of carpal tunnel release in diabetic and nondiabetic patients. Plast Reconstr Surg 2013;131(6):1279–85.

81. Revicki D, Hays RD, Cella D, et al. Recommended methods for determining responsiveness and minimally important differences for patient-reported outcomes. J Clin Epidemiol 2008;61(2):102–9.

82. Rodrigues JN, Mabvuure NT, Nikkhah D, et al. Minimal important changes and differences in elective hand surgery. J Hand Surg Eur Vol 2015;40(9): 900–12.

83. Sorensen AA, Howard D, Tan WH, et al. Minimal clinically important differences of 3 patient-rated outcomes instruments. J Hand Surg Am 2013;38(4): 641–9.

84. Kennedy CA, Beaton DE, Smith P, et al. Measurement properties of the QuickDASH (Disabilities of the Arm, Shoulder and Hand) outcome measure and cross-cultural adaptations of the QuickDASH: a systematic review. Qual Life Res 2013;22(9): 2509–47.

85. Reissner L, Fischer G, List R, et al. Minimal detectable difference of the finger and wrist range of motion: comparison of goniometry and 3D motion analysis. J Orthop Surg Res 2019;14(1):173.

86. Vranceanu A, Ring D, Kulich R, et al. Idiopathic Hand and Arm Pain: Delivering Cognitive Behavioral Therapy as Part of a Multidisciplinary Team in a Surgical Practice. Cogn Behav Pract 2008;15:244–54.

The Burden of Fingertip Trauma on the US Military

Matthew E. Wells, DO[a,b],*, John P. Scanaliato, MD[a,b], Nicholas A. Kusnezov, MD[c],
Leon J. Nesti, MD[d,e], John C. Dunn, MD[a,e]

KEYWORDS

- Fingertip • Military • Finger • Nail • Phalanx

KEY POINTS

- Injuries encountered range from subungual hematomas to finger amputations. Treatment modalities are dictated by injury patterns, anatomic considerations, and the need to return to duty.
- Nail bed injuries should be repaired when possible. Any exposed bone or tendon is treated with appropriate soft tissue coverage.
- If soft tissue coverage is unobtainable, revision amputation should be performed with special attention given to maintaining as much finger length as possible.

ABOUT THE AUTHORS

The authors are active duty US Army surgeons stationed at Fort Bliss located in El Paso, Texas. This base has a sizable restricted airspace containing White Sands Missile Range and Biggs Army Airfield, which are used for missile and artillery training and testing. Fort Bliss is the home of the 1st Armored Division, 32nd Air and Missile Command, 11th Air Defense Artillery Brigade, and the 402nd Field Artillery Brigade of the US Army. The major military treatment facility for the 30,000 soldiers and their dependents stationed at Fort Bliss is William Beaumont Army Medical Center.

BACKGROUND

Deployment readiness is of utmost importance to the US military. Deployment status determines if a soldier is administratively, legally, and medically cleared to be fit for duty. Physical injuries serve as a major limiting factor to the operational fighting force and prevent soldiers from being able to fulfill their given duties. According to Army Directive 2018-22 (Retention Policy for Non-Deployable Soldiers), a soldier must meet physical readiness standards and have the ability to discharge their weapon to be considered deployable and ultimately retainable within the military. There are multiple occupational hazards given the hand-intensive workload of an operational fighting force that warrant consideration.

Finger and hand injuries have a notable burden on the military in stateside and deployment settings. These injuries often remove soldiers from the fight entirely. The Armed Forces Health Surveillance Center tracks inpatient and outpatient encounters among active duty personnel in the Armed Forces. During 2014 alone there were 68,553 ambulatory visit encounters because of a

[a] Department of Orthopaedic Surgery, William Beaumont Army Medical Center, 5005 North Piedras Street, El Paso, TX 79902, USA; [b] Department of Orthopaedic Surgery, Texas Tech University Health Sciences Center, 4801 Alberta Avenue, El Paso, TX 79905, USA; [c] Department of Orthopaedic Surgery, Blanchfield Army Community Hospital, 650 Joel Drive, Fort Campbell, KY 42223, USA; [d] Department of Orthopaedic Surgery, Walter Reed National Military Medical Center, 8901 Rockville Pike, Bethesda, MD 20889, USA; [e] Uniformed Services University of the Health Sciences, Bethesda, MD 20814, USA
* Corresponding author. Department of Orthopaedic Surgery, William Beaumont Army Medical Center, 5005 North Piedras Street, El Paso, TX 79902.
E-mail addresses: matthew.eric.wells@gmail.com; matthew.wells@ttuhsc.edu

Hand Clin 37 (2021) 155–165
https://doi.org/10.1016/j.hcl.2020.09.010
0749-0712/21/Published by Elsevier Inc.

hand-related injury in the nondeployed setting across all branches of the military.[1] Both the stateside and deployed settings bring unique challenges to surgeons and fingertip injuries are a routine consultation.

During Operation Iraqi Freedom, Ibn Sina Hospital served as the US Army's primary trauma receiving center located in Baghdad, Iraq. Over a 2-year period (2007–2009), 7520 patients were seen at the emergency department and 331 cases involved hand injuries.[2] On average, 13.7 noncombat-related hand injuries presented per month accounting for roughly 4.4% of total emergency department visits. Most cases involved finger trauma caused by vehicle doors, hatches, or weapons striking soldiers' fingers. It is likely that these numbers grossly underestimate the finger injury burden on the military in the deployed environment, because there were multiple US military trauma facilities within the combat theater at that time with capabilities to directly evacuate patients to higher echelons of care. Fingertip injuries have similar ramifications among the different branches of the military. The US Navy experiences high proportions of hand injuries during carrier battle group deployments, which contribute to notable impacts on morbidity when compared with other injuries encountered.[3,4] Similar hand injury burden has been reported among other countries' military population.[5]

There is a particular predisposition of hand trauma among combat soldiers, tankers, and engineer mechanics within the military. When compared with artillery, engineer mechanics were 6.5 times more likely to sustain a fracture or dislocation of the hand or fingers.[6] Although some preventative measures, such as required thick glove wear, has notably improved burn injuries to the hand, finger fractures and fingertip injuries have remained problematic in these populations.[7]

Hand and finger injuries have a substantial burden among US military members in the stateside and deployed environments. Military surgeons have the unique responsibility of often having subspecialty fellowship training while still carrying the responsibility of managing any related musculoskeletal trauma in an austere environment. These individuals can expect to see various upper extremity injuries regardless of their subspecialty training. In the setting of fingertip injuries, the goals of treatment may not be dictated by optimal functional outcome, but rather retaining and sustaining the military fighting force. This review serves to outline the burden and type of fingertip injuries experienced within the military and recommended treatment guidelines in austere environments.

ECHELONS OF MILITARY CARE

To better understand military surgeons' role in the deployed environment,[8] a brief overview of the different levels of care, echelons, is prudent. The Joint Health Services simplifies the echelons of care as follows:

- Role 1 (R1) is unit-level medical care responsible for medical treatment, initial trauma care, and forward resuscitation. This involves initial treatment by self-aid, fellow soldiers, or combat field medics known as 68-whiskeys.
- Role 2 (R2) is a forward surgical team located near the front line responsible for damage control and resuscitative surgical management for early patient stabilization. These teams are designed to provide surgical care to bridge the time from wound occurrence to definitive surgical care. However, these stations often have limited equipment and holding capacity.
- Role 3 (R3) is a combat support hospital (referred to as a "cash") medical treatment facility that serves as the highest level of care near combat zones. They are equipped to provide definitive care in addition to damage control procedures when necessary. The R3 medical treatment facility has all the capabilities of an R2 but has a large holding capacity and subspecialty care.
- Role 4 (R4) includes military treatment facilities outside of the combat theater that provide preventative, acute, restorative, curative, rehabilitative, and convalescent care. These are usually found on continental United States bases but also include robust overseas facilities (ie, Landstuhl Regional Medical Center).

CAUSE OF COMBAT FINGER AMPUTATIONS

During the more recent conflicts in Afghanistan and Iraq, injuries from improvised explosive devises were more common than gunshot wounds.[9] The Department of Defense Trauma Registry from 2002 to 2016 showed that the most commonly reported procedures overall for orthopedic surgeons included debridement of open fracture, open reduction internal fixation, and amputations. The upper extremity amputations were primarily located to the distal finger, accounting for 60.5% of upper extremity amputations reported.[10] Blast injuries, in particular, lead to complex injuries requiring multiple surgical procedures before arriving at the echelon required for definitive care.[11] Blast injuries involving the hand are often accompanied by segmental nerve and tendon loss with required serial debridement procedures, flap coverage, and prolonged aggressive occupational therapy.[12] However, most finger injuries and finger amputations within the military involved less extensive trauma from vehicle doors, hatches, or weapons striking soldiers' fingers.[2] These fingertip injuries place significant burden on the US fighting force and warrant treatment guidelines where resources may be scarce. We present our treatment approaches considering the potential challenges of the deployed environment overseas, and the additional focus of expediting return to readiness when possible.

ANATOMY

The distal phalanx lies in the dorsal half of the fingertip with a highly vascular fibroadipose tissue pulp located volarly, whereas perionychium and the nail plate abuts the phalanx dorsally (**Fig. 1**).[13] The nail bed itself consists of the proximal germinal matrix, responsible for most nail growth, and the distal sterile matrix, which serves the role of nail plate adherence to the underlying nail fold; these two structures are clinically distinguished by their juncture at the lunula.[14] The nail plate fulfills a functional role by protecting the dorsal surface of the phalanges, improving sensory perception, and facilitating pinch functions.[15–17] The volar pulp's fibrous septae attach to the volar skin of the fingertip, tethering the tissues together to assist with traction during grip.[18] The pulp also has a high density of pacinian corpuscles that work in conjunction with branches of the palmar digital nerves to provide dynamic two-point discrimination.[16] The radial and ulnar digital arteries meet distal to the terminal insertion of the flexor digitorum profundus to form the distal transverse volar digital arch and branches to the most

distal portions of the fingertip.[19,20] The dorsal veins provide most of the venous outflow for the fingertip.[18]

Nail Bed Injuries

Isolated subungual hematomas
Although isolated nail plate injuries are inconsequential beyond temporary discomfort, damage to the underlying nail bed can result in scarring and permanent deformity to the regenerating nail.[18,21,22] Simon and Wolgin[23] demonstrated that isolated subungual hematomas with less than 50% involvement of the nail surface were unlikely to involve the underlying nail bed, whereas isolated subungual hematomas with greater than 50% involvement of the nail surface or those with an underlying phalanx fracture most often had an underlying nail bed laceration. In this setting, there has been controversy over the management when comparing nail plate removal with underlying nail bed repair versus simple decompression through nail trephination. Trephination of the nail alone has been compared with nail plate removal and underlying laceration repair with equivalent outcomes at follow-up.[24,25] In either case, symptomatic isolated subungual hematomas should be decompressed because it has been shown to provide pain relief for patients.[26] We use nail removal with underlying laceration repair in large (>50%) subungual hematomas based on preferences and outcomes reported next.

Nail bed lacerations
In the setting of concomitant subungual hematoma with obvious nail laceration or disrupted nail margin the nail should be removed, and underlying nail bed lacerations repaired. Lacerated edge approximation should use an absorbable suture, such as 6.0 chromic gut. After nail bed repair is

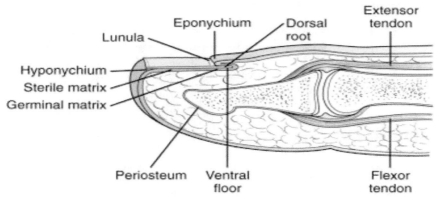

Fig. 1. Illustration demonstrating the anatomy of the distal finger and nail bed. (*From* Kakar S. Digital Amputations. In: Wolfe SW, Hotchkiss RN, Pederson WC, editors. Green's Operative Hand Surgery, 7th Edition. Philadelphia: Elsevier; 2017. P. 1709; with permission.)

complete, the native nail plate or foil of the chromic gut packaging is replaced beneath the eponychial folds and secured using sutures or adhesive glues.[27,28] The importance of meticulous anatomic repair of nail bed lacerations has been established[18,21,22] and ensuring an interposition splint between the eponychial folds and underlying matrix has been used to prevent long-term cosmetic and functional disability adverse outcomes.[29,30] A recent prospective, randomized control trial comparing the outcomes of nail bed repair using 2-octyl cyanoacrylate (Dermabond, Ethicon, Inc, Somerville, NJ) versus primary suture repair showed equivalent long-term outcomes and shorter time to repair when using 2-octyl cyanoacrylate.[31] We advocate that patients with nail bed lacerations be treated with nail plate removal, nail bed repair using 2-octyl cyanoacrylate if available, and apposition of native nail plate or tinfoil beneath eponychial folds (**Fig. 2**).

Distal phalanx fractures

Distal phalanx tuft fractures are commonly experienced in crush injuries. Although highly comminuted, these fractures are stable secondary to the numerous fibrous septae of the surrounding soft tissue and should be managed nonsurgically through finger splint immobilization for 2 to 3 weeks.[32] Conservatively treated distal phalanx fractures that undergo symptomatic nonunion are surgically fixed with or without the use of bone grafting.[33–35] Although rare, if the initial fracture segments are significantly displaced a 1.0-mm Kirschner wire or a 20-gauge hypodermic needle is passed into the bone at the fracture site to ensure stability for 3 to 4 weeks.[36] Recent biomechanical literature supports two crossing 1.0-mm Kirschner wire fixation for greater stability.[37]

Fingertip Amputation

Isolated soft tissue

When fingertip amputations lack exposed bone, healing by secondary intention with regular dressing changes has long been shown to be a simple, inexpensive, and effective treatment method.[38–44] Modern treatment algorithms recommend that smaller wounds (<1.5 cm^2) be treated conservatively, whereas larger defects should be considered for flap coverage.[45] Although various wound dressings have been advocated,[46–51] soft tissue–only fingertip amputations in the military have been treated with topical antibiotics and simple soft dressing coverage for many years.[52] We use simple occlusive dressings with regular dressing changes every 3 to 5 days for smaller soft tissue fingertip amputations without bony exposure.

Exposed bone: revision amputation

Exposed bone brings the unique challenge of determining whether the length of the finger should be preserved, which necessitates coverage, or if the length should be sacrificed to obtain primary closure. Zone 1 revision amputations of the fingertip involve partial removal of the phalanx distal to the insertion of the flexor digitorum profundus to facilitate primary coverage.[53] Replantation of the fingertip has reoperative rates

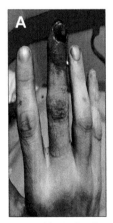 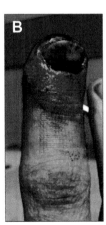 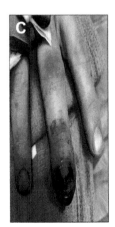 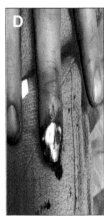

Fig. 2. A 23-year-old 14B (tank crewman) who sustained a crush injury to his right middle finger when closing the driver's hatch on a Stryker tank (*A*). A thin, penetrating laceration was appreciated on the nail plate (*B*) with an underlying distal phalanx fracture. After nail plate removal, a transverse nail bed laceration was repaired using absorbable 6.0 chromic gut because of lack of 2-octyl cyanoacrylate (Dermabond) availability in the field (*C*). The eponychial folds' patency was ensured by using interposition splint from the chromic gut suturing package and secured using the same 6.0 chromic gut in a figure-of-eight pattern (*D*). On subsequent follow-up appointments his nail grew back without deformity.

between 21% and 50%[54,55] and revision amputation has become the more common and often more preferable option.[56,57] Although larger reviews have shown promising outcomes for distal digital amputation replantation, it should be noted these were primarily performed by fellowship-trained hard surgeons and crush-type injuries were not included.[58,59] Furthermore, distal phalanx replantation was shown to have lower success rates when compared with replants at other levels of the finger.[59] Patients undergoing fingertip revision amputation have better sensibility outcomes, faster return to work, and range of motion close to the native finger.[60] These revision amputation procedures are often performed in the emergency department setting because it is more cost-effective than revision amputation performed in the operating room, ultimately with no significant different in secondary revision rates.[61] Because of these findings and the time sensitivity of performing replantation[62] we favor revision amputation with primary closure for fingertip injuries with exposed bone. There should be greater than 20% of the phalanx left in place, or roughly 3 to 4 mm of bone from joint surface, because the flexor digitorum profundus tendon insertion should be maintained to allow continued flexion at the distal interphalangeal joint.[63]

Exposed bone: flap coverage

Flap coverage for larger soft tissue defects or bone exposure has been described and can allow for maintenance of fingertip length with superior aesthetic results.[45] The location of skin loss and geometry of the wound guides flap treatments. Although there are several flaps to choose from, some of the more commonly used flap procedures at our institution and within the military are the V-Y advancement flap, Moberg advanced flap, and cross-finger pedicle flap, discussed next.

In 1970, Atasoy and colleagues[64] described a triangular volar V-Y advancement flap for construction of the distal pad with preservation of length when bone is exposed. A full-thickness triangular "V" flap of skin is formed proximally from the volar digital pulp, advanced distally, and serves as a bridge to approximate the volar and dorsal aspects of the wound. It is indicated for dorsal oblique or transverse distal fingertip amputations with maintenance of the nail bed. The purpose is to use or create an intact volar skin flap to cover the dorsal wound skin loss (**Fig. 3**).

Another commonly used flap is the Moberg advanced flap. Keim and Grantham[65] described a volar advancement flap in the setting of thumb tip amputations. There have been various modifications described on the thumb and other digits

with some expected flexion contracture that can often be treated with aggressive occupational therapy.[66,67] The flap is a bipedicled (served by ulnar and radial digital arteries) cutaneous advancement flap that provides the dermis with sensibility without losing ultimate finger length. Given the thumb's dedicated dorsal vascular supply (princeps pollicis artery) in comparison with the other digits that rely on perforating vessels off the volar digital arteries, some argue against volar flap use in fingers other than the thumb.[45] Although our institution primarily reserves the Moberg advancement flap for volar thumb amputation injuries, there are rare circumstance where its use is appropriate on other digits (**Fig. 4**).

The cross-finger pedicle flap is also commonly used within the military. Gurdin and Pangman[68] originally described using transdigital flaps for volar wounds in 1950. These flaps can provide coverage for exposed bone and tendon with a reliable, durable pad of soft tissue taken from an adjacent digit.[69–71] There are two steps to this procedure: dissection and translation of pedicled full-thickness soft tissue flap from an adjacent digit of the injured finger (**Fig. 5**); and harvest and transfer of a full-thickness skin graft to cover the donor site (**Fig. 6**). It is important that both fingers are immobilized to provide a tensionless repair for the first 2 weeks and to allow unhindered incorporation. After 2 to 3 weeks the cross-finger flap is transected, freeing both fingers for individualized movement. Follow-up studies have shown excellent recovery with nearly normal sensation and minimal morbidity.[72,73] However, this flap is generally contraindicated in patients older than the age of 40 with arthritis because of reported postoperative stiffness and decreased sensation.[69,74] The military population is comprised primarily of young, active patients and thus this flap is maintained within military surgeon's armamentarium.

Distal Interphalangeal Joint/Proximal Interphalangeal Joint Disarticulation

Performing a distal interphalangeal joint disarticulation is a salvage option when finger length maintenance is not possible with flap coverage or revision amputation of the distal phalanx. In all circumstances we prefer to maintain the flexor digitorum profundus when possible; however, severe comminution or extent of injury may preclude treatment options that maintain length. A distal interphalangeal joint disarticulation can be performed or amputation through the middle phalanx with the same principles as discussed previously; soft tissue coverage and maintenance of the flexor digitorum superficialis insertion should be

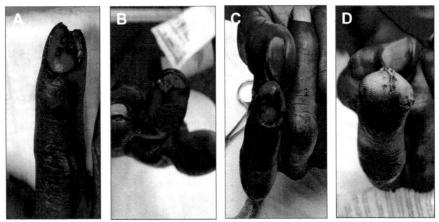

Fig. 3. A 32-year-old 11B (infantryman) who sustained an injury to his right index finger through his distal phalanx when caught between a tank round and the pavement. (*A*). The exit wound led to loss of the central skin on the volar aspect of his finger (*B*). The germinal matrix was removed with a 10 blade and a rongeur was used to trim back the distal phalanx, leaving adequate bone stock ensuring the insertion of the flexor digitorum profundus was not interrupted (*C*). The wound edges were approximated on the volar side of the finger first to form a volar flap that was approximated to the dorsal wound edges, similar to that of the originally described V-Y advancement flap (*D*). On follow-up he had some mild cold insensitivity at the distal fingertip.

priorities for improved function. Although less common, more proximal amputations may be necessary (**Fig. 7**). Certain treatment decisions depend on the finger involved, because a thumb amputation should be considered for replantation, whereas the small finger is perhaps more expendable with much less consequential outcomes.[18]

Antibiotic Prophylaxis

Metcalfe and colleagues[75] performed a systematic review and meta-analysis that pooled 353 open distal phalanx fractures and did not show a significant decrease in superficial infections or osteomyelitis with the administration of prophylactic antibiotics. The authors postulated that the minimal periosteal stripping and contamination associated with finger injuries, digital blocks facilitating prompt irrigation and debridement, and the hand's notable vascularity all contributed to the lack of need for prophylactic antibiotic coverage in open finger fractures. However, given the likely contamination of wounds in the deployed setting, we recommend soldiers receive a single dose of intravenous cefazolin, because infection was cited as a primary reason for poor outcomes after these

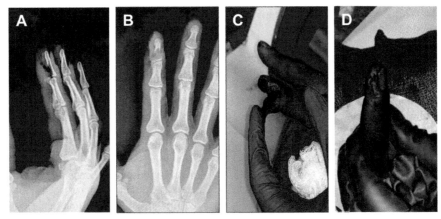

Fig. 4. A 26-year-old 91B (wheeled vehicle mechanic) who sustained a penetrating injury when his right finger was caught in an impact driver and a lug nut while performing vehicle maintenance. The injury penetrated to the distal phalanx with devitalized skin on the fingertip (*A, B*). The devitalized skin was removed and his wound was extended proximally (*C*) to allow for volar flap advancement (*D*). He was able to flex his finger at the distal interphalangeal joint on 2 weeks follow-up in a combat theater setting.

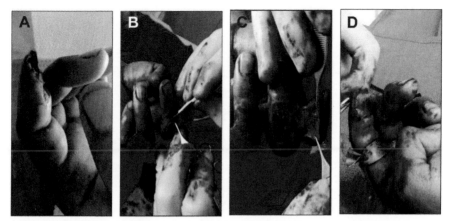

Fig. 5. An 11B (infantryman) who sustained a gunshot wound to his left index finger. The first step in treatment was to remove any devitalized tissue and prepare the accepting site with sharp margins (*A*). The adjacent finger was used as a donor for cross-finger pedicle flap coverage (*B*). With careful dissection, the plane between the paratenon of the extensor mechanism and subcutaneous fat was carefully transected and elevated to form the pedicle flap (*C*). The flap was then reflected and sutured to the accepting site (*D*).

injuries.[21,31] All soldiers in the deployment setting are required to have a tetanus vaccination before deployment and medical records should reflect this accordingly.

COMPLICATIONS ASSOCIATED WITH FINGERTIP INJURIES

When the digital tip is amputated, exposed bone and associated nail matrix injury must be taken into consideration for appropriate treatment. Loss of bony support for the nail bed can lead to the development of a hook nail.[76] The best way to avoid this deformity is excision of the nail bed that extends beyond the limit of the amputated

distal phalanx; ultimately, this may necessitate removing the germinal matrix through excision or ablation if the bone loss occurs at or through the lunula.[77]

Cold Intolerance

Fingertip injuries and amputations often have reported complications of cold intolerance that ranges from 30% to 100%.[18,78–80] It is proposed that the cause is damage to the digital nerves resulting in hypersensitivity[44,81,82] and although cold intolerance typically improves over time, we recommend that patients who sustain fingertip injuries be counseled appropriately for this potential outcome.

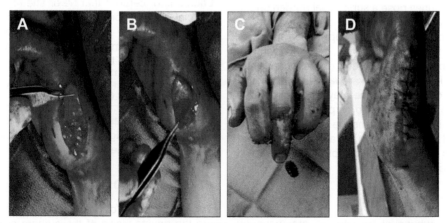

Fig. 6. A hypothenar donor flap was chosen for the 11B infantryman (please see **Fig. 4**). A careful dissection with separation of a subdermal layer was performed (*A*). This flap was then elevated, freed (*B*), and transferred to the dorsal donor site of the previously described cross-finger flap (*C*). The hypothenar donor site was then primarily closed with 3.0 nylon (*D*).

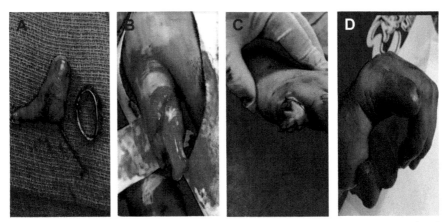

Fig. 7. A civilian contractor who sustained a right small finger ring avulsion injury secondary to her finger being caught in a rotary component of heavy machinery. She arrived to the Combat Surgical Hospital with the amputated digit (*A*) 2 hours after injury. After irrigation and debridement of her finger (*B*) the decision was made to perform revision amputation through the proximal phalanx given inability to salvage the insertion of the flexor digitorum superficialis and specific digit involved (*C*). She had minimal functional deficits at 3-month follow-up except for cosmetic dissatisfaction (*D*).

Lumbrical-Plus Finger

In the native finger, proximal and distal interphalangeal joint flexion occurs in conjunction with simultaneous relaxation of the lumbrical musculature. The paradoxic extension of the distal interphalangeal joint when there is flexion at the proximal interphalangeal joint (the described "lumbrical-plus finger") arises when the flexor digitorum profundus distal to the lumbrical muscle is disrupted causing flexor tendon force to be transmitted through the lumbrical. Although it has been reported in patients with fingertip amputations[83,84] we have not observed this complication.

SUMMARY

Fingertip injuries pose a substantial burden on the US military. Medical providers can expect regular consultations regarding fingertip injuries and management is dictated by nail bed involvement, exposed bone, and geometry of the wound. Nail bed injuries should be repaired, soft tissue coverage of exposed bone may be required, and antibiotics are given based on practitioner discretion. Special considerations are given to thumb injuries and patients should be aware of expected outcomes with possible complications including transient cold intolerance.

CLINICAL CARE POINTS

- Small subungual hematomas are managed conservatively.
- Nail bed injuries should be repaired when possible. This often requires removal of the nail plate and we advocate short-term splinting of eponychial folds to prevent deformities.
- Exposed bone is treated with appropriate soft tissue coverage.
- There are different types of flap coverage. Wound location and geometry dictate which flaps should be considered.
- If soft tissue coverage is unobtainable, revision amputation should be performed with special attention given to maintaining as much finger length as possible.
- Antibiotics are not required, but are often used in the deployed setting.

CONFLICT OF INTEREST

Each author certifies that he or she has no commercial associations (eg, consultancies, stock ownership, equity interest, patent/licensing arrangements) that might pose a conflict of interest in connection with the submitted article.

FINANCIAL DISCLOSURE

Each author certifies that he or she has no financial disclosures that might pose a conflict of interest in connection with the submitted article.

GENERAL DISCLOSURE

The opinions and/or assertions contained herein are the private views of the authors and are not to be construed as reflecting the official position or views of the Department of the Army, the Department of Defense, or the US Government.

REFERENCES

1. AFHSC. Ambulatory visits among members of the active component, U.S. Armed Forces, 2014. MSMR 2015;22(4):18–24.

2. Miller MA, Hall BT, Agyapong F, et al. Traumatic noncombat-related hand injuries in U.S. troops in the combat zone. Mil Med 2011;176(6):652–5.

3. Hebert DJ, Pasque CB. Orthopedic injuries during carrier battle group deployments. Mil Med 2004; 169(3):176–80.

4. Balcom TA, Moore JL. Epidemiology of musculoskeletal and soft tissue injuries aboard a U.S. Navy ship. Mil Med 2000;165(12):921–4.

5. Penn-Barwell JG, Bennett PM, Powers D, et al. Isolated hand injuries on operational deployment: an examination of epidemiology and treatment strategy. Mil Med 2011;176(12):1404–7.

6. Anakwe RE, Standley DM. Hand injuries at a British military hospital on operations. J Hand Surg Br 2006; 31(2):240–3.

7. Dougherty PJ. Armored vehicle crew casualties. Mil Med 1990;155(9):417–20.

8. US Army. Joint publication 4-02: Health service support. United States Department of Defense; 2012. Available at: https://www.jcs.mil/Portals/36/Documents/Doctrine/pubs/jp4_02ch1.pdf.

9. Owens BD, Kragh JF, Wenke JC, et al. Combat wounds in operation Iraqi Freedom and operation Enduring Freedom. J Trauma 2008;64(2):295–9.

10. Stern CA, Stockinger ZT, Todd WE, et al. An analysis of orthopedic surgical procedures performed during U.S. combat operations from 2002 to 2016. Mil Med 2019;184(11–12):813–9.

11. Jacobs N, Taylor DM, Parker PJ. Changes in surgical workload at the JF Med Gp Role 3 Hospital, Camp Bastion, Afghanistan, November 2008-November 2010. Injury 2012;43(7):1037–40.

12. Grewal NS, Kumar AR, Onsgard CK, et al. Simultaneous revascularization and coverage of a complex volar hand blast injury: case report using a contralateral radial forearm flow-through flap. Mil Med 2008;173(8):801–4.

13. Wolfe SW, Hotchkiss RN, Pederson WC, et al. 7th edition. Green's operative hand surgery, Vol. 1. Philadelphia: Elsevier; 2017. p. 590.

14. Peterson SL, Peterson EL, Wheatley MJ. Management of fingertip amputations. J Hand Surg Am 2014;39(10):2093–101.

15. Tos P, Titolo P, Chirila NL, et al. Surgical treatment of acute fingernail injuries. J Orthop Traumatol 2012; 13(2):57–62.

16. Germann G, Rudolf KD, Levin SL, et al. Fingertip and thumb tip wounds: changing algorithms for sensation, aesthetics, and function. J Hand Surg Am 2017;42(4):274–84.

17. Zook EG. Reconstruction of a functional and aesthetic nail. Hand Clin 2002;18(4):577–94, v.

18. Lee DH, Mignemi ME, Crosby SN. Fingertip injuries: an update on management. J Am Acad Orthop Surg 2013;21(12):756–66.

19. Koshima I, Urushibara K, Fukuda N, et al. Digital artery perforator flaps for fingertip reconstructions. Plast Reconstr Surg 2006;118(7):1579–84.

20. Scheker LR, Becker GW. Distal finger replantation. J Hand Surg Am 2011;36(3):521–8.

21. Zook EG, Guy RJ, Russell RC. A study of nail bed injuries: causes, treatment, and prognosis. J Hand Surg Am 1984;9(2):247–52.

22. Fassler PR. Fingertip injuries: evaluation and treatment. J Am Acad Orthop Surg 1996;4(1):84–92.

23. Simon RR, Wolgin M. Subungual hematoma: association with occult laceration requiring repair. Am J Emerg Med 1987;5(4):302–4.

24. Seaberg DC, Angelos WJ, Paris PM. Treatment of subungual hematomas with nail trephination: a prospective study. Am J Emerg Med 1991;9(3):209–10.

25. Meek S, White M. Subungual haematomas: is simple trephining enough? J Accid Emerg Med 1998;15(4): 269–71.

26. Dean B, Becker G, Little C. The management of the acute traumatic subungual haematoma: a systematic review. Hand Surg 2012;17(1):151–4.

27. Stanislas JM, Waldram MA. Keep the nail plate on with Histoacryl. Injury 1997;28(8):507–8.

28. Richards AM, Crick A, Cole RP. A novel method of securing the nail following nail bed repair. Plast Reconstr Surg 1999;103(7):1983–5.

29. Ashbell TS, Kleinert HE, Putcha SM, et al. The deformed finger nail, a frequent result of failure to repair nail bed injuries. J Trauma 1967;7(2):177–90.

30. Stevenson TR. Fingertip and nailbed injuries. Orthop Clin North Am 1992;23(1):149–59.

31. Strauss EJ, Weil WM, Jordan C, et al. A prospective, randomized, controlled trial of 2-octylcyanoacrylate versus suture repair for nail bed injuries. J Hand Surg Am 2008;33(2):250–3.

32. Gaston RG, Chadderdon C. Phalangeal fractures: displaced/nondisplaced. Hand Clin 2012;28(3): 395–401, x.

33. Kim J, Ki SH, Cho Y. Correction of distal phalangeal nonunion using peg bone graft. J Hand Surg Am 2014;39(2):249–55.

34. Meijs CM, Verhofstad MH. Symptomatic nonunion of a distal phalanx fracture: treatment with a percutaneous compression screw. J Hand Surg Am 2009; 34(6):1127–9.

35. Chim H, Teoh LC, Yong FC. Open reduction and interfragmentary screw fixation for symptomatic nonunion of distal phalangeal fractures. J Hand Surg Eur Vol 2008;33(1):71–6.

36. Meals RA, Meuli HC. Carpenter's nails, phonograph needles, piano wires, and safety pins: the history of operative fixation of metacarpal and phalangeal fractures. J Hand Surg Am 1985;10(1):144–50.

37. Wang W, Yu J, Fan CY, et al. Stability of the distal phalanx fracture: a biomechanical study on the importance of the nail and the influence of fixation by crossing Kirschner wires. Clin Biomech (Bristol, Avon) 2016;37:137–40.

38. Bossley CJ. Conservative treatment of digit amputations. N Z Med J 1975;82(553):379–80.

39. Conolly WB, Goulston E. Problems of digital amputations: a clinical review of 260 patients and 301 amputations. Aust N Z J Surg 1973;43(2):118–23.

40. Das SK, Brown HG. Management of lost finger tips in children. Hand 1978;10(1):16–27.

41. Douglas BS. Conservative management of guillotine amputation of the finger in children. Aust Paediatr J 1972;8(2):86–9.

42. Holm A, Zachariae L. Fingertip lesions. An evaluation of conservative treatment versus free skin grafting. Acta Orthop Scand 1974;45(3):382–92.

43. Illingworth CM. Trapped fingers and amputated finger tips in children. J Pediatr Surg 1974;9(6):853–8.

44. Louis DS, Palmer AK, Burney RE. Open treatment of digital tip injuries. JAMA 1980;244(7):697–8.

45. Lemmon JA, Janis JE, Rohrich RJ. Soft-tissue injuries of the fingertip: methods of evaluation and treatment. An algorithmic approach. Plast Reconstr Surg 2008;122(3):105e–17e.

46. Buckley SC, Scott S, Das K. Late review of the use of silver sulphadiazine dressings for the treatment of fingertip injuries. Injury 2000;31(5):301–4.

47. Williamson DM, Sherman KP, Shakespeare DT. The use of semipermeable dressings in fingertip injuries. J Hand Surg Br 1987;12(1):125–6.

48. Fox JW, Golden GT, Rodeheaver G, et al. Nonoperative management of fingertip pulp amputation by occlusive dressings. Am J Surg 1977;133(2):255–6.

49. Lee LP, Lau PY, Chan CW. A simple and efficient treatment for fingertip injuries. J Hand Surg Br 1995;20(1):63–71.

50. Mennen U, Wiese A. Fingertip injuries management with semi-occlusive dressing. J Hand Surg Br 1993;18(4):416–22.

51. Halim S, Stone CA, Devaraj VS. The Hyphecan cap: a biological fingertip dressing. Injury 1998;29(4):261–3.

52. Baker MS. Management of soft-tissue wounds, burns, and hand injuries in the field setting. Mil Med 1996;161(8):469–71.

53. Woo SH, Kim YW, Cheon HJ, et al. Management of complications relating to finger amputation and replantation. Hand Clin 2015;31(2):319–38.

54. Wang H. Secondary surgery after digit replantation: its incidence and sequence. Microsurgery 2002;22(2):57–61.

55. Whitney TM, Lineaweaver WC, Buncke HJ, et al. Clinical results of bony fixation methods in digital replantation. J Hand Surg Am 1990;15(2):328–34.

56. Payatakes AH, Zagoreos NP, Fedorcik GG, et al. Current practice of microsurgery by members of the American Society for Surgery of the Hand. J Hand Surg Am 2007;32(4):541–7.

57. Barzin A, Hernandez-Boussard T, Lee GK, et al. Adverse events following digital replantation in the elderly. J Hand Surg Am 2011;36(5):870–4.

58. Sebastin SJ, Chung KC. A systematic review of the outcomes of replantation of distal digital amputation. Plast Reconstr Surg 2011;128(3):723–37.

59. Dec W. A meta-analysis of success rates for digit replantation. Tech Hand Up Extrem Surg 2006;10(3):124–9.

60. Wang K, Sears ED, Shauver MJ, et al. A systematic review of outcomes of revision amputation treatment for fingertip amputations. Hand (N Y) 2013;8(2):139–45.

61. Gil JA, Goodman AD, Harris AP, et al. Cost-effectiveness of initial revision digit amputation performed in the emergency department versus the operating room. Hand (N Y) 2020;15(2):208–14.

62. Wolfe VM, Wang AA. Replantation of the upper extremity: current concepts. J Am Acad Orthop Surg 2015;23(6):373–81.

63. Chepla KJ, Goitz RJ, Fowler JR. Anatomy of the flexor digitorum profundus insertion. J Hand Surg Am 2015;40(2):240–4.

64. Atasoy E, Ioakimidis E, Kasdan ML, et al. Reconstruction of the amputated fingertip with a triangular volar flap. A new surgical procedure. J Bone Joint Surg Am 1970;52(5):921–6.

65. Keim HA, Grantham SA. Volar-flap advancement for thumb and finger-tip injuries. Clin Orthop Relat Res 1969;66:109–12.

66. O'Brien B. Neurovascular island pedicle flaps for terminal amputations and digital scars. Br J Plast Surg 1968;21(3):258–61.

67. Elliot D, Wilson Y. V-Y advancement of the entire volar soft tissue of the thumb in distal reconstruction. J Hand Surg Br 1993;18(3):399–402.

68. Gurdin M, Pangman WJ. The repair of surface defects of fingers by trans-digital flaps. Plast Reconstr Surg 1950;5(4):368–71.

69. Kleinert HE, McAlister CG, MacDonald CJ, et al. A critical evaluation of cross finger flaps. J Trauma 1974;14(9):756–63.

70. Kappel DA, Burech JG. The cross-finger flap. An established reconstructive procedure. Hand Clin 1985;1(4):677–83.

71. Souquet R, Souquet JR. The actual indications of cross finger flaps in finger injuries. Ann Chir Main 1986;5(1):43–53.

72. Rabarin F, Saint Cast Y, Jeudy J, et al. Cross-finger flap for reconstruction of fingertip amputations: long-term results. Orthop Traumatol Surg Res 2016;102(4 Suppl):S225–8.

73. Megerle K, Palm-Bröking K, Germann G. The cross-finger flap. Oper Orthop Traumatol 2008;20(2): 97–102 [in German].

74. Paterson P, Titley OG, Nancarrow JD. Donor finger morbidity in cross-finger flaps. Injury 2000;31(4): 215–8.

75. Metcalfe D, Aquilina AL, Hedley HM. Prophylactic antibiotics in open distal phalanx fractures: systematic review and meta-analysis. J Hand Surg Eur Vol 2016;41(4):423–30.

76. Kumar VP, Satku K. Treatment and prevention of "hook nail" deformity with anatomic correlation. J Hand Surg Am 1993;18(4):617–20.

77. García-López A, Laredo C, Rojas A. Oblique triangular neurovascular osteocutaneous flap for hook nail deformity correction. J Hand Surg Am 2014; 39(7):1415–8.

78. Han SK, Chung HS, Kim WK. The timing of neovascularization in fingertip replantation by external bleeding. Plast Reconstr Surg 2002;110(4):1042–6.

79. Ni F, Appleton SE, Chen B, et al. Aesthetic and functional reconstruction of fingertip and pulp defects with pivot flaps. J Hand Surg Am 2012;37(9): 1806–11.

80. van den Berg WB, Vergeer RA, van der Sluis CK, et al. Comparison of three types of treatment modalities on the outcome of fingertip injuries. J Trauma Acute Care Surg 2012;72(6):1681–7.

81. Phan TQ, Xu W, Spilker G, et al. Technique and indication of distal arterial-to-proximal venous anastomosis at an amputated distal phalanx. Hand Surg 2012;17(1):135–7.

82. Braun M, Horton RC, Snelling CF. Fingertip amputation: review of 100 digits. Can J Surg 1985;28(1): 72–5.

83. Parkes A. The "lumbrical plus" finger. J Bone Joint Surg Br 1971;53(2):236–9.

84. Lilly SI, Messer TM. Complications after treatment of flexor tendon injuries. J Am Acad Orthop Surg 2006; 14(7):387–96.

Restoring Form and Function to the Partial Hand Amputee
Prosthetic Options from the Fingertip to the Palm

Emily M. Graham, BSN[a], Russell Hendrycks, BS[a],
Christopher M. Baschuk, MPO, CPO[b], Diane J. Atkins, OTR[c,1],
Lana Keizer, OTR, CHT[d], Christopher C. Duncan, MD[e,f],
Shaun D. Mendenhall, MD[a,*]

KEYWORDS

- Partial hand amputee • Hand amputation • Finger amputation • Thumb amputation
- Transmetacarpal amputation • Amputation • Prosthesis

KEY POINTS

- Partial hand amputations include amputations through the fingers, thumb, and transmetacarpal/palm region of the hand.
- Regardless of the amputation level, modern partial hand prostheses can be used to restore form and function to the hand.
- Prosthetic options are categorized into the following classes: passive functional, body-powered, and externally powered prostheses.
- Treatment outcomes are likely maximized when multidisciplinary teams including hand surgeons, prosthetists, occupational and/or certified hand therapists, and physical medicine and rehabilitation physicians collaborate.
- The paucity of published functional outcomes for partial hand prosthesis use is a limitation of this review and of amputee care.

BACKGROUND

Regular use of a prosthetic device increases the health and quality of life in patients with limb loss.[1] Although there are some who learn to adapt and achieve some functional independence without a prosthesis, there are numerous reports highlighting the benefits of consistent prosthesis use.[2,3] These benefits include a greater likelihood of returning to work and increased independence in activities of daily living (ADLs).[4–6] Regular use of a prosthesis is also associated with improvements in phantom limb pain, residual limb pain, and psychological well-being.[7–10]

[a] Division of Plastic Surgery, Department of Surgery, University of Utah School of Medicine, 30 North 1900 East Room 3B400, Salt Lake City, UT 84132, USA; [b] Handspring Clinical Services, 750 East 100 South, Salt Lake City, UT 84102, USA; [c] Department of Physical Medicine and Rehabilitation, Baylor College of Medicine, Houston, TX, USA; [d] Department of Occupational Hand Therapy, University of Utah, 590 Wakara Way, Salt Lake City, UT 84108, USA; [e] Department of Physical Medicine and Rehabilitation, University of Utah School of Medicine, Salt Lake City, UT, USA; [f] Craig H. Neilsen Rehabilitation Hospital, 85 North Medical Drive, Salt Lake City, UT 84132, USA
[1] Present address: 2205 Riva Row #2305, The Woodlands, TX 77380.
* Corresponding author.
E-mail address: Shaun.mendenhall@hsc.utah.edu

Hand Clin 37 (2021) 167–187
https://doi.org/10.1016/j.hcl.2020.09.013
0749-0712/21/© 2020 Elsevier Inc. All rights reserved.

The benefits of regular prosthesis use also apply to those with partial hand (digits, thumb, and transmetacarpal) amputations.[10,11] Notably, partial hand amputations (PHAs) comprise most upper extremity amputations, with 1 in 18,000 individuals affected and an estimated prevalence of 2 million individuals in the United States.[12,13] However, this predicted prevalence is likely conservative because these studies did not clarify whether amputations of the fingertip contributed to the number of finger amputations. Higher rates are also expected for developing countries and regions.[14,15] These epidemiologic findings are understandable considering the frequency of use and vulnerability of the hands. Trauma, vascular compromise, infection, malignancy, and congenital differences may all contribute to the development of a PHA.[13,16–18] These diverse causes create unique population demographics, encompassing a wide spectrum of ages, education levels, and socioeconomic backgrounds.

Despite the large number of individuals affected, those with PHAs are less likely to consistently use a prosthetic device compared with lower limb amputatees.[19] There are many potential explanations for this. Ambulation largely depends on lower limb prostheses and likely motivates individuals with lower limb amputations to consistently use their prostheses. Injuries to nondominant hands may also contribute to the lower rates of prosthetic use in partial hand amputees.[20] Historically, upper limb prostheses were limited in their abilities to restore gross and fine motor function.[7,21] These limitations have been largely overcome by modern engineering advancements in the diversity and functionality of upper extremity prostheses. However, results of a recent survey the authors sent to hand surgery members of the American Association for Hand Surgery (AAHS) revealed that less than 36% of hand surgeons are familiar with these prosthetic options, and that only 24% work in a multidisciplinary upper extremity amputation team (**Fig. 1**).

The purpose of this article is to increase hand provider's knowledge of current prosthetic options for partial hand amputees, including amputations from the fingertip to the palm area of the hand. It discusses the available data and the current barriers to partial hand prosthesis use as well as the role of a multidisciplinary team approach in amputee care. Although it is not feasible to provide a comprehensive list of all the prostheses and companies used to treat PHA, this review provides categories of prosthetic options based on level of amputation and current devices that are readily available. For ease of organization, the authors created the following levels of PHA: (1) distal to distal interphalangeal joint (DIPJ); (2) through the DIPJ and middle phalanx; (3) through the proximal interphalangeal joint (PIPJ) and proximal phalanx; (4) through the metacarpophalangeal joint (MCPJ) and transmetacarpal; and (5) thumb, partial or complete. Each amputation level is marked by unique challenges and requires patient-specific treatment.[22–24] A thorough understanding of these options allows providers to better advocate for patients and help them achieve improved form and function following amputation.

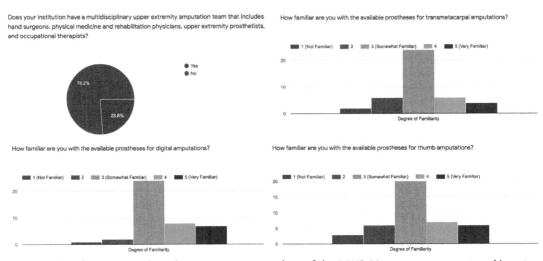

Fig. 1. Results of a survey conducted among surgeon members of the AAHS. Most surgeons report working at an institution without a formal multidisciplinary upper extremity amputation team. In addition, most hand surgeons do not express familiarity with partial hand prostheses.

PROSTHETIC OPTIONS FOR AMPUTATIONS DISTAL TO DISTAL INTERPHALANGEAL JOINT

Amputations of the distal fingertip are the most common amputations treated by hand surgeons.[25] On digits 2 through 5, the fingertip is the portion distal to the insertion of the flexor digitorum profundus (FDP) volarly and the extensor terminal tendon dorsally on the distal phalanx. These amputations cause functional and cosmetic deficits because of loss of digit length, partial or complete loss of the nail bed, reduction in sensation, and decreased perception of body wholeness. These amputations occur globally and are common in developed regions, although surgical management for these injuries varies by location. In the United States, most amputations through the distal tip and DIPJ are treated by revision amputation to expedite functionality of the residuum, whereas many Asian countries are more likely to attempt replantation to improve cosmesis and retain perceptions of body integration.[26–28] The decision to replant or amputate seems to be influenced by cultural norms and perceptions of PHA.[27] However, when attempts to replant are unsuccessful or when replantation is not feasible, prosthetic devices can be used to circumvent distortions of body integration and improve functionality.[29,30] This article presents prosthetic options designed to address the cosmetic and functional deficits caused by these amputations.

Passive Functional Prostheses

Passive functional restorations are among the oldest and most commonly prescribed prostheses used to restore length and improve aesthetic appearance. Within the realm of humanlike passive functional devices are low-definition and high-definition silicone prostheses. Regardless of the PHA level, low-definition and high-definition silicone prostheses can mirror the amputee's unaffected upper extremity and can be fit at any of the amputation levels. Functionally, low-definition and high-definition silicone prostheses behave similarly. As passive prostheses, they are frequently used to supplement movements, including pushing, pulling, and typing, while providing protection to the residuum. However, differences in cosmesis and cost exist between the silicone classes. Low-definition silicone prostheses typically provide less anatomic detail and are available at lower prices. Examples of low-definition prostheses include the readymade and semi–custom-made silicone prostheses by Regal Prosthesis Ltd. (Hong Kong Regal Prosthesis Limited, Hong Kong, China) and custom-rolled

silicone finger extensions made in house at specialty upper extremity prosthetics clinics such as Handspring Clinical Services (Salt Lake City, UT). Note that, although these prostheses are humanlike in appearance, the inability to recreate precise, individual anatomic detail can produce a phenomenon termed the uncanny valley.[31] This phenomenon is frequently referenced by prosthetists and others who work with upper extremity prostheses. First described by Mori[31] in 1970, the uncanny valley describes the feelings of repulsion and eeriness humans feel toward objects that fall just short of appearing completely lifelike, whereas objects with major differences in form but that retain functional similarities to human anatomy are more well perceived. In terms of prosthetic devices, the prostheses that are perfect or near perfect in restoring the form of the amputee's hand, along with prostheses that are robotic in appearance, are generally better perceived by amputees, and by those with whom they associate, compared with the prostheses that are mannequinlike in appearance.[31–33] Thus, although low-definition prostheses may provide similar functional benefits to high-definition silicone prostheses, clinicians should discuss the uncanny valley with patients to ensure that psychological well-being and quality of life are maximized.

High-definition silicone prostheses include brands such as Livingskin (Össur Americas, Foothill Ranch, CA) and Prosthetic Artworks (Prosthetic Artworks LLC, Northeastern, PA). These prostheses can be painted to uniquely match individual skin tones, hair patterns, freckles, scars, and tattoos (see **Fig. 7**). The precise recreation of anatomic detail makes these prostheses an attractive option for amputees desiring to restore the form of an affected hand. Even amputees with primary goals to improve hand function may still appreciate a passive functional high-definition prosthesis during certain social events and occasions.

Limitations to low-definition and high-definition silicone restorations include diminished tactile sensation and heat dissipation caused by the encapsulation of the residuum. Silicone restorations are also less durable than other prosthetic options and may be susceptible to damage and staining. As such, patient education regarding appropriate use and care of the prostheses before and after delivery is critical. In our experience, the passive functional prostheses serve users best when the primary goal is to conceal the injury and not draw attention to the finger difference or loss. Examples of where this has proved useful is for school teachers in classrooms full of younger children and for any jobs that have a high degree of customer interaction. They are also frequently used for social and religious engagement.

Body-powered Prostheses

To our best knowledge, there are no body-powered prostheses available for amputations distal to the DIPJ.

Externally Powered Prostheses

Like body-powered prostheses, there are no externally powered prosthetic options for amputations distal to the DIPJ.

PROSTHETIC OPTIONS FOR AMPUTATIONS THROUGH THE DISTAL INTERPHALANGEAL JOINT AND THE MIDDLE PHALANX

Similar to amputations of the distal tip, PHA through the DIPJ and middle phalanx can result in challenging cosmetic and functional impairments. Because the flexor digitorum superficialis (FDS) inserts on the mid–middle phalanx, amputations proximal to this can decrease grip strength, and limit pincer grip and other fine motor movements. Loss of flexion at the DIPJ is a major source of disability and early retirement, placing a major burden on individuals and society.[34–36] Thus, careful consideration is needed to ensure motor function and independence are maximized, especially if the amputation resides on the dominant hand.

Passive Functional Prostheses

The same classes of low-definition and high-definition silicone passive functional prostheses available to PHA distal to the DIPJ are also available to PHA through the DIP and middle phalanx (**Fig. 2**). These prostheses are especially useful because amputations at this level produce more notable changes in digit length, which can negatively affect whole-body perception and function. The use of a passive functional prosthesis can thus restore cosmesis and improve overall hand functionality.

Body-Powered Prostheses

In addition to passive functional prostheses at this level and proximal, body-powered (BP) partial hand prostheses are available. Mechanical in appearance, BP prostheses harness the amputee's remaining joints and anatomy to restore range of motion (ROM), including flexion and extension, along with restoration of digit length (**Figs. 3** and **4**). BP prostheses function independent from external batteries and electricity. Advantages of BP prostheses include improved sensory and positional feedback, decreased rate of amputee fatigue, and synchronous movement with natural hand movements.[37,38] In amputations through the middle phalanx not including the insertion site of the FDS, BP prostheses use the remaining middle phalanx and PIPJ to restore length of the missing digit and function of the lost DIPJ.

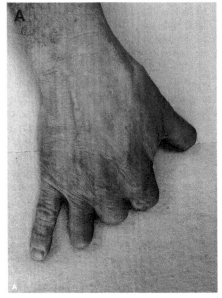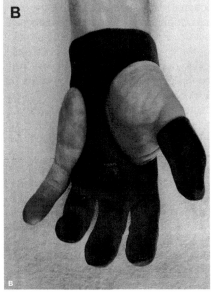

Fig. 2. An example of a custom silicone heavy-duty passive functional prosthesis that was created to be easy to use, durable, and cover less of the hand to improve heat dissipation. (*A*) The patient's hand in the pronated position without the prosthesis. (*B*) The patient wearing the prosthesis with his hand supinated.

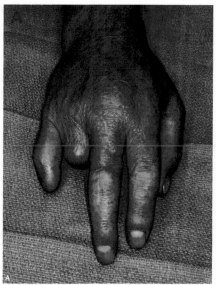
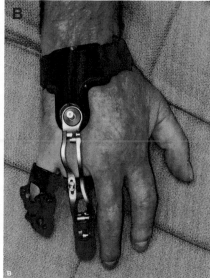

Fig. 3. (*A*) This patient experienced partial hand amputations to the fourth digit through the proximal phalanx and the fifth digit through the middle phalanx. Dorsal view of hand without his prostheses. (*B*) Patient wearing his prostheses. He was fitted with a Naked Prosthetics MCPDriver on the fourth digit and a Naked Prosthetics PIP-Driver on the fifth digit.

One BP prosthetic option for this level is the PIP-Driver by Naked Prosthetics (Naked Prosthetics Inc., Olympia, WA). Although functional outcomes are forthcoming, our experience is remarkable. Many patients report significant decreases in pain in the wrist, elbow, and shoulder after being fitted with the prosthesis because they are no longer required to make compensatory motions to grasp objects. The roll-cage–style design also lends itself to protecting the frequently hypersensitive distal end of the residual digit, which may further enable amputees to engage with their environments. Because of the intuitive nature of this prosthesis, acceptance and integration into ADLs is rapid. Even individuals with long-standing PHAs express high levels of satisfaction after being fitted with the PIPDriver. Tasks requiring grip strength and motor control, such as retrieving

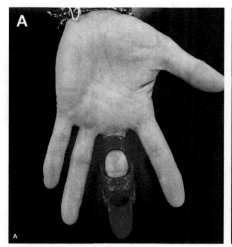
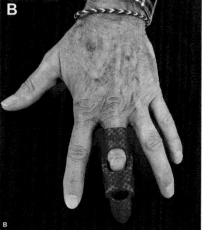

Fig. 4. (*A*) Volar perspective of a patient wearing a Naked Prosthetics PIPDriver on the third digit. (*B*) Dorsal perspective of PIPDriver on third digit.

keys from pockets and pulling credit cards out of a wallet, are reportedly easier while using this prosthesis. The authors have witnessed patients returning to play musical instruments such as the piano and saxophone, file papers, open envelopes, use utensils, and tie shoelaces (**Fig. 5**). The improvement and ease of performing ADLs with the PIPDriver is especially notable when amputations at this level reside on the index finger, because it can restore up to 10% of hand function.[39]

Limitations to BP prostheses are primarily cosmetic. The design surrounds the digit, increasing the width around the remaining anatomic joints. If a glove is needed to cover the prosthesis for work-related activities, a larger size is typically needed on the affected side compared with the sound side.

Externally Powered Prostheses

To the best of our understanding, there are no externally powered prostheses available for PHA through the DIPJ and middle phalanx.

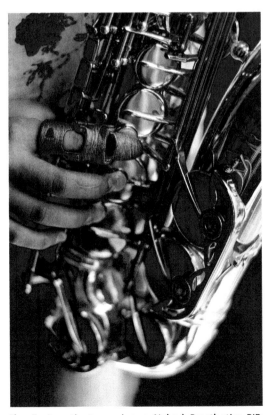

Fig. 5. A patient wearing a Naked Prosthetics PIP-Driver to restore digit length and functionality to play the saxophone. Image courtesy of Naked Prosthetics.

PROSTHETIC OPTIONS FOR AMPUTATIONS THROUGH THE PROXIMAL INTERPHALANGEAL JOINT AND PROXIMAL PHALANX

The more proximal the transphalangeal amputation occurs, the more pronounced the deficits become. Impairment ratings for PHA of the proximal phalanx are often classified as moderate with a 16% loss in total hand function when the index finger and/or middle finger is involved.[39] When the amputation occurs through the proximal phalanx, the actions of the FDS and FDP are lost, leaving the residuum under the control of the extensor digitorum communis for extension and the intrinsic hand muscles for flexion. Because the intrinsic hand muscles are susceptible to fatigue, it can be challenging finding a prosthesis that restores functionality without exhausting the capabilities of these muscles.[40,41] Although low-definition and high-definition silicone prostheses are used to rehabilitate amputations at this level (see **Figs. 2,6,7**), emphasis is often placed on supplementing with a prosthesis that can restore length and mimic the functions of the FDS and FDP to maximize gross and fine motor function.

Passive Functional Prostheses

Passive articulating (PA) prostheses are widely available and include the Point Partial (Point Designs LLC, Lafayette, CO), Titan Partial (Partial Hand Solutions, LLC, Warren, MI), and Vincent Partial Passive (Vincent Systems GmbH, Karlsruhe, Germany). Point Partial and Titan Partial are better suited for amputations through or proximal to the PIPJ, whereas Point Digit, GripLock, and Vincent Partial Passive are designed for amputations through or proximal to the MCPJ. Independent of amputation level, PA prostheses restore

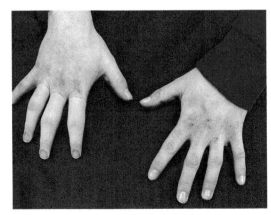

Fig. 6. An example of a high-definition silicone passive functional prosthesis on a partial hand amputee.

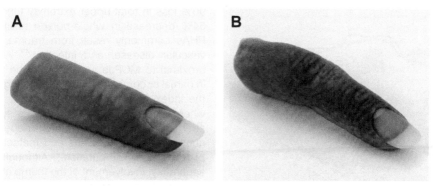

Fig. 7. (*A, B*) Examples of high-definition silicone passive functional prostheses used on separate patients. Images courtesy of Össur.

function by using a passive ratcheting mechanical mechanism to lock the prosthesis into various degrees of flexion to enhance functionality and overall movement. Use of the unaffected hand is common for positioning but is not necessary for adjusting the degree of flexion. When extension of the prosthesis is desired, the amputee can touch a button or use the spring-loaded release mechanism to reset the prosthetic to its normal resting position. Although changing the degree of flexion is simple, the inability of these prostheses to automatically flex and extend with movement of the residuum may be a limitation for some amputees. This type of prosthesis is ideal when heavy-duty bimanual tasks are required. Construction work, landscaping, welding, and automotive repair are a few examples of successful applications. Eating, food preparation, holding plates, holding grocery bags, and self-grooming are some of the ADLs where these prostheses are most useful.

Body-Powered Prostheses

Comparable to the PIPDriver, Naked Prosthetics (Naked Prosthetics Inc., Olympia, WA) also manufactures a BP prosthesis that uses the strength of an intact MCPJ to restore the length and functionality of the middle and distal phalanges. The MCPDriver restores finger flexion, extension, abduction, and adduction (**Figs. 8** and **9**). Another BP prosthesis option for this level includes the Partial M-Finger (Partial Hand Solutions, LLC, Warren, MI), which functions similarly to the MCPDriver. The primary difference between the M-Fingers and the MCPDriver are the mechanisms for capturing the motion of the intact MCPJs. The MCPDriver relies on a mechanical linkage for both flexion and extension, whereas the M-Fingers rely on a mechanical linkage for flexion but use spring-assist cable mechanism for extension.

Although the cable system of the M-Fingers can be lower profile, the mechanical advantage of the MCPDriver is greater than that of the M-Fingers and facilitates higher overall grip strength. However, the M-Fingers make it easier to adjust the ROM and mechanical advantage than the MCPDriver, which has a fixed mechanical ratio that cannot be adjusted without ordering new custom-made linkages. Ideal candidates for these prostheses should have an intact MCPJ to power the prosthetic PIPJ and DIPJ, have enough residuum in the proximal phalanx to engage with the ring and/or harness, and be able to perform a minimum 60° of active ROM at the MCPJ.

Although randomized controlled clinical trials evaluating the effectiveness of these devices are forthcoming, our clinical experience with the MCPDriver is remarkable. This device has opened a new realm of functional possibilities that were not previously available to individuals with this amputation level. One anecdotal example from our practice includes a retired Air Force mechanic who had his thumb amputated proximal to the interphalangeal joint (IPJ) and middle finger amputated proximal to the PIPJ in a table saw accident. He was fitted with 2 custom MCPDrivers. Since his original fitting, he reports consistent, daily use of his prostheses. Through his prostheses, he can continue his passion of restoring classic cars. He recently reported that he was able to independently finish a hot rod remodel, which included a complete engine out overhaul and rebuild. He stated that he would not have been able to do all of the work himself had he not had his prostheses. The dexterity and grip strength provided by the MCPDriver, as well as the protection to his sensitive distal residual digits, are the factors that contributed to his success. Thus, the potential of this device to restore overall hand function and quality of life should not be overlooked by clinicians or insurers.

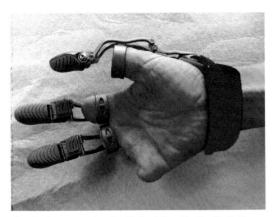

Fig. 8. An example of a Naked Prosthetics 3-digit system with a metacarpophalangeal (MCP) ThumbDriver and 2 MCPDrivers. The residual digits on digits 4 and 5 are not long enough to be used with the Naked Prosthetics MCPDrivers. Provision of point digits for digits 4 and 5 were considered; however, with input from the patient and a trial fitting, it was determined that the MCPDrivers alone provided the best functional return in this case.

Externally Powered Prostheses

There are no externally powered prostheses for this amputation level currently available.

PROSTHETIC OPTIONS FOR AMPUTATIONS THROUGH THE METACARPOPHALANGEAL JOINT AND TRANSMETACARPAL

Injuries that result in amputations through or proximal to the MCPJ result in significant functional losses caused by destruction of intrinsic hand muscles, flexor and extensor tendons, MCPJ, and neurovascular structures. Transmetacarpal amputations immediately distal to the wrist often produce severe impairments, with an estimated 90% loss in total upper extremity function and a 54% decrease in whole-person ability.[39] These PHAs commonly result from trauma, peripheral vascular disease, and infection.[42] Amputations proximal to MCPJs and distal to the wrist result in partial or complete loss of grip strength because the index and middle fingers permit fine grasp, whereas the ring and small fingers support grip strength. Severity of impairment depends on the number of affected digits and metacarpals, and proximity of the amputation.[43] Although discussed separately, involvement of the thumb also contributes greatly to overall hand function. Because of the severity of this level of amputation and the accompanying decreased hand function, the prosthetic interventions are more involved to mitigate deficits. There is a greater variety of prosthetic options available at this amputation level. The more proximal the amputation, the more space available for prosthetic technology, including motors, batteries, and joints.

Passive Functional Prostheses

PA prostheses designed to treat proximal hand amputations include Point Digit (Point Designs LLC, Lafayette, CO), GripLock (Naked Prosthetics Inc., Olympia, WA), Titan Full (Partial Hand Solutions, LLC, Warren, MI), and Vincent Passive (Vincent Systems GmbH, Karlsruhe, Germany) (**Figs. 10** and **11**). These prostheses use a passive ratcheting mechanism to lock the prosthesis into various degrees of flexion, similar to the Point Partial and Titan Partial. Some of these prosthetics are touchscreen compatible, allowing amputees to interact with various modern touchscreen devices for additional functional use. The strength and carrying capacity of these prostheses are also reportedly higher compared with Point Partial, with

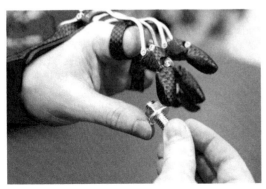

Fig. 9. An example of the fine motor restoration that can be provided to amputees with amputations through the proximal phalanx. Image courtesy of Naked Prosthetics.

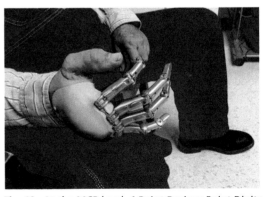

Fig. 10. At the MCP level, 4 Point Designs Point Digits are used to create a robust, heavy-duty prosthesis for this farmer.

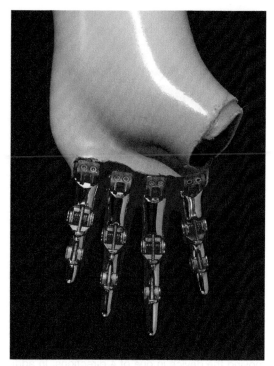

Fig. 11. Volar aspect of the 4 Point Designs Point Digits.

carrying capacities near 90 kg (200 lb). The high strength and carrying capacities are advantageous compared with low-definition and high-definition silicone passive functional prostheses and externally powered prostheses because these classes of prostheses would fail under similar strenuous applications. In addition, PA prostheses are resistant to muscle fatigue because they do not depend on active muscle contraction to maintain flexion and grip, as do externally powered prosthetic devices. However, a limitation to these prostheses is a lack of spontaneous, natural body movement because the amputee must individually set the desired degrees of flexion for each prosthetic digit.

Body-Powered Prostheses

At this amputation level, BP prostheses are commonly referred to by their historical names, Robin-Aids, by the Medicare Healthcare Common Procedural Coding System (HCPCS) and by clinicians who work with upper extremity prostheses. Invented by George Robinson in the 1950s, this prosthesis consisted of a set of individual fingers linked together on a shared axis that are spring loaded and can be voluntarily opened by putting tension on a cable extending up the arm and looped around the contralateral shoulder. Although this device is no longer available, the concept used by the Robin-Aids prosthesis can still be used with commercially available components (**Fig. 12**). For transradial and more proximal level amputations, a wrist unit is typically used to attach various terminal devices depending on the desired function. These wrist units often allow quick changing between the different terminal devices. Two companies, Texas Assistive Devices (Brazoria, TX) and TRS Prosthetics (Boulder, CO), have developed quick-disconnect wrist units that have been adapted for the use at this partial hand level. The quick-disconnect unit is mounted either on the palmar surface of the residual hand or on a cuff on the residual wrist. The appropriate attachment is then connected to the quick-disconnect unit. This arrangement allows for use of traditional voluntary opening and voluntary closing terminal devices, as well as activity-specific terminal devices such as utensils and sport and recreational attachments, both also available from Texas Assistive Devices and TRS Prosthetics, respectively. For these devices to work, a custom silicone interface and laminated composite frame are necessary. This prosthesis is functionally robust and retains full ROM at the wrist. In addition, recent advances in the quality and strength of additive manufacturing materials has increased the opportunity for innovation in this space.

The M-Fingers by Partial Hand Solutions (Partial Hand Solutions, LLC, Warren, MI) is an additional BP prosthesis that is specifically marketed and manufactured for this level. The M-Finger prosthesis is designed to mimic tenodesis by flexing the fingers with wrist extension and allowing the prosthesis to extend the finger with wrist flexion. This prosthesis is larger than BP prostheses designed for more distal PHAs to maximize the movements of the remaining MCPJ and intrinsic hand muscles. However, similar to all BP

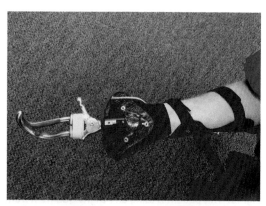

Fig. 12. An example of a BP prosthesis used for a transmetacarpal partial hand amputation.

prostheses, this device restores length and the ability to grip, and naturally extends and flexes the digits with movement. One advantage to this design is that the control does not require a cable and harness that run up the arm and around the contralateral shoulder. Partial Hand Solutions also carries Pediatric M-Finger, which is a BP prosthesis uniquely designed to rehabilitate children with PHAs and those born with congenital differences.

Externally Powered Prostheses

Externally powered prostheses become an option at this amputation level. Myoelectric (MYO) prostheses are externally powered prosthetic devices that function by recording surface electromyography (EMG) signals from muscle contraction of the residual intrinsic hand muscles to move the prosthetic digits (**Figs. 13** and **14**). If insufficient surface EMG signals are present in the intrinsic hand muscles, then the extrinsic hand muscles in the forearm can be used to control the device. However, use of the extrinsic muscles is not ideal because wrist motion can inadvertently cause undesired activation of the powered digits. MYO devices are powered by a battery and microprocessor located in the amputee's device wristband. These prostheses have several advantages, including the ability to achieve various grip postures through independent and synchronous control of the affected digits. At present, the control of the digits produces a composite grasp, opening and closing the digits in a preprogrammed pattern selected by the user.

The i-Digits Quantum (Össur, Reykjavik, Iceland) is an example of an MYO hand prosthetic for individuals with partial hand amputation or deficiency distal to the wrist and proximal to the MCPJ and can include loss of 1 to 5 digits. The i-Digits Quantum has up to 32 automated grips and has features

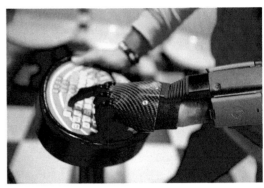

Fig. 14. MYO options are often capable of sustaining various grip postures in addition to providing restoration of fine motor movement. Image courtesy of Össur.

including i-MO Gesture Control, Vari-Grip and Auto Grasp to enhance grip strength and functional use. Vari-Grip allows adjustable digit-by-digit strength and autograsp prevents objects from slipping. Gesture control is unique because it enables an automated grip to be accessed by moving the device in one of 4 directions. In addition, the amputee can enhance the speed and strength of the prosthetic and choose between several different preset grips by using the Biosim My i-limb app on a smartphone device. The i-Digits Access is a device that functions similar to the i-Digits Quantum except it only has 12 grips available and does not have as many functional enhancing features. The i-Digits Access was specifically developed for use with patients who have limited funding resources. This device is appropriate for low-impact to moderate-impact functions that do not exceed the maximum device load of 20 kg for the total hand and 5 kg for the digits. In addition to the i-Digits Quantum and Access, the Vincent Partial 3 Active (Vincent Systems GmbH, Karlsruhe, Germany) is the only other externally powered MYO digit system available for PHA.

When all 5 digits are involved in a transcarpal amputation or an extremely proximal transmetacarpal amputation, the option exists to use a full prosthetic hand that has a specially adapted lamination collar. There are multiple prosthetic hands that have this option, including the Transcarpal Hand and the Bebionic Short Wrist (Ottobock, Duderstadt, Germany), the Vincent Evolution 3 and Vincent Young (Vincent Systems GmbH, Karlsruhe, Germany), the Motion Hand, ETD, and ETD2, all with the short wrist option (Motion Control, Salt Lake City, UT), and the i-Limb Quantum, i-Limb Ultra, and i-Limb Access all with the wrist disarticulation option (Össur, Reykjavik, Iceland).

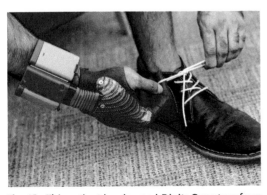

Fig. 13. This patient is using an i-Digits Quantum from Össur to accomplish ADLs independently. Image courtesy of Össur.

Fabrication for these devices requires a custom silicone interface with a rigid carbon fiber shell for the terminal device to mount properly. The custom silicone interface allows for retention of the anatomic motions of the wrist joint. Pockets in the silicone forearm portion can be created to house the electronics and batteries.

Several studies report functional outcomes and cosmetic appeal of BP and MYO prostheses in upper extremity amputees. Although many of these studies are not specific to PHA, they may provide insight while specific studies relating to PHA are forthcoming. MYO options are reportedly more aesthetically pleasing than BP prostheses because they better resemble the natural form of the hand.[37,44] BP prostheses are usually more mechanical and hooklike in appearance because these prostheses generally leave the harness and cables exposed. However, some individuals prefer the distinct appearance of a BP prosthetic to more traditional-appearing MYO devices. Exploring preferences in cosmesis should be performed before selecting a class of prostheses.[38]

MYO prostheses are also more commonly associated with improvements in phantom limb pain.[37,45,46] This association may be because of how the MYO prostheses are activated using the same muscles that would activate the anatomic digits. This feature creates a greater sense of embodiment of the device, which may contribute to the reduction in phantom limb pain. BP prostheses are activated using gross body motions, which may not reproduce the same level of embodiment. In terms of functionality, both are associated with advantages, and neither prosthetic has consistently shown superior outcomes. This finding continues to show that neither device category should be considered in opposition to one another. Each device type has its own unique purpose and function. No single prosthesis can make up for the deficits associated with upper limb loss.[47]

However, an advantage of BP prostheses includes improved sensory feedback compared with MYO devices.[37,48,49] Both MYO and BP prostheses use visual feedback as a means to control the prosthetic device. Proprioception and tactile feedback may be additional sensory modes available to amputees with BP prostheses through the external harness and cables.[37] BP prostheses are also thought to be more durable and easier for amputees to maintain, and require less specificity during fittings.[37,48–50] Rather than being joint driven and cable controlled like BP prostheses, MYO devices require stimulation from proximal muscles. Establishing a stable connection between the

muscles and the prosthesis requires precise, patient-specific fittings. The time required to precisely fit the MYO device, along with the increased time needed to achieve success in performing ADLs, is another disadvantage of MYO devices. MYO devices may thus be better suited for amputees hoping to improve the natural form of the hand, for those only needing a prosthesis for light-intensity work, and for those with primary goals of alleviating phantom limb pain.[37] However, research on functional outcomes specific to PHA are needed to validate these conclusions.

PROSTHETIC OPTIONS FOR AMPUTATIONS THROUGH THE THUMB

The thumb is the most important digit of the hand. Although loss of the index or long finger can result in up to a 20% loss in total hand function, loss of the thumb results in a 40% reduction in total hand function and a 22% reduction in whole-person function.[39,51] The significance of the thumb is largely attributed to its ability to serve as a sensate post, enabling the hand to grip in multiple positions for gross and fine motor function.[52] Often quoted, the hand without the thumb is nothing more than an animated spatula, serving little to perform ADLs and maintain independence.[53] The thumb is also one of the most humanistic features of the body.[54] Loss of the thumb can impede social interactions and decrease self-esteem.[55] Whether the amputation to the thumb is partial, complete, or part of a polytrauma to the hand, restoring the length and actions of the thumb should remain a priority. Several surgical approaches are available, including toe to thumb transfers, pollicization, metacarpal lengthening, web space deepening, various flaps, and potentially osseointegration.[56] However, these procedures have contraindications and complications.[57–59] Often, the use of a prosthetic device may serves as a straightforward solution to correcting an amputation through the thumb.

Passive Functional Prostheses

One of the primary functions of the thumb is to serve as a post to allow opposition. Although flexion at the IPJ is important for fine motor tasks, restoring thumb length and rotation at the MCPJ can greatly improve overall hand function. For this reason, low-definition and high-definition silicone prostheses can be used for partial and complete thumb amputations (**Figs. 2** & **15**). Vincent Passive Thumb (Vincent Systems GmbH, Karlsruhe, Germany) is another passive functional prosthesis designed for thumb amputations through

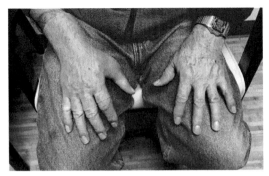

Fig. 15. A medium-definition silicone passive functional prosthesis used to restore the form and length of an amputated thumb.

the MCPJ that restores thumb length and can serve as a post (**Fig. 16**). An advantage of this prosthesis includes a rotating base near the MCPJ that allows thumb rotation and 2 degrees of freedom. The capability to rotate at the base can promote additional gripping positions. However, like silicone prostheses, this prosthesis cannot provide flexion of the IPJ. Titan Thumb and M-Thumb by Partial Hand Solutions (Partial Hand Solutions, LLC, Warren, MI) are PA prostheses that are better suited for movements requiring pincer grasp. Both prostheses are designed for thumb amputations at or proximal to the MCPJ and carry the same advantages as other PA prostheses previously mentioned. An added advantage of the M-Thumb is an artificial fingernail that allows amputees to pick up small objects and perform other fine motor movements. Although the Titan Thumb and M-Thumb are better at

restoring hand function than low-definition and high-definition silicone prostheses, all prostheses in this class are unable to restore natural thumb flexion and extension.

Body-Powered Prostheses

ThumbDriver by Naked Prosthetics (Naked Prosthetics Inc., Olympia, WA) is one of the only BP prostheses available for thumb amputations (**Figs. 17** and **18**). Ideal candidates for this device are individuals with amputations occurring distal to the thumb MCPJ but proximal to the IPJ. Advantages of using a BP prosthesis on the thumb include synchronicity with the natural flexion and extension of the hand to rapidly interact with the environment. Gross and fine motor tasks such as catching and throwing a ball, playing a musical instrument, and opening and closing zip-lock bags are made possible by the intrinsic nature of BP prostheses. A limitation of the ThumbDriver is that it is not designed for distal partial thumb amputations. To combat this limitation, the authors occasionally use a custom variant of the PIPDriver (Naked Prosthetics Inc., Olympia, WA) for amputees with more distal thumb amputations and who desire a BP prosthesis. Although our implementation of the PIPDriver for distal partial thumb amputations is an off-label use of the prosthesis, we have seen remarkable improvements in total hand function.

Externally Powered Prostheses

Thumb amputations proximal to the MCPJ may benefit from MYO prostheses (**Fig. 19**). Both the i-Digits and Vincent Partial Active can be used to restore functional grasp in both lateral and opposition postures. However, for implementation of these devices to be successful, a sufficient amount of the ray needs to be resected. Also, as previously

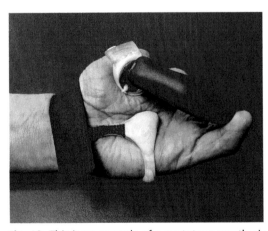

Fig. 16. This is an example of a prototype prosthesis created with an opposition post. Thermoplastics, epoxy, and Velcro are all used in this important diagnostic phase of the fitting protocol in order to optimize the fit and very function before committing to the definitive prosthesis.

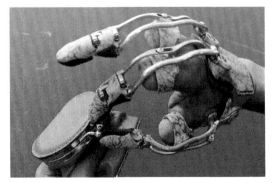

Fig. 17. A demonstration of the dexterity and pinch force that can be generated with the Naked Prosthetics MCPDrivers and MCP ThumbDriver. The patient was able to easily open and close this coin purse using this custom prosthesis.

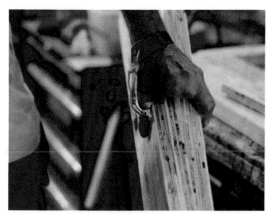

Fig. 18. The restoration of gross motor function and thumb strength through the Naked Prosthetics MCP ThumbDriver. (Image courtesy of Naked Prosthetics.)

described, the use of an MYO partial hand prosthesis is for low-duty to moderate-duty tasks.

ACTIVITY-SPECIFIC PROSTHESES

A separate class of prostheses that can be described for many amputation levels is an activity-specific prosthesis (**Fig. 20**). As the name implies, this type of prosthesis is designed to assist with a particular function and is more of an assistive device or tool than a replacement. Unlike the previously described prostheses, these devices are not used for extended periods of time. They may be used only a few times per week. However, this does not detract from their importance in the overall prosthetic rehabilitation of an individual with a PHA.

Initial activity-specific prostheses can be made simply using Aquaplast (Performance Health, Warrenville, IL), a low-temperature thermoplastic. They are often fitted by a certified hand therapist (CHT) or occupational therapist (OT) during an inpatient rehabilitation stay. These prostheses tend to be beneficial in the short term but are not suitable as long-term use devices because of degradation over time. They can be beneficial as prototypes of a permanent long-term activity-specific device made from composites, leather, and/or from additive manufactured materials. Examples include a device made to specifically help with dressing and doing up buttons or a comb integrated into a mitt that allows easier grooming. They can also be more recreational, such as a prosthesis to hold onto handlebars, grasp a bow, or throw a ball (**Fig. 21**). A single activity-specific prosthesis can be made to perform a variety of activities through the use of a quick-disconnect unit, as previously described from TRS or Texas Assistive Devices. This device allows the attachment of any number of individual terminal devices.

A summary of the available prosthetic devices by level of amputation is provided in **Table 1**.

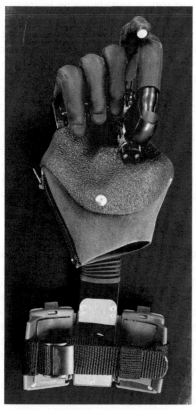

Fig. 19. A full 5-digit Össur i-Digits system used for a patient with amputation of all digits proximal to the MCPJs.

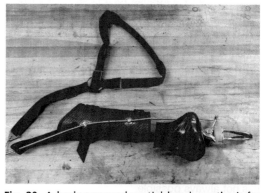

Fig. 20. A body-powered partial hand prosthesis for the same patient that uses the prosthesis in **Fig. 12**. This prosthesis uses a quick disconnect palmar wrist unit. The forearm shield and cable can be removed from this prosthesis and different activity specific terminal devices can be connected to the remaining palmar portion of the prosthesis.

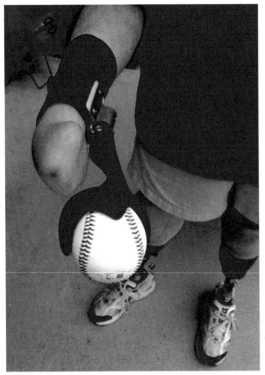

Fig. 21. Example of an activity specific prosthesis for throwing a baseball. The patient and his son were overjoyed when they were able to play catch together for the first time.

SURGICAL INTERVENTIONS TO IMPROVE PROSTHETIC FUNCTION

Having a working understanding of partial hand prostheses, such as those mentioned in this review, can guide hand surgeons in initial treatment and secondary surgeries for PHAs. Furthermore, building a relationship with a specialized upper extremity prosthetist can prove invaluable when working with patients with PHA. Our survey of AAHS members showed that slightly more than a quarter of hand surgeons regularly consult with a prosthetist before performing revision surgeries on the PHA. This finding could be caused by the low number of upper extremity–focused prosthetists or simply by a lack of surgeon understanding of prosthetic options. Working in a multidisciplinary upper extremity limb loss team is the ideal scenario to maximize patient outcomes, although it is not always possible.

Surgical interventions to maximize prosthetic possibilities for PHA include performing procedures at the time of the initial injury and secondary revision surgeries. Examples of primary operative interventions include preserving or decreasing length to enable specific prosthetic use. As an

example, a patient presented to us with a mutilating 5-finger saw injury. The thumb and index finger were salvaged and replanted, but the middle, ring, and small fingers were nonsalvageable. We chose to perform filet flaps to preserve as much length of the proximal phalange as possible and fitted MCPDrivers to the unsalvageable fingers, rather than disarticulating at the MCPJ (**Fig. 22**).

Examples of secondary revisions to optimize partial hand prosthesis fitting include digit shortening, lengthening, flap revisions/debulking, and muscle and nerve procedures. Gaston and colleagues[60] recently described a technique of dissecting and translocating the interosseous muscles of a PHA superficially for stronger EMG signals, allowing individual digit MYO function in the starfish procedure. Nerve procedures such as targeted muscle reinnervation and the regenerative peripheral nerve interface have also been described for improving prosthetic control in the setting of more proximal amputations and hold potential for improving prosthetic EMG signals and decreasing neuroma pain.[61–65]

As an example of a secondary revision to optimize prosthetic fitting in our practice, a patient presented with a crush/avulsion injury to his left hand in an industrial accident resulting in dorsal hand degloving with nonsalvageable amputations to the index through small fingers through the proximal phalanges. He was treated with groin flap coverage to preserve length. At the recommendation of the prosthetist, he underwent multiple debulking procedures and syndactyly releases of the second, third, and fourth web spaces (**Fig. 23**) to be fitted with MCPDrivers. In our practice, considering partial hand prosthetic devices and maintaining open discussion with the multidisciplinary team results in effective surgical planning and improved patient outcomes.

ROLE OF HAND THERAPY

As expressed throughout this review, the importance of the loss of a hand, or part of the hand, cannot be overstated. In addition to the necessary ADLs, the hand is also an organ of performance. It serves as eyes for the blind and enables the deaf to speak. It has become a symbol of salutation, supplication, and condemnation. The hand plays a significant role in the creative life of every known society. It has come to be symbolic of the whole person in art, drama, and dance.[66] Thus, the background and training of OTs and/or CHTs is critical in enabling individuals with PHAs to adapt and resume independence. Ideally, the relationship between the patient and OT/CHT should be

Table 1
Summary of partial hand prosthetic options by level of amputation

Amputation Level	Prosthesis Class	Prosthetic Options
Distal to DIPJ	Passive functional	Low-definition silicone High-definition silicone
DIPJ and middle phalanx	Passive functional	Low-definition silicone High-definition silicone
	Body powered	PIPDriver
PIPJ and proximal phalanx	Passive functional	Low-definition silicone High-definition silicone Point Partial Titan Partial Vincent Partial Passive
	Body powered	MCPDriver Partial M-Finger
MCPJ and transmetacarpal	Passive functional	Low-definition silicone High-definition silicone Point Digit GripLock Titan Full Vincent Passive
	Body powered	M-Fingers and Pediatric M-Finger Palmar Quick Disconnect Pro Cuff
	Externally powered	i-Digits Quantum Vincent Partial 3 Active
Thumb, partial or complete	Passive functional	Low-definition silicone High-definition silicone Vincent Passive Thumb Titan Thumb M-Thumb
	Body powered	ThumbDriver PIPDriver
	Externally powered	i-Digits Vincent Partial Active

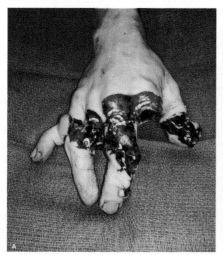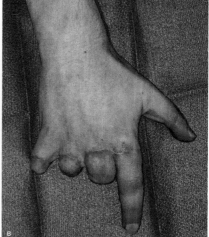

Fig. 22. After a traumatic partial hand injury, reconstruction with filet flaps was chosen to maximize residuum length on the middle, ring, and small fingers for later fit with MCPDrivers.

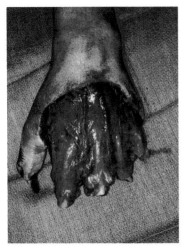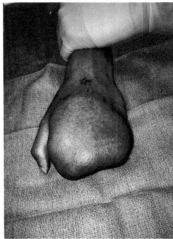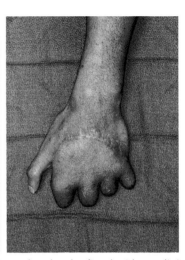

Fig. 23. A series of surgical revisions were completed to prepare the patient's hand to be fitted with a 4-digit Naked Prosthetics MCPDriver custom prosthesis after an industrial crush avulsion of the hand that was reconstructed with a groin flap.

established no later than 3 to 5 days after the initial presentation of PHA. Establishing an early patient-therapist relationship likely contributes to improved short-term and long-term outcomes because the OT/CHT serves to educate and support the patient and act as a liaison for the multidisciplinary team.

Preprosthesis Care

OT/CHT awareness of the preprosthetic principles of care is critical to the successful management of individuals who have sustained traumatic PHA. During the healing phase, emphasis is placed on providing wound care and teaching the patient how to maintain hand hygiene, control edema, stump shaping, promote hand desensitization, and perform active ROM (AROM) and passive ROM (PROM) exercises. Comprehensive hand therapy during the healing phase helps maintain skin mobility and muscle strength. Mirror therapy and laterality awareness are also used early to diminish phantom limb pain.[67] The time spent with an OT/CHT affords patients opportunities to express current and future hand function goals and time to explore prosthetic device options. During this time, OTs/CHTs are also able to evaluate patient needs for functional independence and can strategize which 1-hand techniques and adaptive equipment are needed. If a prosthesis is desired, an experienced OT and CHT can fabricate protective splinting and preprosthetic devices such as a thumb post to mimic future prosthetic use and can determine potential EMG sites if an MYO prosthesis is being considered.

During the time the partial hand prosthetic prescription is being discussed, there are many factors that the OT/CHT should document and explore with the patient to determine the best prosthetic option. Physical characteristics, including amputation level, amount of soft tissue coverage, AROM/PROM and muscle strength of the remaining hand, status of the unaffected extremity, presence and quality of remaining sensation, and the presence of adherent scars, should be noted on the physical examination during therapy. Social factors, including patient goals, attitude and motivation, ability to learn and adapt, vocational and avocational interests, and third-party payer considerations, should also be discussed with the multidisciplinary team.[68]

Postprosthesis Care

Once the multidisciplinary team, patient, and family decide on a type of prosthesis, successful outcomes can be attributed to early posttraumatic intervention, experienced team approach, patient-directed prosthetic training, patient education, patient monitoring, and follow-up. Regardless of the device, the following keys should be included in every partial hand prosthetic training program: (1) independence in donning and doffing; (2) orientation to a gradual prosthetic wearing program and monitoring skin status; (3) orientation to prosthetic controls training when an electric partial hand prosthesis is prescribed; (4) prosthetic practice in grasp and release function; (5) functional use training with an emphasis on bilateral tasks that will be possible with the partial hand prosthesis. Of these training principles, the most important is the emphasis placed on bilateral tasks that are considered important for the individual with partial hand loss to accomplish. These tasks should be practiced sitting and standing. Unless these tasks are identified, practiced, and reinforced, the true value of the partial hand prosthesis will not be experienced or appreciated. Successful use training is achieved when the amputee uses the prosthesis spontaneously and effectively for most daily activities.[69]

ROLE OF PHYSICAL MEDICINE AND REHABILITATION PHYSICIANS IN PARTIAL HAND AMPUTEE CARE

Physical medicine and rehabilitation (PMR) physicians, or physiatrists, are integral to the multidisciplinary team. Although hand surgeons readily value the contributions of prosthetists and OTs/CHTs, our recent AAHS survey revealed that many surgeons do not fully appreciate the contributions of PMR physicians. Note that, although hand surgeons provide amputee care initially, PMR physicians often provide short-term and long-term care throughout the amputee's life. Highlighting their role in the multidisciplinary team may thus improve outcomes and increase quality of life for patients with PHAs.

PMR physicians are trained in diagnosing, assessing, and treating patients with physical disabilities. Although their profession is frequently associated with caring for chronic neurologic conditions, their training also prepares them to manage amputees. Within the multidisciplinary team, their role is to maximize physical, psychological, social, and occupational independence by restoring hand function. This goal is often accomplished through prescribing pharmacologic agents, teaching therapeutic exercises, and engaging amputees in holistic therapies, including cold, heat, massage, traction, electrical stimulation, and biofeedback. These interventions are frequently used to improve functionality in addition to alleviating pain. Pain at the residuum is a frequent obstacle to amputee care. Pain often decreases mobility and return to normal ADLs and increases prosthetic abandonment. PMR physicians are invaluable to combatting these sequelae. Managing amputee pain is complex and patient specific; however, physiatrists often provide relief using local and/or regional injections and other pharmacologic agents. Examples of common injection classes include local anesthetics (lidocaine), steroid injections (methylprednisolone acetate), and neuromuscular junction toxins (botulinum toxin type A). Other pharmacologic classes used in amputee pain management include N-methyl-D-aspartate (NMDA) receptor antagonists, opioids, anticonvulsants, antidepressants, and calcitonin.[70] Another important role PMR

physicians play at our institution is in identifying and referring amputees who have failed standard pain management strategies for targeted muscle reinnervation to treat their neuroma and phantom limb pains. This role has become an important part of the multidisciplinary approach at the University of Utah.

Perhaps more valuable than their knowledge of pharmacologic pain management is the physiatrists' ability to prevent the development of pain and promote wellness. PMR physicians with clinical interests in limb rehabilitation often have extensive knowledge of prostheses and are proficient amputee educators. Prevention and early detection of poor prosthesis fit and/or pressure ulceration can prevent prosthetic abandonment and other negative sequelae. Ultimately, PMR physicians serve as powerful liaisons to multidisciplinary teams and as advocates for patients. As institutions expand and create upper extremity care teams, the role of the PMR physician should not be overlooked.

BARRIERS TO PROSTHETIC REHABILITATION

There are multiple factors that create impediments to the provision of prosthetic rehabilitation for partial hand amputees. Time from injury to provision of a prosthesis, patient involvement in prosthesis selection, perceived need, functionality, and comfort of the prosthesis were the top contributing factors in achieving a successful functional outcome.[71,72] Clinically, a perceived lack of options and poor outcomes historically have dissuaded many physicians and surgeons from prescribing PHA prostheses. It is the hope of the authors that the information provided in this review will change that perspective, noting that there are now many different options available for the different levels of amputation that can produce successful functional outcomes. There is a pervasive misapprehension that prosthetic technology is responsible for the success or failure of the outcome. It is easier to blame the device and technology than it is to introspectively assess the way in which the prosthesis was provided. It has been our experience that many users who have rejected the use of a prosthesis have done so because they were not fitted with the appropriate prosthetic technology. Even when amputees may have been fitted with the most appropriate prosthesis, not having a proper fit by a prosthetist that has experience in upper limb prostheses can also lead to subsequent prosthetic abandonment. According to the most recent clinical practice survey of all certified prosthetists in the United States, on average prosthetists only spend 2% of their time caring for individuals with PHA.[73] Most of their time is spent caring for individuals with lower limb absence or difference. Because the functional restorative needs for the upper and lower limbs are distinct, so is the expertise to be able to properly treat and care for these different patient populations. Fortunately, there are prosthetists that have dedicated most of their practices to the care and provision of upper limb prostheses. These upper limb prosthetic specialists tend to work in and around regional metropolitan centers. It is critical for the prosthetic outcome that individuals needing a partial hand prosthesis be cared for by a prosthetist with extensive experience in treating this level of amputation, which may mean the individual seeking care having to travel to regional centers. An inexperienced prosthetist may not be able to provide an objective clinical evaluation to determine the most appropriate prosthetic recommendation. An inexperienced prosthetist may also not be able to produce a well-fitting prosthetic socket, which can contribute to discomfort, pain, and potentially skin breakdown, all factors highly likely to contribute to abandonment.

Insurance authorization and reimbursement for partial hand prostheses can be a barrier to a successful outcome, but it is possible to achieve. Over the past several years, payers have become increasingly aware of some of the newer technologies and have begun to provide coverage with appropriate clinical justification. However, the established HCPCS L-Codes used by Medicare and private insurance to describe and reimburse for prostheses are often outdated and limited in scope. For this reason, miscellaneous codes are often necessary in billing. Any time miscellaneous codes are used, the burden of documentation of medical necessity increases. Also, many insurance policies include language deeming prostheses distal to the wrist as experimental and investigational, which is no longer accurate.

A collaborative team approach including a surgeon, physiatrist, OT/CHT, and upper limb prosthetist is the most effective way to overcome reimbursement barriers.[74] When members of the multidisciplinary team are unified in outcome objectives, a comprehensive rehabilitation plan can be formulated and implemented. It is important to document all clinical decisions during treatment and collaboration sessions. This documentation shows that a process was followed, and that the recommended treatment plan is based on solid clinical practices rather than simple appeal to novelty. When possible, prototype prostheses should be constructed and trialed to prove clinical viability and functionality. When a prosthesis is provided within the golden window of 6 months after amputation, there is a significant increase in the probability of successful integration of the prosthesis into ADLs, a reduction in the likelihood of abandonment, and a drastically improved likelihood that the individual will be able to return to work and active participation in society.[71,72] The authors' combined experience shows that the sooner an upper limb prosthesis is fitted and delivered, the better the outcome and likelihood of use in daily activities. Prosthetic training by a skilled OT/CHT in amputee rehabilitation is of paramount importance in ensuring success.

For insurance authorization purposes, the prescribing physician's documentation must include medical necessity and justification. Other members of the rehabilitation team can help produce this documentation, but it ultimately needs to be included in the prescribing physicians' clinical progress notes. The prescribing physician must be prepared to defend this clinical justification in a peer-to-peer session with the medical reviewers from the payer. When this model is implemented, the authors have seen success in having medical policies overturned and the various described devices authorized.

SUMMARY

PHAs are the most common upper extremity amputation. Because the fingers, thumb, and transmetacarpal regions can be affected, treatment options restoring form and function are essential to alleviating the burdens on individuals and communities. Through recent advancements in engineering, prosthetic devices are increasingly available and provide straightforward solutions for partial hand amputees. To enhance clinician familiarity and promote patient care, this article highlights many of the current prosthetic options by amputation level, as well as some of the critical elements to successful prosthetic fitting. Understanding the application of these devices allows more proficient amputee care, especially while working within a multidisciplinary team. As partial hand amputee care expands, this article may provide a foundation for future research and serve clinicians during patient care and advocacy.

DISCLOSURE

D.J. Atkins is a former consultant at Össur and Touch Bionics. C.C. Duncan is partially funded by a National Science Foundation grant. S.D. Mendenhall is a consultant for PolyNovo. The other authors have no disclosures.

REFERENCES

1. Akarsu S, Tekin L, Safaz I, et al. Quality of life and functionality after lower limb amputations: comparison between uni- vs. bilateral amputee patients. Prosthet Orthot Int 2013;37(1):9–13.

2. Durmus D, Safaz I, Adiguzel E, et al. The relationship between prosthesis use, phantom pain and psychiatric symptoms in male traumatic limb amputees. Compr Psychiatry 2015;59:45–53.

3. Pasquina CP, Carvalho AJ, Sheehan TP. Ethics in Rehabilitation: Access to Prosthetics and Quality Care Following Amputation. AMA J Ethics 2015; 17(6):535–46.

4. Burger H, Marincek C. Return to work after lower limb amputation. Disabil Rehabil 2007;29(17): 1323–9.

5. Craig M, Hill W, Englehart K, et al. Return to work after occupational injury and upper limb amputation. Occup Med (Lond) 2017;67(3):227–9.

6. Sheikh K. Return to work following limb injuries. J Soc Occup Med 1985;35(4):114–7.

7. Raichle KA, Hanley MA, Molton I, et al. Prosthesis use in persons with lower- and upper-limb amputation. J Rehabil Res Dev 2008;45(7):961–72.

8. Dietrich C, Nehrdich S, Seifert S, et al. Leg prosthesis with somatosensory feedback reduces phantom limb pain and increases functionality. Front Neurol 2018;9:270.

9. Bouma SE, Postema SG, Bongers RM, et al. Musculoskeletal complaints in individuals with finger or partial hand amputations in the Netherlands: a cross-sectional study. Disabil Rehabil 2018;40(10):1146–53.

10. Grob M, Papadopulos NA, Zimmermann A, et al. The psychological impact of severe hand injury. J Hand Surg Eur Vol 2008;33(3):358–62.

11. Kuret Z, Burger H, Vidmar G, et al. Adjustment to finger amputation and silicone finger prosthesis use. Disabil Rehabil 2019;41(11):1307–12.

12. Varma P, Stineman MG, Dillingham TR. Epidemiology of limb loss. Phys Med Rehabil Clin N Am 2014;25(1):1–8.

13. Ziegler-Graham K, MacKenzie EJ, Ephraim PL, et al. Estimating the prevalence of limb loss in the United States: 2005 to 2050. Arch Phys Med Rehabil 2008; 89(3):422–9.

14. Chang DH, Ye SY, Chien LC, et al. Epidemiology of digital amputation and replantation in Taiwan: A population-based study. J Chin Med Assoc 2015; 78(10):597–602.

15. Panagopoulou P, Iakovakis I, Mentis AFA, et al. Epidemiology and Prevention of Hand Amputations in Greece: Data from the Emergency Department Injury Surveillance System. Inj Prev 2010;16:A173.

16. Bahar Moni AS, Hoque M, Mollah RA, et al. Diabetic Hand Infection: An Emerging Challenge. J Hand Surg Asian Pac Vol 2019;24(3):317–22.

17. Shale CM, Tidwell JE 3rd, Mulligan RP, et al. A nationwide review of the treatment patterns of traumatic thumb amputations. Ann Plast Surg 2013;70(6):647–51.

18. Clasper J, Ramasamy A. Traumatic amputations. Br J Pain 2013;7(2):67–73.

19. Davidson J. A comparison of upper limb amputees and patients with upper limb injuries using the Disability of the Arm, Shoulder and Hand (DASH). Disabil Rehabil 2004;26(14–15):917–23.

20. Adamo DE, Taufiq A. Establishing hand preference: why does it matter? Hand (N Y) 2011;6(3):295–303.

21. Burger H, Maver T, Marincek C. Partial hand amputation and work. Disabil Rehabil 2007;29(17): 1317–21.

22. Kearns NT, Jackson WT, Elliott TR, et al. Differences in level of upper limb loss on functional impairment, psychological well-being, and substance use. Rehabil Psychol 2018;63(1):141–7.

23. Imbinto I, Peccia C, Controzzi M, et al. Treatment of the partial hand amputation: an engineering perspective. IEEE Rev Biomed Eng 2016;9:32–48.

24. Imbinto I, Peccia C, Controzzi M, et al. Corrections to "treatment of the partial hand amputation: an engineering perspective. IEEE Rev Biomed Eng 2018; 11:322.

25. Wang K, Sears ED, Shauver MJ, et al. A systematic review of outcomes of revision amputation treatment for fingertip amputations. Hand (N Y) 2013;8(2): 139–45.

26. Sebastin SJ, Chung KC. A systematic review of the outcomes of replantation of distal digital amputation. Plast Reconstr Surg 2011;128(3):723–37.

27. Shauver MJ, Nishizuka T, Hirata H, et al. Traumatic finger amputation treatment preference among hand surgeons in the United States and Japan. Plast Reconstr Surg 2016;137(4):1193–202.

28. Payatakes AH, Zagoreos NP, Fedorcik GG, et al. Current practice of microsurgery by members of the American Society for Surgery of the Hand. J Hand Surg Am 2007;32(4):541–7.

29. Ozer K, Kramer W, Gillani S, et al. Replantation versus revision of amputated fingers in patients air-transported to a level 1 trauma center. J Hand Surg Am 2010;35(6):936–40.

30. Soucacos PN. Indications and selection for digital amputation and replantation. J Hand Surg Br 2001; 26(6):572–81.

31. Mori M. Bukimi no tani [The uncanny valley]. Energy 1970;7(4):33–5.

32. Buckingham G, Parr J, Wood G, et al. Upper- and lower-limb amputees show reduced levels of eeriness for images of prosthetic hands. Psychon Bull Rev 2019;26(4):1295–302.

33. MacDorman KF, Ishiguro H. The uncanny advantage of using androids in cognitive and social science research. Interact Stud 2006;7(3):297–337.

34. Fujioka M, Hayashida K. Proximal interphalangeal replantation with arthrodesis facilitates favorable esthetics and functional outcome. J Trauma Manag Outcomes 2015;9:7.

35. Sears ED, Chung KC. Replantation of finger avulsion injuries: a systematic review of survival and functional outcomes. J Hand Surg Am 2011;36(4): 686–94.

36. Sprague BL. Proximal interphalangeal joint injuries and their initial treatment. J Trauma 1975;15(5): 380–5.

37. Carey SL, Lura DJ, Highsmith MJ, et al. Differences in myoelectric and body-powered upper-limb prostheses: Systematic literature review. J Rehabil Res Dev 2015;52(3):247–62.

38. Whelan L, Flinn S, Wagner N. Individualizing goals for users of externally powered partial hand prostheses. J Rehabil Res Dev 2014;51(6):885–94.

39. Rondinelli RD. American Medical Association's guides to the evaluation of permanent impairment. Chicago: American Medical Association; 2008.

40. Danion F, Latash ML, Li ZM, et al. The effect of a fatiguing exercise by the index finger on single- and multi-finger force production tasks. Exp Brain Res 2001;138(3):322–9.

41. Danna-Dos Santos A, Poston B, Jesunathadas M, et al. Influence of fatigue on hand muscle coordination and EMG-EMG coherence during three-digit grasping. J Neurophysiol 2010;104(6):3576–87.

42. Maduri P, Akhondi H. Upper limb amputation. Treasure Island (FL): StatPearls; 2020.

43. Landi AA, Leti A, Rosa ND. The historical odyssey of the mutilated hand. In: Weinzweig N, Weinzweig J, editors. The mutilated hand. Mosby; 2005. p. 3–14.

44. Meredith JM. Comparison of 3 myoelectrically controlled prehensors and the voluntary-opening split hook. Am J Occup Ther 1994;48(10):932–7.

45. Mioton LM, Dumanian GA. Targeted muscle reinnervation and prosthetic rehabilitation after limb loss. J Surg Oncol 2018;118(5):807–14.

46. Lotze M, Grodd W, Birbaumer N, et al. Does use of a myoelectric prosthesis prevent cortical reorganization and phantom limb pain? Nat Neurosci 1999; 2(6):501–2.

47. Passero TD, K. Aesthetic prostheses. In: Smith DG, Michael JW, Bowker JH, editors. Atlas of amputations and limb Deficiencies: surgical, prosthetic and rehabilitation Principles. 3rd edition. Rosemont (IL): American Academy of Orthopedic Surgeons; 2004. p. 303–10.

48. Williams TW 3rd. Progress on stabilizing and controlling powered upper-limb prostheses. J Rehabil Res Dev 2011;48(6):ix–xix.

49. Uellendahl JE. Upper extremity myoelectric prosthetics. Phys Med Rehabil Clin N Am 2000;11(3): 639–52.

50. Kejlaa GH. Consumer concerns and the functional value of prostheses to upper limb amputees. Prosthet Orthot Int 1993;17(3):157–63.

51. Flatt AE. Our thumbs. Proc (Bayl Univ Med Cent) 2002;15(4):380–7.

52. Duncan SF, Saracevic CE, Kakinoki R. Biomechanics of the hand. Hand Clin 2013;29(4):483–92.

53. Napier JR, Tuttle R. Hands. Rev. ed. Princeton (NJ): Princeton University Press; 1993.

54. Marzke MW. Evolutionary development of the human thumb. Hand Clin 1992;8(1):1–8.

55. Snoek GJ, MJ IJ, Hermens HJ, et al. Survey of the needs of patients with spinal cord injury: impact and priority for improvement in hand function in tetraplegics. Spinal Cord 2004;42(9):526–32.

56. Li Y, Kulbacka-Ortiz K, Caine-Winterberger K, et al. Thumb amputations treated with osseointegrated percutaneous prostheses with up to 25 years of follow-up. J Am Acad Orthop Surg Glob Res Rev 2019;3(1):e097.

57. Lin PY, Sebastin SJ, Ono S, et al. A systematic review of outcomes of toe-to-thumb transfers for isolated traumatic thumb amputation. Hand (N Y) 2011;6(3):235–43.

58. Goldfarb CA, Monroe E, Steffen J, et al. Incidence and treatment of complications, suboptimal outcomes, and functional deficiencies after pollicization. J Hand Surg Am 2009;34(7):1291–7.

59. Kumar B, Acharya A, Bhat AK. A re-look at pollicization. Indian J Plast Surg 2011;44(2):266–75.

60. Gaston RG, Bracey JW, Tait MA, et al. A novel muscle transfer for independent digital control of a myoelectric prosthesis: the starfish procedure. J Hand Surg Am 2019;44(2):163.e1-5.

61. Kuiken TA, Li G, Lock BA, et al. Targeted muscle reinnervation for real-time myoelectric control of multifunction artificial arms. JAMA 2009;301(6):619–28.

62. Daugherty THF, Mailey BA, Bueno RA Jr, et al. Targeted muscle reinnervation in the hand: an anatomical feasibility study for neuroma treatment and prevention. J Hand Surg Am 2020;45(9): 802–12.

63. Chepla KJ, Wu-Fienberg Y. Targeted muscle reinnervation for partial hand amputation. Plast Reconstr Surg Glob Open 2020;8(6):e2946.

64. Vu PP, Vaskov AK, Irwin ZT, et al. A regenerative peripheral nerve interface allows real-time control of an artificial hand in upper limb amputees. Sci Transl Med 2020;12(533):eaay2857.

65. Hooper RC, Cederna PS, Brown DL, et al. Regenerative peripheral nerve interfaces for the management of symptomatic hand and digital neuromas. Plast Reconstr Surg Glob Open 2020;8(6):e2792.

66. Alpenfels EJ. The anthropology and social significance of the human hand. Artif Limbs 1955; 2(2):4–21.

67. Ramachandran VS, Rogers-Ramachandran D. Synaesthesia in phantom limbs induced with mirrors. Proc Biol Sci 1996;263(1369):377–86.

68. Atkins DJ. Postoperative and preprosthetic therapy programs. In: Atkins DJ, Meier RH, editors. Comprehensive management of the upper-limb amputee. New York: Springer New York; 1989. p. 11–5.

69. Meier RA, Atkins DJ. Functional restoration of adults and children with upper extremity amputation. 2nd edition. New York: Demos Medical Publishing; 2004.

70. Hsu E, Cohen SP. Postamputation pain: epidemiology, mechanisms, and treatment. J Pain Res 2013;6:121–36.

71. Biddiss E, Chau T. Upper-limb prosthetics: critical factors in device abandonment. Am J Phys Med Rehabil 2007;86(12):977–87.

72. Biddiss EA, Chau TT. Upper limb prosthesis use and abandonment: a survey of the last 25 years. Prosthet Orthot Int 2007;31(3):236–57.

73. Whiteside SA, MJ, Bick JA, et al. Practice analysis of certified practitioners in the disciplines of orthotics and prosthetics. Alexandria (VA): American Board for Certification in Orthotics, Prosthetics & Pedorthics, Inc.; 2015.

74. Dolhi CD. Comprehensive Management of the Upper-Limb Amputee - Atkins, Dj, Meier, Rh. Am J Occup Ther 1990;44(10):955.

Moving?

Make sure your subscription moves with you!

To notify us of your new address, find your **Clinics Account Number** (located on your mailing label above your name), and contact customer service at:

Email: journalscustomerservice-usa@elsevier.com

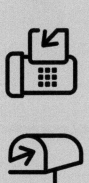

800-654-2452 (subscribers in the U.S. & Canada)
314-447-8871 (subscribers outside of the U.S. & Canada)

Fax number: 314-447-8029

Elsevier Health Sciences Division
Subscription Customer Service
3251 Riverport Lane
Maryland Heights, MO 63043

*To ensure uninterrupted delivery of your subscription, please notify us at least 4 weeks in advance of move.

ELSEVIER